Quality in Laboratory Hemostasis and Thrombosis

To Mo, Lorrie and Di

Quality in Laboratory Hemostasis and Thrombosis

Steve Kitchen
Clinical Scientist
Sheffield Hemophilia and Thrombosis Centre
Royal Hallamshire Hospital
Sheffield
and
Scientific Director, UK National External Quality Assessment Scheme (EQAS) for Blood
Coagulation
Scientific Director, WHO and WFH International External Quality Assessment Programs for
Blood Coagulation
Sheffield
UK

John D. Olson
Professor and Vice Chair for Clinical Affairs
Department of Pathology
University of Texas Health Science Center
San Antonio, Texas
USA

F. Eric Preston
Emeritus Professor of Hematology
University of Sheffield
and
Director, WHO and WFH International External Quality Assessment Programs for Blood
Coagulation
Sheffield
UK

Foreword by Professor Dr Frits R. Rosendaal, Leiden University Medical Center

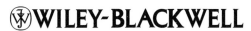
A John Wiley & Sons, Ltd., Publication

This edition first published 2009 © 2009 by Blackwell Publishing Ltd
Blackwell Publishing was acquired by John Wiley & Sons in February 2007. Blackwell's publishing program has been merged with Wiley's global Scientific, Technical and Medical business to form Wiley-Blackwell.

Registered office: John Wiley & Sons Ltd, The Atrium, Southern Gate, Chichester, West Sussex, PO19 8SQ, UK

Editorial offices: 9600 Garsington Road, Oxford, OX4 2DQ, UK

          The Atrium, Southern Gate, Chichester, West Sussex, PO19 8SQ, UK

          111 River Street, Hoboken, NJ 07030-5774, USA

For details of our global editorial offices, for customer services and for information about how to apply for permission to reuse the copyright material in this book please see our website at www.wiley.com/wiley-blackwell

Library of Congress Cataloging-in-Publication Data

Quality in laboratory hemostasis and thrombosis / edited by Steve Kitchen, John D. Olson, Eric Preston.

     p. ; cm.

  Includes bibliographical references and index.

  ISBN 978-1-4051-6803-8 (hardcover : alk. paper)

  1. Blood coagulation disorders–Diagnosis.   2. Blood–Analysis–Laboratory manuals.   3. Hemostasis.   4. Thrombosis.   I. Kitchen, Steve, Dr.   II. Olson, John David   III. Preston, F. E., 1944–

  [DNLM: 1. Hemostatic Techniques.   2. Anticoagulants.   3. Blood Coagulation Disorders, Inherited–diagnosis.   4. Blood Coagulation Factors.   5. Clinical Laboratory Techniques.   6. Thrombophilia–diagnosis. WH 310 Q11 2009]

  RC647.C55Q38 2009

  616.1´57075–dc22

  2008024092

ISBN: 978-1-4051-6803-8

A catalogue record for this book is available from the British Library.

Set in 9 on 11.5 pt Sabon by SNP Best-set Typesetter Ltd., Hong Kong
Printed in Singapore by Fabulous Printers Pte Ltd

1   2009

Contents

Contributors, vii

Foreword, x
Frits R. Rosendaal

Preface, xii

1 General Quality Planning in the Hemostasis Laboratory, 1
John D. Olson

2 Hemostasis Test Validation, Performance and Reference Intervals, 9
Richard A. Marlar

3 International Standards in Hemostasis, 19
Trevor W. Barrowcliffe

4 Sample Integrity and Preanalytical Variables, 31
Dorothy M. Adcock

5 Internal Quality Control in the Hemostasis Laboratory, 43
Steve Kitchen, F. Eric Preston, John D. Olson

6 External Quality Assessment in Hemostasis: Its Importance and
Significance, 51
F. Eric Preston, Steve Kitchen, Alok Srivastava

7 Initial Evaluation of Hemostasis: Reagent and Method Selection, 63
Wayne L. Chandler

8 Point-of-Care Testing in Hemostasis, 72
Chris Gardiner, Samuel Machin, Ian Mackie

9 Assay of Factor VIII and Other Clotting Factors, 81
Steve Kitchen, F. Eric Preston

10 Application of Molecular Genetics to the Investigation of Inherited Bleeding
Disorders, 90
Stefan Lethagen, Marianne Schwartz, Lars Bo Nielsen

11 Standardization of D-dimer Testing, 99
Guido Reber, Philippe de Moerloose

12 Diagnostic Assessment of Platelet Function, 110
Paquita Nurden, Alan Nurden

13 Laboratory Evaluation of von Willebrand Disease: Phenotypic Analysis, 125
Emmanuel J. Favaloro

14 Laboratory Analysis of von Willebrand Disease: Molecular Analysis, 137
Anne Goodeve, Ian Peake

CONTENTS

15 Dilemmas in Heritable Thrombophilia Testing, 147
   Isobel D. Walker, Ian Jennings

16 Evaluation of Antiphospholipid Antibodies, 160
   Michael Greaves

17 Monitoring Heparin Therapy, 170
   Marilyn Johnston

18 Monitoring Oral Anticoagulant Therapy, 179
   Armando Tripodi

19 Monitoring New Anticoagulants, 190
   Elaine Gray, Trevor W. Barrowcliffe

20 Detecting and Quantifying Functional Inhibitors in Hemostasis, 198
   Bert Verbruggen, Irena Nováková, Waander van Heerde

Index, 209

Contributors

Dorothy M. Adcock MD
Esoterix Coagulation
Englewood, Colorado
USA

Trevor W. Barrowcliffe PhD
Formerly National Institute for Biological Standards
 and Control
Potters Bar
UK

Wayne L. Chandler MD
Department of Laboratory Medicine
University of Washington
Seattle, Washington
USA

Emmanuel J. Favaloro PhD
Department of Hematology
Institute of Clinical Pathology and Medical
 Research
Westmead Hospital, NSW
Australia

Chris Gardiner PhD
Hematology Department
University College London Hospitals NHS Trust
London
UK

Anne Goodeve PhD
Academic Unit of Hematology
Henry Wellcome Laboratories for Medical Research
Sheffield
UK

Elaine Gray PhD
National Institute for Biological Standards and
 Control
Potters Bar
UK

Michael Greaves MD, FRCP, FRCPath
School of Medicine
University of Aberdeen
Aberdeen
UK

Ian Jennings PhD, CSci
UK NEQAS (Blood Coagulation)
Rutledge Mews
Sheffield
UK

Marilyn Johnston ART
Hemostasis Reference Laboratory
Henderson Research Centre
Hamilton, Ontario
Canada

Steve Kitchen PhD
Sheffield Hemophilia and Thrombosis Centre
Royal Hallamshire Hospital
Sheffield
UK

Stefan Lethagen PhD, MD
Copenhagen Hemophilia Center
Thrombosis and Hemostasis Unit
Department of Hematology
Copenhagen University Hospital (Rigshospitalet)
Copenhagen
Denmark

Samuel Machin FRCP, FRCPath
Hematology Department
University College London Hospitals NHS Trust
London
and
Hemostasis Research Unit
Hematology Department
University College London
London
UK

Ian Mackie PhD
Hematology Department
University College London Hospitals NHS Trust
London
and
Hemostasis Research Unit
Hematology Department
University College London
London
UK

Richard A. Marlar PhD
Pathology and Laboratory Medicine
Oklahoma City VA Medical Center
and
Department of Pathology
University of Oklahoma Health Sciences Center
Oklahoma City, Oklahoma
USA

Philippe de Moerloose MD
Hemostasis Unit
University Hospital Geneva
Geneva
Switzerland

Lars Bo Nielsen MD, PhD, DMsc
Department of Clinical Biochemistry
Copenhagen University Hospital (Rigshospitalet)
and
Department of Biomedical Sciences
University of Copenhagen
Copenhagen
Denmark

Irena Nováková MD, PhD
Department of Hematology
Radboud University Nijmegen Medical Center
Nijmegen
The Netherlands

Alan Nurden PhD
Centre de Référence des Pathologies Plaquettaires
Plateforme Technologique d'Innovation
  Biomédicale
Hôpital Xavier Arnozan
Pessac
France

Paquita Nurden MD, PhD
Centre de Référence des Pathologies
  Plaquettaires
Plateforme Technologique d'Innovation
  Biomédicale
Hôpital Xavier Arnozan
Pessac
France

John D. Olson MD, PhD
Department of Pathology
University of Texas Health Science Center
San Antonio, Texas
USA

Ian Peake PhD
Academic Unit of Haematology
Henry Wellcome Laboratories for Medical
  Research
Sheffield
UK

F. Eric Preston MD, FRCPath, FRCP
WHO/WFH EQA
Rutledge Mews
Sheffield
UK

Guido Reber PhD
Hemostasis Unit
Department of Internal Medicine
University Hospital and Faculty of Medicine
Geneva
Switzerland

Frits R. Rosendaal MD
Department of Clinical Epidemiology and
  Department of Thrombosis and Hemostasis
Leiden University Medical Center
Leiden
The Netherlands

Marianne Schwartz PhD
Department of Clinical Genetics
Copenhagen University Hospital (Rigshospitalet)
Copenhagen
Denmark

Alok Srivastava MD
Department of Hematology
Christian Medical School
Vellore
India

Armando Tripodi PhD
Angelo Bianchi Bonomi Hemophilia and
    Thrombosis Center
Department of Internal Medicine
University School of Medicine and IRCCS Maggiore
    Hospital, Mangiagalli and Regina Elena
    Foundation
Milan
Italy

Waander van Heerde PhD
Central Laboratory for Hematology
Radboud University Nijmegen Medical Center
Nijmegen
The Netherlands

Bert Verbruggen PhD
Central Laboratory for Hematology
Radboud University Nijmegen Medical Center
Nijmegen
The Netherlands

Isobel D. Walker MD
Department of Hematology
Glasgow Royal Infirmary
Glasgow
UK

Foreword

Thou art always figuring diseases in me,
but thou art full of error: I am sound.
(William Shakespeare. Measure for
Measure (1604); Act I, Scene II)

A correct diagnosis is the cornerstone of medicine. Without it, no remedy can be prescribed, or prognosis given. Although laboratory tests are only a part of the diagnostic arsenal, together with history taking, clinical examination and imaging techniques, few diagnoses are arrived at without some form of laboratory test. Inadequate tests may lead to either false reassurance, or false alarm. They may lead to the erroneous choice not to give treatment when treatment would be beneficial, or even to prescribe the wrong treatment, which is likely to be harmful. It is therefore of the utmost importance that whenever laboratory tests are performed, the results are reliable.

Laboratory tests in the field of thrombosis and hemostasis are notoriously difficult, which is related to the large variety in techniques that are used, and the sensitivity of many assays to small preanalytical and analytical variation. Therefore, quality assurance is crucial, and no hemostasis laboratory can afford not to invest in internal and external quality control. The book *Quality in Laboratory Hemostasis and Thrombosis*, edited and written by authorities in the field, will become an indispensable help for those who wish to set up a hemostasis laboratory, as well as those who already work in such a place. For, to quote from the first chapter: "Process is never optimized; it can always be improved."

The book has two parts: the first eight chapters give a scholarly overview of the concepts that underlie quality assurance, explaining the various aspects of test validation, with its components, of which accuracy and precision are the most important: does a test measure what it is supposed to measure, and does it do so with acceptable reproducibility. Subsequent chapters in this first part explain in detail how internal quality control deals with precision and external quality control with accuracy. The development of international standards is an important and ongoing

development in improving accuracy and comparability of hemostasis laboratory tests. Here, the Scientific and Standardization Committee of the International Society on Thrombosis and Haemostasis, working together with the World Health Organization, has played a major role. Over the years we have witnessed the emergence of large external quality assurance programs, in which samples are sometimes sent to more than a thousand participating laboratories. Such programs not only allow laboratories to evaluate their performance, but also to group results by reagent or instrument, which leads to valuable insights, and further quality improvement.

In the second part of the book, Chapters 9 through 20, a detailed description is given of all major assays in hemostasis, ranging from classical clotting factor assays to genetic analyses in the hemophilias, and tests for the immunologic abnormalities that lead to the antiphospholipid syndrome. These chapters give the reader invaluable information on the performance and interpretation of these tests.

The ultimate test for a laboratory test is whether it improves medical care, i.e., reduces morbidity and mortality, which depends on the effect a negative or positive test result has on the treatment of a patient. A test that does not affect clinical management is a waste of resources. Both at the beginning and the end of laboratory tests there is usually a clinician, who first makes the decision to order a test, and subsequently has to interpret the test result. Although these clinical decisions and interpretation are not part of the content of this book, which would have made it unwieldy to say the least, these are of obvious importance, and one of the tasks of individuals working in hemostasis laboratories is to educate clinicians about the clinical value of the various assays. This education will usually lead to a reduction in the number of tests ordered. The practice of medicine knows a wide variety of tests, which generally serve three purposes, either to diagnose a disease, or to test for a risk factor for disease, or to screen for either of these. This distinction is rarely sharply made, while it seems that clinically one type (diagnosing a disease) is almost always indicated and useful, and another type (testing for risk factors) only rarely is. While it is logical to find out which disease a patient with complaints has, it is not so logical to try and identify the causes of that disease, or even to try and identify those risk factors in non-diseased individuals, such as relatives of individuals with thrombosis. The reason the distinction between diagnosing a disease and identifying a risk factor is not always sharply made, is possibly because in some diseases in the field, notably bleeding disorders, there is an almost one-to-one relationship between the cause of the disease and the disease itself. While excessive bleeding is the disease, and the clotting factor level a cause, individuals with no factor VIII or IX will invariably have the clinical disease of hemophilia, and therefore measuring the clotting factor level has become synonymous to diagnosing hemophilia. This is quite different for thrombosis. Thrombosis (deep vein thrombosis or pulmonary embolism) is a disease, whereas thrombophilia is not. Given the multicausal nature of the etiology of thrombosis, in which multiple risk factors need to be present to lead to disease, it is far from self-evident that testing for thrombophilic abnormalities has any clinical value. So far, there are no clinical studies that show a benefit of such testing, although it is performed on a broad scale.

The reliability of a particular assay should be viewed in the context in which the test is ordered. Suppose one would order a test for high factor VIII as a prothrombotic risk factor, the abovementioned notwithstanding, an error of 5 IU/dL would be irrelevant, since the purpose is discriminate between levels of over 150 or 200 IU/dL versus plasma concentrations around 100 IU/dL. The same error in a factor VIII assay to diagnose hemophilia A could be disastrous.

A clinician, when ordering a test, will have to deal with so-called prior probabilities, which is of particular relevance in screening tests. A slightly prolonged aPTT has a vastly different meaning when found in a healthy woman who had four uneventful deliveries who has come to the hospital for a tubal ligation, than in an 18-month-old boy who needs to undergo a duodenoscopy with possible biopsies. She is unlikely to have a bleeding tendency, even when the aPTT is prolonged, while the young boy may suffer from hemophilia. Screening tests affect the likelihood of disease, which, according to Bayes' theorem, is also a function of the prior probability of disease. Virtually all tests that use reference ranges based on statistical cut-off values, such as the population mean plus or minus two standard deviations, are screening tests, that do neither establish a risk factor or a disease, but only, when abnormal, affect the likelihood of that state. Nature does not use standard deviations, and using a cut-off of two standard deviations by definition finds 2.5% of the population below, or over, such a cut-off. In reality, diseases and risk factors may have prevalences that exceed, or, more usual, lie far below this figure. Tests using "normal ranges" therefore can never establish an abnormality, and should be followed by more specific tests, such as clotting factor assays or genetic tests.

Over the last decades, major progress has been made in quality assurance of hemostatic laboratory assays. This book will be an indispensable part of every hemostasis laboratory, where, given its hands-on nature, it will rarely sit to get dusty on the shelves.

Frits R. Rosendaal
September 2008

Preface

In the past two to three decades, few disciplines, if any, in Laboratory Medicine have seen the growth in the number of tests and complexity of testing as that experienced in the discipline of Hemostasis and Thrombosis. These rapid changes have presented challenges for laboratories as they develop quality programs for the oversight of this testing. The quality issues extend across all levels of testing and all sizes of laboratories. In the USA alone, there are thousands of locations performing the prothrombin time (INR) for the monitoring of oral anticoagulant therapy. In contrast, the number of laboratories employing highly sophisticated methods is measured in dozens worldwide.

While considering the title for this book we had an interesting discussion regarding the possibilities of "... the Hemostasis and Thrombosis Laboratory" and "... Laboratory Hemostasis and Thrombosis". The distinction is subtle but relevant, the former being a place and the latter a discipline. Quality issues in this discipline extend well beyond the walls of the laboratory. In this book we have included contributions from recognized experts. They have provided information on elements of managing quality as it relates to individual tests or groups of tests extending from nuances of internal quality control to the challenges in the many areas where standardization may be absent or inadequate. There is information on all aspects of testing from preanalytic to analytic and result reporting as well as external quality assurance. In addition, chapters are included regarding the development of international guidelines for methods as well as the preparation of international standard plasmas and reagents.

Quality is a changing process, continually striving to improve the product while reducing errors and improving safety. This book represents an event in this continuum, and is intended to capture the elements of quality at all levels of the practice of Laboratory Hemostasis and Thrombosis, as they exist in 2008. We believe that it will provide a useful guide for those involved Hemostasis and Thrombosis testing, whether very simple, like the point of care, or complex, like the major reference laboratory.

John Olson
Eric Preston
Steve Kitchen
August, 2008

1 General quality planning in the hemostasis laboratory

J.D. Olson

"So", you might ask, "What is quality, anyway?" The word quality repeatedly infiltrates our discussions and interactions as we work to produce or choose a product. The *Oxford English Dictionary* devotes more that 3000 words in its effort to define the many variations on the use of this word. We may all have difficulty with a definition, but we do know what we mean. The customer of the product or service defines many aspects of its quality while those who are producing define many others. Stated in its simplest terms, quality is the condition or state of a person, thing or process.

Elements of quality management systems began with a publication by Shewhart in 1931[1] providing a footing for quality processes based on a scientific and/or statistical footing. He stated: "A phenomenon will be said to be controlled when, through the use of past experience, we can predict, at least within limits, how the phenomenon may be expected to vary in the future. Here it is understood that prediction means that we can state, at least approximately, the probability that the observed phenomenon will fall within given limits."[1]

The evolution of quality management systems were influenced by experiences in World War II. During the war, individuals involved in the production of reliable devices (weapons and other implements to support a war effort) for the consumer (soldier) to do their job effectively tied the entire system from raw material to the use of the finished product in a unique "team" from start to finish. Few circumstances can link the person in production so directly to the importance of the outcome. The success of the soldier was tied to the long-term well-being of the person making the weapon or other defense device. This ability to build the tight feeling of kinship and team on the part of people in production to the quality of the product is the goal of quality programs in all sectors of the economy today. It is, of course, very difficult to achieve this attitude in the workplace in the same way that it could be when the outcome could so directly benefit the producers.

Following World War II, the effort of reconstruction of the industry and economy of the affected countries became a major international effort and influenced the evolution of quality programs. The work of Deming[2] and Juran,[3,4] both associates of Shewhart, extended his work. In 1951, Juran[3] published a seminal book that proposed the key elements for managing quality: quality planning, quality control and quality improvement. Following World War II, Deming proposed a significant departure from the "standard" thinking about quality, proposing that modification to the real relationships of quality, costs, productivity and profit. The different approach to quality espoused by Deming is compared with the "standard" thinking in Table 1.1.[5] Thus, anything that improves the product or service in the eyes of the customer defines the goals of the quality program.

Organizations that follow Deming principles find that good quality is hard to define, but the lack of quality is easily identified. In the "standard" management of a system, the workers ultimately pay for

Quality in Laboratory Hemostasis and Thrombosis, 1st edition. By Steve Kitchen, John D. Olson and F. Eric Preston. Published 2009 by Blackwell Publishing. ISBN: 978-1-4051-6803-8

Table 1.1 Comparison of Deming and traditional management principles.[5]

Common company practices
- Quality is expensive
- Inspection is the key to quality
- Quality control experts and inspectors can ensure quality
- Defects are caused by workers
- The manufacturing process can be optimized by outside experts with little or no change in system afterwards
- Little or no input from workers
- Use of work standards, quotas and goals can help productivity
- Fear and reward are proper ways to motivate
- Employees can be treated like commodities – buying more when needed, laying-off when needing less
- Rewarding the best performers and punishing the worst will lead to greater productivity and creativity
- Buy one supplier off against another and switch suppliers based only on price
- Profits are made by keeping revenue high and costs down

"Deming" company practices
- Quality leads to lower costs
- Inspection is too late. If workers can produce defect-free goods, eliminate inspections
- Quality is made in the boardroom
- Most defects are caused by the system
- Process is never optimized; it can always be improved
- Elimination of all work standards and quotas is necessary. Fear leads to disaster
- People should be made to feel secure in their jobs
- Most variation is caused by the system
- Buy from vendors committed to quality and work with suppliers
- Invest time and knowledge to help suppliers improve quality and costs. Develop long-term relationships with suppliers
- Profits are generated by loyal customers

management failure; when profits are reduced, then management reduces labor costs. In contrast, moving quality programs as close to the worker as possible will ultimately lead to lower cost and improved consumer and worker satisfaction.

The clinical laboratory has three "consumers" of their product:

1 The patient who benefits from the best possible result.

2 The ordering clinician who depends upon the right test, at the right time, with an accurate result in order to make a clinical decision.

3 The hospital, clinic or other entity that depends upon the laboratory for a positive margin when comparing cost with revenue.

All three consumers benefit when the quality program drives the best possible practice.

Many different quality practices and/or programs have evolved in the decades since the original work of Shewhart, Juran and Deming. They all have acronyms (e.g. TQM, CQI, ISO, IOP, ORYX, Six Sigma®) and a common goal of improving the quality of the performance (and product) of an organization. The discussion of these individual programs is beyond the scope of this chapter, but many of the principles are addressed below and in other chapters of this book. All programs have great strength, but they also suffer from being proscriptive, an issue that is discussed later in this chapter.

Elements of quality in the hemostasis laboratory

At the moment that a clinician orders a laboratory test, he/she sets in motion a complex process that involves many individuals. More than two dozen individual actions, involvement of sophisticated instruments and multiple interfaces of computing devices encompass three phases: preanalytic phase (order, collection and transport); analytic phase (making the correct measurement); postanalytic phase (formulating and delivering the data and the action of the clinician in response to the result). Figure 1.1 is a graphic depiction of this process. Examining the figure, one might think of each arrow representing an opportunity for error that could effect the final result. A quality program must encompass all of these events with process to prevent errors and to detect an error if it occurs.

Internal quality control

The control of the testing procedure (quality control) evolved with the transition of research testing into the

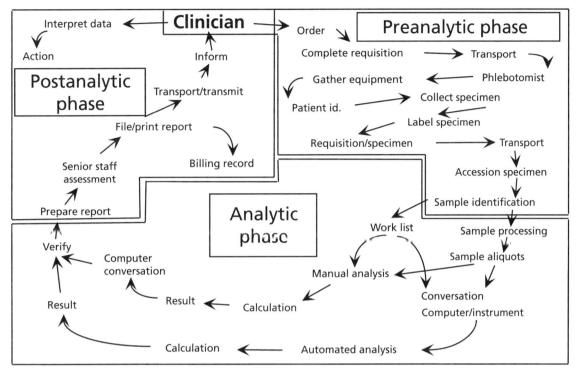

Fig. 1.1 The laboratory cycle. Depicted are the steps needed to complete a laboratory test, beginning with the ordering clinician and ending with the response of the ordering clinician to the result. Preanalytic, analytic and postanalytic parts of the process are indicated. More that two dozen steps, indicated by arrows, are involved, each of which may be the source of an error. Monitoring by a quality program is required.

clinical arena. To be confident that the method returns the correct result requires that steps be taken to assure all elements are within the control of the operator. Technologists are taught that instruments/methods are designed to fail and that they can rely upon results only if the entire method performs within defined limits with specimens of known value. The frequency of these control events are method specific and a function of the stability of all of the elements (reagent, specimen, instrument) and must be driven by historical data from the method itself. Internal quality control is the grandfather of quality programs in the laboratory and is detailed elsewhere in this book (Chapter 5).

Many industries and some laboratories have adopted control processes that focus on quantifying and reducing errors called Six Sigma®.[6] Six Sigma® was developed by an engineer (Bill Smith) at the Motorola company and the company began using the program in the mid 1980s. Six Sigma® is a registered trademark of the Motorola Corporation. Application of the process has become very popular among companies internationally. Six Sigma® processes can be applied to discrete events (e.g. mislabeled specimens, clerical errors) and to variable events (i.e. variance of a method like the fibrinogen assay). Elements of these activities are depicted in Table 1.2. Discrete elements are expressed in defects per million events (DPM). Achieving the Six Sigma® goal means that defects are less than $1:1,000,000$, a level achieved in the airline industry. Errors in the healthcare industry are much more frequent, with errors causing injury to hospitalized patients at 10,000 DPM (3.8 σ), errors in therapeutic drug monitoring 244,000 DPM (2.2 σ) or errors of laboratory reporting much better at 447 DPM (4.8 σ).[7]

Other aspects of the laboratory activity rely on analysis of the variability of data. This variability can be measured at several levels. The greatest variability is seen in External Quality Assessment (EQA) data

Table 1.2 Six Sigma® metrics.[6]

Measure outcomes
Inspect outcomes and count defects
Calculate defects per million
Convert DPM to sigma metric

Measure variation
Measure variation of a process (SD)
Calculate sigma process capability
Determine QC design metric

DPM, defects per million events; QC, quality control; SD, standard deviation.

Table 1.3 Sigma metrics for common coagulation tests.[8]

Test	Sigma metric			
	TEa	NTQ	NMQ	LMQ
Prothrombin time	15%	na	1.77	5.35
INR	20%	na	2.39	3.52
Fibrinogen assay	20%	1.78	2.01	3.24

INR, international normalized ratio; LMQ, Local Method Quality (single laboratory); na, not available; NMQ, National Method Quality (within method); NTQ, National Total Quality (all methods); TEa, total acceptable error.

regarding the all method variance, referred to as the National Total Quality (NTQ). EQA programs also report data for an analyte comparing many laboratories using the same method, referred to the National Method Quality (NMQ). NMQ is frequently significantly better because variability is only among laboratories using the same methods, but not among methods. The lowest variability is seen with a single method in a single laboratory, referred to as the Local Method Quality (LMQ).[8] Thus, the degree of variability is best controlled at the local level, method-specific interlaboratory variability is greater variability and the greatest is the variability examining across all methods. Examples of this degree of variability are shown for prothrombin time, international normalized ratio (INR) and fibrinogen assay in Table 1.3.[8] The data in Table 1.3 are very specifically based on the data from the 2004 EQA data of the College of

American Pathologists, as reported by Westgard.[8] Should a number of different EQA data sets be analyzed, there would be a range of sigma statistics of a similar magnitude. The low sigma values shown mean that adequate control will demand more rigorous attention to control procedures, often necessitating multiple control rules. Common goals in industry are to strive for 6 σ processes and to accept 3 σ. At 3 σ or below, effective error detection could not be achieved, even with as many as six quality control rules. There is much progress yet to be made in the quality of many coagulation procedures.

Quality Assurance

During the 1980s, laboratories began looking beyond the analytic procedure with quality programs called Quality Assurance. Quality control remained a part of the Quality Assurance program, but the program expanded to consider such items as laboratory orders, requisitions, collections techniques and other issues directly impacting the result of the test but not always directly in the control of the laboratory. Preanalytic issues are detailed elsewhere in this book (Chapter 4). Postanalytic issues also became a part of quality initiatives this same era. Such issues as reporting formats, verification of calculated results, timely reporting and even action taken as a result of the data reported. It was during this period that computer applications in both the laboratory and the clinical environments began to grow, requiring the validations and continued verification of computer function and interfaces for electronic result reporting between computers as well as between instruments and computers. Encouraged (or demanded) by accreditation and/or regulatory agencies, laboratory professionals also began asking questions of and listening to clinicians regarding the quality of service, needs to provide new tests shown to have clinical value and to remove antiquated tests that no longer offer added clinical information. These activities started the interaction of the quality programs in the laboratory with similar programs in the rest of the healthcare institution.

External Quality Assessment

In the 1930s,[9] the need for interlaboratory standardization for public health programs led to early efforts at EQA. The concept of an unknown specimen being sent from a central EQA agency to the laboratory for testing with the results sent back to the agency for evaluation added an important new level of assurance for the quality of analysis. In addition, results were reported in a way that allowed a laboratory to compare their performance with other laboratories using the same or similar methods. Laboratory participation in EQA programs grew rapidly in the 1950s and 1960s. In large part this growth was due to the development of accreditation and regulatory programs requiring EQA; however, the recognition by unregulated laboratories that EQA was vital to the quality of their own programs has also led to widening acceptance. Detailed discussion of EQA programs is addressed elsewhere in this book (Chapter 6).

Error detection and correction

McGregor[10] contrasted two theories of company management which he referred to as X and Y. A company following theory X assumes that the worker prefers to be directed and wants to avoid responsibility. In contrast, a company that is following theory Y assumes that the workers enjoy what they do and, in the right conditions, will strive to do their very best. In general, the company that follows theory X manages from the "top down" with dependence of the worker upon management as he/she performs tasks. A hallmark of theory X is toughness, the rules are laid out and every employee must "obey." The workplace has an element of fear that an error might occur and that reprimand will result. The style of the company that follows theory Y is different. Management works from the "bottom up." The workplace is configured to satisfy the worker and to encourage commitment to the organization. Workers are encouraged to be self-directed and the management and supervisory style is supportive. Theory Y has been described as operating with a "velvet glove." Stated in another way, one can think of management under theory X strives to "drive" the organization and the workers to success, while the management under theory Y strives to "lead" the organization and the workers to success. The goal in both cases is essentially the same, but the means are very different. This brief description of diverging management styles can impact process improvement within the laboratory.

In order for any method, process or laboratory to improve, it is paramount to correct and understand the cause of the errors that interfere with productivity. The laboratory needs a system for capturing and categorizing errors. Such a system becomes the infrastructure for improvement in a quality program. It is obvious that for such a system to be successful, there needs to be an aggressive program to identify all errors, optimally at the time of the occurrence and the ideal process is one that is looking prospectively at processes, seeking to prevent. Deming[5] pointed out that inspection after the fact is too late. The airline industry provides an example. Considerable effort is applied to understanding what causes the big error, an airplane crash. However, great efforts are now directed at the near misses both in the air and on the ground, a proactive effort to understand the "close call" to help prevent the major event. The laboratory needs a similar aggressive approach that must begin with each individual owning their part of the process and identifying the problems as they occur, or seeing ways to prevent problems by changing process. In order for such a process to be most efficient, the worker cannot be threatened by the mechanism to report errors. The examples regarding the differing approaches may be useful.

First, a technologist has just completed a run on an automated instrument using expensive reagents and many patient results. He/she notices that two required reagents were placed in the wrong position, causing them to be added in the wrong order. The error caused erroneous patient results, but not to the degree that it would be easily detected. The consequence of repeating the run is twofold: the cost of the reagent and time of the technologist are expensive and the delay in completing the testing resulting in complaints from clinicians. In this scenario, management under theory X results in a reprimand from the supervisor and a letter being placed in the technologist's personnel file for consideration at the next performance evaluation. The consequences may be severe enough for the technologist to consider not reporting the error. In contrast, management under theory Y would result in the supervisor complementing the technologist for detecting the problem and engaging the technologist in an investigation of the reason that the error occurred. The supervisor and the technologist understand that the goal is to prevent this from happening in the future, whether this person or another performs the procedure.

Second is a case in which the error that occurred above was not detected by the technologist performing the test, but at a later time during the supervisor's inspection of reported results. Managing under theory X, the supervisor will confront the technologist with the data and, just as in the prior example, will issue a reprimand and a letter. Managing under theory Y, the supervisor will present the information to the technologist and ask the technologist to assist in understanding how the problem occurred and how it might be avoided in the future.

Errors like those described that are detected and investigated are most frequently found to be problems in the process, not exclusively with the individual carrying out the procedure at the time. Improving the process to help workers prevent errors is the goal, which can only be achieved if all errors are detected and investigated. Contrasting the approaches, one can see that punishing the worker and failing to examine process will not improve the quality and the worker will not be enthused about reporting future errors. The second approach engages the workers and rewards activities that improve quality in the laboratory.

Quality System Essentials

Development and maintenance of a quality program in a laboratory requires that there be an infrastructure of support in order for internal and external quality control and quality assurance to be successful. The field of hemostasis provides an excellent example of this issue. The hemostasis laboratory has the entire spectrum of testing from the highly automated to the complex manual tests that are time-consuming and demand a different skill set. Thus, in addition to a good quality control program, there is need for an effective program for development and continuing education of the staff. The same can be said of a host of essential activities in the laboratory including such things as: acquisition and maintenance of capital equipment; supply inventory; safety of staff and patients; and others. In the late 1990s and early 2000s, recommendations began to appear for the comprehensive management of the quality of all aspects of the laboratory operations. International Standards Organization (ISO) developed the ISO 17025 (primarily a laboratory management program)[11] and ISO 15189 (a program specifically for clinical

Table 1.4 Quality System Essentials (CLSI 1999).[11]

Purchasing and inventory
Organization
Personnel
Equipment
Document and records
Process control
Information management
Deviations, non-conformance
Assessments: internal and external
Process improvement
Customer service
Facilities and safety

laboratories).[12] The Clinical Laboratory Standards Institute (CLSI), at the time named NCCLS, published the Quality System Essentials (QSE).[13] The ISO programs have achieved acceptance in Europe, while the QSE programs are more commonly in use in North America. Both approach the issues of quality with a very broad perspective, covering all elements of laboratory operations. There is a brief description of some aspects of QSE below.

The list presented in Table 1.4 is an example of the QSE for a given laboratory. The list is not intended to be the list for use in every laboratory. Each laboratory needs to develop its own essentials, formulated to help manage issues within their own laboratory. The list is ordinarily 9–12 items in length and the types of issues to be addressed are encompassed in Table 1.4. Each of the item on this list will be controlled by a set of three levels of documents:

Policies
Statement of intent with regards to rules and requirements of regulations, accreditation and standards. Each QSE will have one or a small number of policies that will provide the framework for all activities within the QSE. In the case of test development, policies may address such things as validation, quality control, EQA and others.

Process descriptions
This is a description of how the policies are implemented. Process descriptions will often cross more than one department, section of departments and procedures within a department. Flowcharts and tables

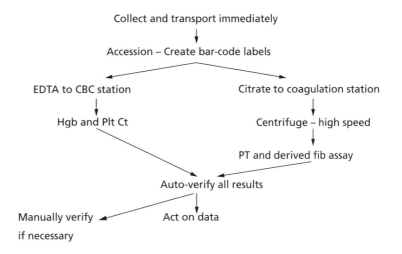

Fig. 1.2 Process for the bleeding profile. This process for reporting the results of the prothrombin time (PT), fibrinogen assay (fib assay), platelet count (Plt Ct) and hemoglobin (Hgb) involves the activity of at least four different units in the health system and execution of as many as 10 standard operating procedures (SOPs). As a part of the Quality System Essentials (QSE), a process description would be needed to assure return of results rapidly enough for clinician action when managing an actively bleeding patient.

are often used to describe processes. An example of a process requiring control is given below.

Procedures and related forms

The standard operating procedure (SOP) is a step-by-step description of how to perform an individual method or task.

The policy and the SOP are commonly used documents in all laboratories; however, the process description may not be as familiar. An example is shown in Fig. 1.2. The purpose of this process is to provide the surgeon and anesthesiologist with information needed to manage blood transfusion therapy in the rapidly bleeding patient. The data needed are the prothrombin time, fibrinogen, hemoglobin and platelet count. The process needs for an order, specimen collection, transport, laboratory receipt/accession, testing in two separate sections of the laboratory, reporting and delivery of the data to the clinician. Ownership of the various steps in this process are in the control of the physician, nurse and three different sections of the laboratory. In order for this to occur in a meaningful time frame in the clinical setting (less than 15 minutes), there must be well-understood coordination among all of those involved. Each step in the process described has its own SOP for the action taken. In this case, there are at least 10 SOPs supporting a single process.

Implementation of a program can be challenging. Most laboratories have a quality program that can provide the beginning for the development of QSE.

Most laboratories also have most of the essentials that they will define in their QSE, they are just not under the umbrella of the program and not easily identified. Thus, an initial step in changing the program will be gathering key individuals with knowledge and energy for the process to identify the QSE for the organization. Technologists should also be represented in this process. Once the QSE are identified, teams can be formed to begin drafting of policies. Leadership from the highest levels, supporting the changes that need to be made and leading the infrastructure of a management structure based upon McGregor's theory Y is a crucial element. Possibly the most important issue is putting reality into fault-free reporting of errors, followed by an investigation to improve process to prevent future occurrences.

For many laboratories, instituting the concepts that are described in this chapter would necessitate significant change in the quality program, the perspective of the manager and the attitude of the employee. Such a change in the culture is difficult. It is tempting to try to "buy, install and run" a program from a quality vendor. Such an approach is likely to meet with resistance, with workers viewing it as "just another of those quality things that the administration is going to force on us." In the past two decades (or more) most laboratories have instituted more than one new quality program in an effort to find a solution that works well in their setting. One possible difficulty in such an approach is the proscriptive nature of the process. They provide everything that is needed:

policies, forms, SOPs, etc. What they do not provide is the personal ownership that can come from the internal development of the quality process. Managers may find a smoother and more lasting solution in providing policies that allow for each unit to develop their own approach to the gathering of data, the identification of errors and the many other elements of the quality program.

Conclusions

Over the course of the past 70 years or more, elements of the quality program have evolved in a somewhat stepwise fashion, beginning with internal quality control and progressing to more comprehensive programs that encompass all activities in the workplace. In the remainder of this book you will find information regarding quality in all aspects of the hemostasis laboratory. Experts provide information regarding the highest level of development of standards (both methods and materials) to the finest details of the nuances of selected methods. Integrated into a comprehensive quality program, similar to that described above, the information should help in the development of a "quality hemostasis laboratory."

References

1 Shewhart WA. *Economic Control of Quality of Manufactured Product*. New York: D. Van Nostrand, 1931.
2 DeAguayo R. *Deming: The American Who Taught the Japanese About Quality*. New York: Simon and Schuster, 1990: 1–66.
3 Juran JM. *Juran's Quality Control Handbook*, 4th edn. New York: McGraw-Hill, 1988.
4 Juran JM. *Juran on Leadership for Quality: An Executive Handbook*. New York: Collier Macmillan, 1989: 1–80.
5 Travers EM, McClatchy KM. Basic laboratory management. In *Clinical Laboratory Medicine*, 2nd edn. McClatchy KM (ed.). Philadelphia: Lippincott, Williams and Wilkins, 2002: 3–31.
6 Westgard JO. *Six Sigmas Quality Design and Control*. Madison, WI: Westgard QC, 2001: 11–22.
7 Nevalainen D, Berte L, Kraft C, Leigh E, Morgan T. Evaluating laboratory performance on quality indicators with the Six Sigma scale. *Arch Pathol Lab Med* 2000; **124**: 516–519.
8 Westgard JO, Westgard SA. The quality of laboratory testing today: an assessment of σ metrics for analytic quality using performance data from proficiency testing surveys and the CLIA criteria for acceptable performance. *Am J Clin Pathol* 2006; **125**: 343–354.
9 Cumming HS, Hazen HH, Sanford FE, *et al*. Evaluation of serodiagnostic tests for syphilis in the United States: report of results. *Vener Dis Inf* 1935, **16**: 189.
10 McGregor D. *The Human Side of Enterprise*. New York: McGraw-Hill, 1960: 1–58.
11 International Organization for Standardization. ISO/IEC 17025:2005: General requirements for the competence of testing and calibration laboratories. http://www.iso.org/iso/catalogue_detail?csnumber=39883
12 International Organization for Standardization. ISO 15189. 2007: Medical Laboratories: Particular requirements for quality and competence. http://www.iso.org/iso/iso_catalogue/catalogue_tc/catalogue_detail.htm?csnumber=42641
13 National Committee for Clinical Laboratory Standards. *A Quality System Model for Health Care: Approved Guidelines*. NCCLS Document GP26-A. Wayne, PA: NCCLS, 1999.

2

Hemostasis test validation, performance and reference intervals

R. A. Marlar

The clinical hemostasis laboratory is a complex testing arena that does not fit well into the mold of hematology ("counting" of particles – red blood cells or platelets) or chemistry with known concentrations of analytes (sodium charge, albumin mass). The hemostasis assay inventory spans multiple tests types (from clotting tests to chromogenic and immunologic assays to specialized tests such as electrophoresis, aggregation and radioactive-based tests) and results are expressed in a wide variety of units: time, percentage, units, mass, radioactivity and even visual interpretation. The majority of these values are without established international standards. These parameters complicate the development, validation and performance of methods for both routine coagulation laboratory and the complex methods in the "special" coagulation laboratory.

Modifications such as using one manufacturer's kit on another manufacturer's instrument or in-house ("home-brew") tests or components lead to many challenges of standardization and validation of methods to produce accurate diagnostic or therapeutic information. Before a new method can be introduced into clinical use, both analytical and clinical performance must be verified under the operating parameters of the laboratory. This chapter is intended to review the validation procedure and outline a systematic approach for validation of hemostatic assays helping laboratories to meet the daily needs of

Quality in Laboratory Hemostasis and Thrombosis, 1st edition. By Steve Kitchen, John D. Olson and F. Eric Preston. Published 2009 by Blackwell Publishing. ISBN: 978-1-4051-6803-8

internal quality standards and external certification requirements.

The general and continuing assessment of clinical coagulation falls to one or more accrediting agencies sanctioned by each country. The accreditation requirements of "good laboratory practices" for each oversight group are varied but specific to each agency. For a number of hemostatic tests, significant problems are encountered including differences in reagents generating results in arbitrary units (Pro Time and activated partial thromboplastin time [aPTT]); hemostatic tests with multiple protocols (Bethesda vs. Nijmegen inhibitor assays) and tests with results reported based on experience or visual interpretation (platelet aggregation or von Willebrand factor [VWF] multimers).

A general introduction to the processes of validation and performance evaluation is presented followed by a discussion of the reference interval. The use of validation protocol will objectively evaluate the performance of the method and must be established prior to any studies to define the limits of the method (Table 2.1). Validation is the process of proving that a procedure, process, system, the equipment and methods work singly and together as expected to achieve the intended result. Validation of a method investigates the major characteristics of the method with continued performance evaluation over time maintaining assurance that the method has the same characteristics as initially assigned. After the assay has been deemed valid and the performance characteristics established, the final aspect is to determine the range of the values present in the populations in which the assay will be used.

Table 2.1 Types and requirements for reference intervals in coagulation.

Reference interval	Criteria definition
New analyte	Measurement of reference interval is difficult, lack of established data on physiology and medical aspects
New analyte method	Measurement of reference interval is easier as physiologic and medical information is established
Transference of reference values	Same analyte with same method utilizing new lot or instrument, however difficult to establish evaluation of standards

This concept of population and sampling along with the basic establishment of reference interval is discussed.

Hemostatic tests validation concepts

The purpose of validating test methods is to ensure the generation of high quality data for the accurate diagnosis of disease. The time invested in validating analytical methods will ultimately provide the necessary diagnostic advantages in the long run. Procedural, methodologic or instrumentation validation will demonstrate that the procedure, method or instrument, respectively, is acceptable for the overall intended use. These steps must be thorough for all aspects of the process and should include specificity, accuracy, precision, limits, linearity and robustness. Validation of coagulation assays, instruments or reagents is the cornerstone of laboratory diagnostics for the coagulation laboratory and is the process to demonstrate acceptability of the analytical method.

The validation procedure is necessary for the determining of performance characteristics. A working written procedure (protocol) detailing the validation should include the procedural steps necessary to perform the test, the necessary instrumentation, reagents and samples, the method for calibration, formulae for generating results, and source of reference standards and controls. In addition, the common statistics (see chapter appendix) used in coagulation

testing is presented. The typical validation parameters are discussed below using descriptions from formal definitions and slanted toward hemostatic testing.[1,2] These include **specificity, accuracy, precision, linearity, limit of detection, limit of quantitation and robustness.**

A validation process must be designed to ensure that the result of a method will correctly support the diagnosis of patients with coagulation defects. The samples, reagents, controls, calibrators and instruments to be used for validation purposes should be carefully selected. Samples and specimens for validation must be collected, processed and stored by established guidelines and identical to routine collection methods.[3] In the validation process for diagnostic and/or therapeutic control methods, the reagent lots and instruments must be those that will be used in the laboratory when the methods are put in place.[2,3]

Specificity

Specificity is the ability to unequivocally assess the analyte in a standard specimen in the presence of components that may be expected to be present.[2,4] Typically, this includes such components as the matrix (plasma) and degraded or inactive components. The method should be capable of differentiation of similar analytes or interference that could have significant effect on the value. In commercially available methods (especially Food and Drug Administration [FDA] approved methods) these evaluations should have been performed by the manufacturer. In "home-brew" assays, specificity must be demonstrated by the user, a task that may be very difficult.

Accuracy

Accuracy is the closeness of agreement between the test value and the true value.[5] In hemostasis testing, this can be one of the most difficult or impossible parameters to determine; in fact, the concept of "true value" may not even apply to many coagulation tests especially those that report results as time values (prothrombin time [PT], aPTT, thrombin time).[2,6] In a like manner, the majority of hemostasis tests have no "gold" standard or even established true value. This concept is changing as international standards are developed (fibrinogen, factor VIII, protein C, antithrombin and VWF).[7,8] For some standards (fibrinogen, protein C, antithrombin, factor VIII), accuracy issues arise because of differences in the methods used. The laboratory must make certain that their standards are linked to the international standard through secondary standards of the manufacturer.[2,6] Preparation of international standards is addressed elsewhere in this book (Chapter 3).

Precision

Precision is the closeness of agreement (degree of variability) among a series of measurements obtained from multiple sampling from a single sample or reference material.[2,9] Precision includes within-assay variability (intra-assay) and day-to-day variability (inter-assay). Intra-assay precision or repeatability is precision under the same operating conditions. Inter-assay precision or reproducibility is the imprecision of the method when the assay components may be different (different days, different operators and different equipment). Precision is established without accuracy because it is the closeness of the data that is important. The precision is usually expressed as coefficient of variation (CV).

Precision evaluation consists of a two-prong assessment: within-run precision and between-run or day-to-day variation. The within-run variation is determined by performing the assay on the same specimen or control within a single run using the same reagent batch for a minimum of 20 measurements. The CV should be <10% but usually 3–6% for clotting, chromogenic and most immunologic analytes. For the more complex assays (platelet aggregation, VWF and lupus anticoagulant), the imprecision in terms of CV may be 10–20%.

Between-run precision is evaluated by repeating the same specimens (usually controls) on the same instrument but other variables for a minimum of 10 runs. In general, the imprecision for between-run studies are greater than observed for within-run precision studies. For some of the more complex assays, the precision can increase to a significant 30–40%. The acceptable limits of imprecision during validation is difficult to define and will vary among laboratories. No hard and fast rules apply for coagulation testing precision acceptability; however, the laboratory should decide acceptable limits of imprecision based on publications, manufacturer's data or published guidelines. At least three samples that cross the range to be validated are part of the precision study. The acceptable levels of imprecision may be different between normal and abnormal samples, the type of assay and the reagent–instrument combination. The precision results should mirror the values reported by the reagent and/or instrument manufacturer. Precision within the manufacturer's reported limits is acceptable. If the obtained value is greater than the manufacturer, the laboratory may still accept the results if they feel their method parameters justify the increased imprecision.

Limits

In the evaluation of an assay's performance, two types of limits must be considered: limit of detection and limit of quantitation.[2,6,10]

Limit of detection

The limit of detection (LOD) of a method is the level that can be distinguished from a sample without analyte present (blank), but not necessarily sufficient to be precisely or accurately quantified.[10] The LOD is usually defined as 3 standard deviations (SD) above the mean of the blank so the limit is above the "noise" of the method and the probability of a false positive is small (<1%). Both the accuracy and precision of the method (including all components and preanalytical variables) have an important role in determining this limit. Although these classic aspects are important in the coagulation laboratory, an added layer of assay complexity with time-based results (PT and aPTT) is found, because these methods have no specific analytes to determine. Many coagulation methods have poor limits of detection because of imprecision or no differentiation at levels that are clinically relevant. The standard protocol for determining the lower limit of detection is to measure a zero standard (no analyte present) multiple times (20 replicates) and calculate the standard deviation. The 3 SD range is considered noise and the value at 3 SD is the lower limit of detection. In the coagulation laboratory, this lower limit is sometimes difficult to ascertain because finding a true zero standard that is plasma-based is not available. It is important to understand the lower limit of detection of the assay in relation to the clinical use of the assay. A good example of this relationship is associated with hemophilia testing in which it is important to distinguish clinically between a level of <1% and 3%. If the lower LOD is only 3%, then patients with severe bleeding symptoms cannot be differentiated from milder bleeding forms. The laboratory must decide what level of detection is necessary clinically for each method and then determine the level of detection for their method.

There are a number of different "detection limits" that must be taken into account in the overall evaluation of the coagulation method (instrument LOD, method LOD, reagent and plasma substrates LOD). Both the instrument detection limit and method detection limit are the main parameters for evaluations of a new method or new reagent–instrument system. This information is usually supplied by the manufacturer but should be verified by the laboratory prior to using the assay.

Limits of quantitation

The limits of quantitation (LOQ) defines the lowest amount of analyte to be quantified and the level at which two values can be distinguished with acceptable precision and accuracy.[10] Usually, the lower LOQ is statistically defined as 5–10 SD from the negative control value; however, each method must be evaluated to determine the lowest level.

The laboratory, in consultation with the clinical staff, must determine the clinically necessary lower LOQ for each assay. The LOQ can be drastically different among methods, type of method, result reported and among laboratories. Coagulation assays such as the PT, aPTT and some lupus anticoagulant tests have a large difference in LOQ because they are global-based assays measuring multiple factors.

Range

The range of an analytical method is the interval between the upper and lower analyte concentration for which the analytical method has demonstrated a suitable level of precision, accuracy and linearity.[2,10] The range of each assay is dependent on the clinical needs of the specific analyte. The lower end of the linear range is usually the most important but

may be the most difficult to establish. The laboratory cannot report values lower than the lowest standard of the calibration curve. If the test method cannot be reported to the level necessary for clinical utility, then alternative methods or modifications of the method must be undertaken to achieve the desired level including curves established for lower ranges, different dilutions of the standards or other methods.[2,11]

Linearity

The linearity is the ability to obtain results that are directly proportional to the concentration of analyte within a given range.[2,12] Mathematical transformations of data can help to promote linearity if there is scientific evidence that transformation is appropriate for the method. A good example is the factor assay that may use semi-log or log–log transformations. Linearity acceptance criteria are usually based on the correlation coefficient of linear regression. It is important not to force the origin to zero in the calculation as this may skew the actual best-fit slope through the range of use. For quantitative coagulation methods used for diagnosis and monitoring, the analytical method must have a good proportional relationship between analyte concentration and instrument response. The limit for the upper range must not exceed the level of the highest linear standard.

Methods for linearity determination of a coagulation quantitative method have changed over the last decade.[2] Linearity computations have evolved from visual assessment of the line to statistical analysis via linear regression.[2] However, linear regression will not readily define acceptable limits because many of the quantitative coagulation assays are somewhat imprecise and have a poor linear fit. In the future, refined statistical methods including polynomial analysis will become a standard linearity assessment tool.

Robustness

The robustness of an analytical procedure is a measure of its capacity to remain unaffected by small variations in method parameters and provides an indication of its reliability during normal usage.[13,14] The important parameters include different machines, operators, reagent lots and sample preparation, among a host of others.

Robustness is difficult to assess truly and generally has more problems with increasing complexity of the analytical system. The majority of the analysis for robustness is determined by the manufacturer and usually approved by a regulatory agency such as the FDA. However, if the reagents are not designed and evaluated by the manufacturer, then stated claims of the method are not validated. In this case, the coagulation laboratory must assume responsibility for determining robustness. The parameters that the laboratory must evaluate are those encountered in the clinical setting.

Ideally, robustness should be explored during the development of the assay method through the use of a protocol. For such a protocol, one must first identify variables in the method that may influence the results. One might expect storage conditions and processing of the sample, minimal and maximal dilution and type of diluant; level of interference (e.g. hemolysis, lipemia). Preanalytic issues are addressed elsewhere in this book (Chapter 4). This type of method manipulation will ensure that the system components are robust.

Protocol

Prior to initiating any validation study, whether establishing a new test, changing reagents or instruments, or changing methodology, a well-planned validation protocol is instituted for scientific and clinical soundness.[2,15] Protocol outlines are typically provided by commercial companies who supply the reagents and/or instruments. The protocol must describe in detail the planned studies including the statistics and defined acceptance criteria.[15] The protocol must be performed in a timely manner with adequate samples, standards and calibrators. Much of this information is described in documents provided by accrediting and standards organizations.[1,2,6,15]

After performing the validation protocol, the data must be analyzed with predetermined statistical methods such that the results and conclusions are presented in a validation summary report. If the defined criteria established in the protocol are met and any variations affecting the overall conclusions justified, then the method can be considered valid. The final validation report, along with all of the data,

statistical analyses and the signatures and titles of all participants, including supervisors, administrators, consultants and reviewers are placed in the official standard operating procedure (SOP).

Performance of hemostasis assays

To ensure the continued proper diagnosis and treatment of hemostatic disorders, long-term consistent precise and accurate laboratory testing is necessary. For each assay, consistency and reproducibility over time with continued accurate results are required objectives. This requires ongoing evaluation of the method, not only during each performance run (internal quality control) but also periodic comparison with others laboratories for continual accuracy (external quality assurance).

Internal quality control

A good quality control program maintains an ongoing statistical analysis for each method. This is usually mandated by regulatory agencies, government and/or standards institutes. The main aim of an internal quality assessment program is to confirm that generated results remain consistent over time. Internal quality control is discussed in detail elsewhere in this book (Chapter 5).

External quality assessment

External quality assessment is a critical element in any laboratory quality program and today, in many countries, laboratories are required to participate in external programs to promote accurate and consistent test results. External quality assessment is discussed in detail elsewhere in this book (Chapter 6).

Reference interval

The interpretation of coagulation test data from a patient is a comparative decision-making process, i.e. patient results are compared with a "reference interval" for making diagnostic and/or therapeutic decisions. Therefore, the determination of the correct reference interval is of the utmost importance. In the past, ranges have been poorly defined without a consistent process for determination. With the broad spectrum of coagulation testing methods, a systematic and consistent process must be utilized to establish the proper reference interval for the population in question. Reference interval criteria and methodology can be found in a variety of publications and guidelines from standardization organizations.[16,17] The criteria and protocols for reference interval determination fall into three categories (Table 2.1), each requiring different method requirements. A therapeutic reference interval such as for heparin therapy must be determined in a similar manner as the reference interval.

For reference intervals, definitions of the terminology have a very special place. A *reference population* is the population consisting of all of the *reference individuals*.[18] This is usually very large and hypothetical group. The *reference sample group* is a selected group of individuals representing the reference population. The *reference distribution* is the range of reference values with the *reference limits* determined by a statistical evaluation of the reference sample group and the *reference interval* is the set of values between the upper and lower reference limits.[17,18] Reference intervals can be associated with normal or good health, pathologic conditions and therapeutic interventions.

To establish a reference interval, a well-defined protocol must be utilized. An outline of a protocol for new analytes and/or new methods is presented in Table 2.2; however, more detailed protocols for general laboratory reference intervals have been published elsewhere.[16–18] These can be tailored to coagulation testing using published protocols.[2,6]

One of the most difficult aspects of reference interval determination for coagulation testing is the inclusion and exclusion of potential individuals. Many factors influence the levels of hemostatic parameters and factors. In addition, changes in these individual factors will influence the results of global type assays. As an example: exercise, hormonal therapy and pregnancy can increase factor VIII levels to an extent that the aPTT value can be shortened. It is important to develop a questionnaire to exclude inappropriate reference individuals. The individuals utilized to establish the reference interval should reflect the population that will be the primary group being evaluated. Also important is consideration of pre-

Table 2.2 Basic protocol for establishing reference interval for a new analyte or new analyte method.

1 Establish biologic variations and analytic interferences from literature
2 Establish selection (or exclusion) criteria and develop questionnaire and consent form
3 Determine potential reference individuals (exclude as necessary)
4 Determine appropriate number of reference individuals
5 Collect appropriate samples under appropriate preanalytical conditions
6 Determine reference values and review for data distribution, errors or outliers
7 Analyze reference values into appropriate categories and determine reference interval(s) as predefined in protocol
8 Document all of the steps and procedures

analytical and analytical variables. The results from the reference population values must reflect the variables encountered in the determination of patient values.[2,3] The same considerations for sample collection, processing and storage must be utilized.[3] It is unacceptable to determine the reference interval using a different method, protocol, manufacturer and even reagent lots than what will be used for patient testing.[2,3,6]

The reference interval is defined as the interval between the upper and lower reference limits. The assignment of those limits is established as an a priori statistical value. For most coagulation testing, those limits are 2 SD from the mean for a normally distributed (Gaussian or parametric) population. Limits for non-Gaussian distribution are established by more complex methods. The reference limits become more accurate and closer to the true reference population values with a larger sample group. In practice, it is difficult to procure a large set of qualifying reference individuals.[2,6] A minimum of 40 individuals should be used to establish the reference interval. If that is too difficult or impossible, then a group as few as 20 individuals may be tested but greater care must be taken when comparing the values and determining the limits.[2,6] The calculated reference limits should be compared with other laboratories using the same method, reagents and instruments. For some coagulation reference intervals, subdivisions of specific groups may be necessary, such VWF and blood type. It is the responsibility of the laboratory to set the appropriate number of samples for each subgroup to establish these ranges.

Establishing a new reference interval for a new test or change in methodology can be difficult and costly; therefore, significant pressure can be applied to the coagulation staff to just "transfer" the reference interval from their previous method, another laboratory, manufacturer or the literature. The methods to transfer reference values are not soundly established.[2,17] Much effort has been attempted in the establishment of protocols for transference; however, a variety of scenarios makes the effort complex: different reference group from another laboratory, literature or manufacturer, slightly different analytical methods and different preanalytical problems.[17,18] Although not recommended, transference has two major issues that must be taken into account: comparability of analytical methods and comparability of test population.[17] Even using the same population (age, gender, regional location, demographics and preanalytical variables), it may be very difficult and it may not be possible to arrive at the same reference interval. If the method has the same characteristics and values (imprecision, interferences, standards, secondary reference standards, calibrators and units) then the assay method can be considered *similar* and possibly the same range. Several approaches can be utilized to judge the acceptability of reference interval transference:[16]

1 Use inspection and subjectivity of the original method reference range (demographics and preanalytical variables) and the new method. Based on judgment of consistent method similarities, then the reference interval can be transferred without validation studies. This is unfortunately performed by many coagulation laboratories that do not have the ability to acquire appropriate samples from the population. However, this method is not recommended.

2 Validation of the reference range provided by the manufacturer or other laboratory using a small number of reference individuals (minimum of 20 from the same population) to compare with a larger study performed by the original laboratory or manufacturer. Again, problems are created because of the differences in preanalytical variables, population and regional demographics. After testing the 20 speci-

mens, if the results are statistically evaluated with no outliers then the reference interval can be accepted. If values are outside of the reference range, then the outlier should be evaluated for cause but in all likelihood the reference interval should not be accepted and a complete determination of a reference interval must be undertaken.

The majority of information and theory dealing with transference of reference intervals has been established for analytes with established quantities such as cell number per volume and mass per volume.[16,17] For such analytes as clotting factors and coagulation tests reported in time intervals, transference methods have not been validated.[6] More detailed methodology for transference of reference intervals can be found in general standards guidelines.[16,17] As with any established reference interval, they must be periodically reevaluated.[2,16]

The majority of reference intervals are established to compare a patient's value with the population. The patient result is usually reported as: *within normal limits*, *high* (above the reference interval) or *low* (below the reference interval). Clinical interpretation of the value as either above or below the reference interval is the responsibility of the health care provider; however, it may be the responsibility of the laboratory director to assign the importance of a value that does not fall within the reference interval. In consultation with clinical staff, the levels that are critical for disease diagnosis or therapeutic use must be established and designated in the computer system and/or a written report.

Acknowledgments

This work was supported in part by a MERIT Review grant from the Department of Veteran's Affairs.

References

1 CLSI Evaluation Protocols (EP05 through EP21). Wayne, PA: Clinical and Laboratory Standards Institute, 2004. www.nccls.org

2 Clinical and Laboratory Standards Institute (CLSI). *Protocol for the Evaluation, Validation, and Implementation of Coagulometers*. H57-P, 2008.

3 Clinical and Laboratory Standards Institute (CLSI). *Collection, Transport, and Processing of Blood Specimens for Testing Plasma-Based Coagulation Assays and Molecular Hemostasis Assays*. H21-A5. 2008.

4 McPherson RA. Laboratory statistics. In *Henry's Clinical Diagnosis and Management by Laboratory Methods*. McPherson RA, Pincus MR (eds.) Philadelphia, PA: Saunders, 2007: 91–98.

5 Clinical and Laboratory Standards Institute (CLSI). *User Demonstration of Performance for Precision and Accuracy*. EP15-A. 2001.

6 Clinical and Laboratory Standards Institute (CLSI). *One-Stage Prothrombin Time (PT) Test and Activated Partial Thromboplastin Time (aPTT) Test*. H47-A2. 2008.

7 Hubbard AR. International biological standards for coagulation factors and inhibitors. *Semin Thromb Hemost* 2007; **33**: 283–289.

8 Hubbard AR, Heath AB. Standardization of factor VIII and von Willebrand factor in plasma: calibration of the WHO 5th International Standard. *J Thromb Haemost* 2004; **2**: 1380–1384.

9 Clinical and Laboratory Standards Institute (CLSI). *Evaluation of Precision Performance of Quantitative Measurement Methods*. EP5-A2. 2004.

10 Clinical and Laboratory Standards Institute (CLSI). *Protocols for Determination of Detection and Limits of Quantitation*. EP17-A. 2004.

11 Clinical and Laboratory Standards Institute (CLSI). *Statistical Quality Control for Quantitative Measurement Procedures: Principles and Definitions; Approved Guideline*, 3rd edn. C24-A3. 2004.

12 Clinical and Laboratory Standards Institute (CLSI). *Evaluation of the Linearity of Quantitative Measurement Procedures*. EP6-A. 2003.

13 Kroll M, Gilstad C, Gochman G, *et al.* (eds.) *Laboratory Instrument Evaluation, Verification and Maintenance Manual*, 5th edn. Northfield, IL: College of American Pathologists, 1999.

14 Clinical and Laboratory Standards Institute (CLSI). *Method Comparison and Bias Estimation Using Patient Samples*. EP9-A2. 2002.

15 Lott JA. Process control and method evaluation. In *Management in Laboratory Medicine*, 3rd edn. Snyder JR, Wilkinson DS (eds.) Philadelphia, PA: Lippincott, 1998: 293–325.

16 Clinical and Laboratory Standards Institute (CLSI). *How to Define and Determine Reference Intervals in the Clinical Laboratory*. C28-A2. 2000.

17 Daniel WW. *Biostatistics: A Foundation for Analysis in the Health Sciences*, 7th edn. New York: John Wiley & Sons, 1999.

18 Dawson B, Trapp RG. *Basic and Clinical Biostatistics*, 3rd edn. London: Lange Medical/McGraw-Hill, 2001.

Appendix

Standards and guideline developing organizations

A number of international organizations, usually non-profit-making, develop consensus guidelines and standards as a concise and cost-effective laboratory medicine process to improve patient testing. Most of these organizations base their guidelines and standards on an initial consensus document written by experts followed by open and unbiased input from the general laboratory community. "Standards" documents are developed through the consensus process to clearly identify *specific and essential requirements* for the material, method or practice. Whereas "guideline" documents are developed through the consensus process for *general criteria* of a material, method or practice that may be used as written or modified to fit the user's needs upon validation. The most well-known organization is the Clinical Laboratory Standards Institute which is an international non-profit-making organization that uses voluntary experts and laboratory community input to develop guidelines and standards in all areas of patient testing and other healthcare issues.

Statistics

The assembly, evaluation, comparison and interpretation of coagulation assay data increase the clinician's ability to diagnose patients with hemostatic disorders. Evaluation and subsequent interpretation of a variety of coagulation data (reference intervals, standard curves, comparison of patients) encompasses the field of statistics. In general, statistical evaluations are divided into two groups: descriptive statistics that define a population based on data from a sample set, and comparative statistics that evaluates the difference or similarity of two groups. Different types of data call for different statistical evaluations. This appendix summarizes the basic statistical methods used in the coagulation laboratory. More in-depth information on statistical methods is available in many books and computer programs.[17,18]

Descriptive statistics are used to "describe" the data, i.e. evaluate the sample to assess the representation of the population. The **mean, standard deviation (SD), range** for minimum and maximum values, the **95.0% confidence interval** and **coefficient of variation (CV)** are the most important descriptive statistics. This summary information provide an initial assessment of the test data compared to the population. In addition, these statistics may indicate outliers or data entry errors.

The concept of **comparative statistics** is to compare and contrast differences between two sets of data. In the comparison of two groups, the data are the same (termed the *null hypothesis*) or statistically significantly different. Usually, the 95% confidence limit is used as the differentiating point, i.e. if greater than 95% then the two means are considered different between the two groups or populations. In a cautionary note, it is very easy to read too much into the term *significant*. As an example, two groups of data may be statistically significantly different, but are not clinically different. Statistical significance and clinical significance are two unrelated interpretations of the data. Asking how the data will be used from a clinical perspective (will this data change the treatment plan?) may be as important as statistical significance.

Statistics are as important for evaluation and performance of methods and instruments as it is for determining reference intervals. The laboratory personnel must be able to analyze the results using the proper statistical methods. The *P* **value**, which stands for probability, has a value ranging from 0 to 1.0. It is useful in the interpretation of many statistical tests such as the Student's *t*-test. If the *P* value is small (usually <0.05), the difference between sample means are not likely the same population. Again, the *P* value is a statistical result and does not necessarily reflect the "clinical difference."

The **Student's *t*-test** compares the means of two groups of data. For example, comparison of the PT/international normalized ratio (INR) results obtained between two reagent–instrument combinations. To use the Student's *t*-test, the same variables must be compared. The result is a *P* value that determines if the comparison is statistically the same or different.

Regression and **linear regression** are the statistical methods used to describe the "best fit" of two sets of continuous data. For example, linear regression is used to find the relationship between two instruments when comparing a large number of patient coagulation values over a wide range. For these types of method comparisons, theoretically the slope should be $1.0 \pm 5\%$ with the "best-fit" line crossing the y axis at 0. When the slope is outside the range of 0.95–1.05, a true difference or bias between the methods being compared is a possibility. It is the responsibility of the laboratory to determine if this difference is important clinically.

Linear regression is used to create a standard curve for clotting factor, enzyme-linked immunosorbent assay (ELISA) or chromogenic assays. Standards with known values are analyzed and the instrument data is recorded. These two data sets (concentration and instrument output data) are compared to generate the "best-fit" line. The instrument output data for an unknown sample can be used to find the unknown sample's concentration or activity from this curve. **Linear correlation** quantifies how well two sets of data vary together. The statistical correlation coefficient (r value between 0.0 and 1.0) indicates the amount of random error (variation) between the two sets of data. The correlation coefficient is a semi-quantitative indication of imprecision. These r values are helpful with standard curves, such as clotting factor or ELISA assays. For most coagulation studies, an r value of <0.9 is not optimum.

From the laboratory perspective, one of the best statistical methods for comparing two measurements techniques, instruments or methods is the **Bland–Altman plot**, a graphic representation of the absolute differences, or differences as percentage of the mean, or ratios of different comparisons of methods and/or components. The results are a scatter diagram of the differences plotted against the average. This evaluation will elucidate the differences in means and determine systematic bias and identify outliers. If there is no detectable statistical bias and no *clinical* differences, then the two methods can be considered the same.

From a clinical or disease-related perspective, sensitivity and specificity are two of the most widely used statistics describing a diagnostic test, but must be interpreted with caution. **Clinical sensitivity** is defined as the probability of a positive test among patients with disease; whereas **clinical specificity** is the probability of a negative test present in patients without disease. Measurements of test performance may not take into account the level at which a test is clinically positive. **Receiver operator characteristics (ROC) curves,** a complex statistical analysis that is underutilized in coagulation work, assess the performance of a test throughout the assay's range of values observed in disease states. As the ROC curve approaches 1.0, the better the clinical diagnostic ability. While a truly random test parameter for predicting disease has the ROC curve of 0.5.

3 International Standards in hemostasis

T. W. Barrowcliffe

Assays of most components of the hemostatic system, and of many therapeutic materials used to treat disorders of hemostasis, are carried out on a comparative basis, relative to a standard of known potency. This is true of many other biologic materials such as hormones and cytokines, and such comparative assays have many advantages over direct determinations without reference to a standard, which in any case are either difficult or impossible in complex biologic matrices such as plasma.

In order to relate results in one laboratory to those in other laboratories there must be some means of linking the standards used in local laboratory assays. The concept of a single biologic standard that could provide such a link was first established for insulin in the early 20th century by Sir Henry Dale,[1] and this has been developed into a well-established international system for many biologic components under the auspices of the World Health Organization (WHO).

The first International Standard in the area of hemostasis was for heparin, established in 1942 by the League of Nations, which subsequently became WHO.[2] In the 1960s, work commenced on establishing WHO Reference Preparations for thromboplastin reagents, because of their widespread use in control of oral anticoagulation,[3] and this was soon followed by establishment of the first International Standard

for one of the clotting factors, factor VIII (FVIII).[4] Since then, International Standards have been established for most of the components of the hemostatic system; Tables 3.1–3.4 give an up-to-date summary of the International Standards that are currently available. Further information about these and other standards can be found on the WHO website (www. who.int/biologicals).

This chapter describes the establishment and use of International Standards in the field of hemostasis and thrombosis, with particular emphasis on their role in quality control of clinical samples.

International Standards and International Units

Units of activity

For most biologic materials, including those involved in hemostasis, units of biologic activity are defined soon after their discovery, and well before the establishment of International Standards. The definition of the unit is usually related to the type of activity, e.g. anticoagulant or procoagulant, and the method of measurement. Thus, the unit of activity for heparin was first defined in terms of its ability to delay clotting of cats' blood,[5] and that for thrombin in terms of the clotting time of a preparation of fibrinogen.[6] For most clotting factors in plasma, the unit of activity was first defined as the amount in "average normal plasma." Such units may have practicability initially, but are not a very good basis for standardization of results among different laboratories.

Quality in Laboratory Hemostasis and Thrombosis, 1st edition. By Steve Kitchen, John D. Olson and F. Eric Preston. Published 2009 by Blackwell Publishing. ISBN: 978-1-4051-6803-8

Table 3.1 World Health Organization (WHO) Standards for therapeutic concentrates of coagulation factors and inhibitors.

Clotting factor	Current Standard
Factors II & X	3rd
Factor VII	1st
Factor VIIa	1st
Factor VIII	7th
Fibrinogen	1st
von Willebrand factor	1st
Factor IX	3rd
Antithrombin	2nd
Protein C	1st

Table 3.2 World Health Organization (WHO) Standards for coagulation factors and inhibitors in plasma.

Clotting factor	Current Standard
Factors II, VII, IX, X	3rd
Factor V	1st
Factor VIII/VWF	5th
Factor XI	1st
Factor XIII	1st
Fibrinogen	2nd
Antithrombin	2nd
Protein C	2nd
Protein S	2nd

Table 3.3 Other WHO Standards and reference reagents used in hemostasis.

Material	Current Standard or reference reagent
Ancrod	1st
β-Thromboglobulin	1st
Factor IXa	1st
Thrombin	2nd
Factor V Leiden (DNA reference panel)	1st
Prothrombin mutation G20210A (DNA reference panel)	1st
Heparin	5th
LMW heparin	2nd
Platelet factor 4	1st
Thromboplastin, human	3rd
Thromboplastin, rabbit	4th
Thromboplastin, bovine	2nd

LMW, low molecular weight.

Table 3.4 Standards in fibrinolysis.

Material	WHO Standard or reference reagent
Plasmin	3rd
PAI-1	1st
Streptokinase	3rd
Streptodornase	1st
tPA	3rd
Urokinase	1st

PAI-1, plasminogen activator inhibitor-1; tPA, tissue plasminogen activator; WHO, World Health Organization.

International Units

When International Standards have been established for the first time they are usually calibrated using the pre-existing units in order to provide continuity of measurement. Once the first International Standard has been calibrated it is assigned a value in International Units, and from then on the unit of activity for that particular parameter is defined only in terms of the amount of activity in the International Standard. Subsequent batches of International Standards are calibrated in International Units against the previous Standard, although there may be ongoing studies of the relationship between the International Unit and the pre-existing unit, as has been the case

for several of the clotting factor plasma standards (see p. 25).

Establishment of International Standards

The procedure for establishment of International Standards has evolved over the last 60 years and, although it has tended to become more complex and sophisticated in recent years, many of the basic principles remain unchanged. The process is described in detail by WHO,[7] but a brief outline is given here because it is common to many of the Standards in hemostasis.

Choice of materials

For establishment of the first International Standard for any parameter, it may be necessary to investigate a number of potential candidate materials in preliminary studies, and to include more than one candidate in the collaborative study. The type of material is chosen on the basis of its intended use, with application of the "like vs. like" principle (see below), and consideration of its stability. For replacement standards it is usually possible to select only one candidate on the basis of previous experience, although there are exceptions, notably low molecular weight (LMW) heparin (see p. 23).

"Like vs. like"

A basic tenet of biologic standardization is the principle of "like vs. like", i.e. the test sample should be of similar composition to that of the standard against which it is assayed. This follows from one of the assumptions of comparative bioassays, namely that the test sample should behave like a dilution of the standard. This is most likely if the standard and test are very similar to one another. Differences in composition would have little impact if coagulation assays were completely specific and unaffected by the type of matrix, but in practice this is not the case, and comparison of unlike materials, such as plasma and concentrates, tends to give high variability and differences among methods. Therefore, for most coagulation factors, International Standards have been established for both plasma and concentrates (see p. 20).

Physical attributes

Certain physical requirements must be fulfilled for preparations to serve as International Standards. These include homogeneity (inter-ampoule variability) of the preparation and characteristics consistent with long-term stability, such as low residual moisture and oxygen content.[8,9] International Standards exist as multiple sealed glass ampoules containing the freeze-dried physical material (the standard), and it is essential that all ampoule contents must be as near identical as possible. This is achieved by extremely precise liquid filling, which is monitored through numerous check-weights evenly spaced throughout the total fill. Although the WHO guidelines quote inter-ampoule variability (coefficient of variation [CV]) of <0.25% for liquid fills and <1% for viscous fills (e.g. plasma), CVs below 0.2% are routinely achieved for both plasma and concentrates. In practice, this corresponds to an extreme range of liquid filling weights less than ±1% of the mean filling weight.

Low residual moisture and low oxygen content, which improve long-term stability, are controlled during the manufacturing process by the use of efficient freeze-drying cycles, which routinely achieve residual moisture levels below 0.2% w/w (considerably below the WHO recommendation of <1% w/w) and by the back-filling of ampoules with nitrogen gas before sealing. Sealed glass ampoules are preferred for most International Standards to ensure no ingress of atmospheric gases during long-term use, which may be over 10 years, but for materials that are very stable and are replaced over a shorter time frame, stoppered vials may be acceptable (e.g. FIX concentrate).

Collaborative study

International Standards undergo calibration in extensive multicenter international collaborative studies, often involving more than 20 laboratories. Collaborative studies are planned carefully to include relevant expert laboratories (clinical, academic and commercial) and to represent the current methodologies.

Organization and analysis of such studies is quite complex and time consuming, and it is essential to have an experienced central organization to undertake this. For virtually all WHO Standards in the hemostasis area, this task has been undertaken by the National Institute for Biological Standards and Control (NIBSC), which also acts as the custodian for the great majority of WHO Standards (for further details and information on ordering standards see the website: www.nibsc.ac.uk).

Proposed assigned potencies are usually based on the consensus overall mean estimates, and these require endorsement by study participants and by the Scientific and Standardization Committee (SSC) of the International Society on Thrombosis and Haemostasis (ISTH) before they are submitted to the WHO Expert Committee on Biological Standardization for formal establishment of the standard.

In some cases, excessive variability in the estimates from different laboratories that contribute to the consensus mean, or significant differences between methods, can preclude the assignment of a mean value. This was found to be the case for the calibration of the first International Standard for LMW heparin against the unfractionated heparin standard. Fortunately, such occurrences are rare and it is usually possible to assign a single value acceptable for all methods relating to a given analyte (e.g. FVIII:coagulant activity, protein S function).

Stability studies
International Standards may be used for many years, and it is therefore essential that the preparations remain stable and the assigned values are valid for the period of use. This property is also critical for maintaining the continuity of the International Unit, given that replacements are calibrated relative to previous standards. Assessment of stability relies on two approaches: the accelerated degradation study and real-time stability.

Accelerated degradation studies have been used to predict the degradation rates of lyophilized coagulation factors for more than 30 years.[10,11] These studies are based on the measurement of residual potency of ampoules stored at elevated temperatures (e.g. 4, 20, 37 and 45°C) relative to ampoules stored at the bulk storage temperature (e.g. −20°C). The predictive model is based on the assumption that degradation is caused by unimolecular decay, with the probability of any intact molecule changing state in any unit of time remaining constant. In addition, the degradation rate must also follow a fixed law of temperature dependency, as described in the Arrhenius equation; hence, the degradation occurring at higher temperatures only differs from the degradation at lower temperatures in terms of rate. This allows the measured relative loss of activity observed for samples stored at elevated temperatures to be used to predict the degradation rate for samples stored at the bulk storage temperature of −20°C.

Results from accelerated degradation studies have indicated that the International Standards for coagulation factors should be remarkably stable when stored at −20°C. For example, studies on even the more labile factors, FV:C and FVIII:C, have returned extremely low predicted losses of <0.1% per year.[12]

Real-time studies provide a more objective assessment of the stability of ampoules in bulk storage by direct comparison with ampoules stored at lower temperatures (e.g. −70 or −150°C), and are most useful when performed after several years of storage or when the current International Standard is due for replacement. Acceptable data from both approaches increases confidence that the International Standards have remained stable throughout their lifetime and the assigned values are valid for the direct calibration of replacement preparations.

Usage
For practical reasons the number of ampoules comprising a batch of material for an International Standard has in the past been limited to around 4000. Therefore it is impractical to use International Standards as working standards in laboratories, as the whole batch would be used very quickly. It is desirable to avoid too frequent replacements of International Standards, as the replacement process is time consuming, hence the main use of International Standards is to calibrate national, regional or local standards. For plasma assays, most reagent manufacturers issue commercial plasma standards that are calibrated in International Units against the appropriate International Standard. The considerable quality control requirements for manufacturers of plasma standards could lead to excessive demand on the supply of WHO Standards, and in order to mitigate this a secondary plasma standard, calibrated for multiple parameters and available in large quantities, has been developed under the auspices of the ISTH.

For assays of therapeutic concentrates, working standards are issued in the USA by the Food and Drug Adminstration's Center for Biologics Evaluation and Research (FDA/CBER), and in Europe, European Pharmacopeia (EP) Standards by the European Department for the Quality of Medicines (EDQM). These are calibrated against the appropriate International Standard in multicenter studies. However, as the number of manufacturers is not large it is feasible for manufacturers to calibrate their in-house standards directly against WHO standards – this is preferable to using an intermediate working standard as it shortens the pathway between the International Standard and the product.

Heparin and low molecular weight heparin

The first International Standard for unfractionated heparin (UFH) was established by WHO in 1942, and this has been replaced at regular intervals – the current WHO Standard is the fifth.[13] The EP and the US Pharmacopoeia (USP) both issue working standards; the EP Standard is calibrated in International Units against the current WHO Standard, but the USP unit, as defined by the USP Standard, differs from the International Unit by approximately 7%.[14]

Despite the considerable technical differences, when different methods have been compared in international collaborative studies of UFH, the potencies given by the various methods have agreed to within a few percent.[13] This is a corroboration of the principle of "like vs. like", in that the potencies are largely independent of the method used. However, when the first samples of LMW heparin were assayed against the UFH Standard this was clearly not the case – there was large variability between laboratories, even when ostensibly using the same method. For instance, the CV among seven laboratories carrying out a chromogenic method on the same LMW heparin sample was 43%.[15] There was also a tendency to non-parallelism between the log dose–response lines of the LMW heparin and UFH Standard, rendering many of the assays statistically invalid. In addition, as expected from the known properties of LMW heparin, there was a large difference in potency between methods based on inhibition of FXa, and those based in thrombin inhibition or delay of clotting times. The anti-Xa : anti-IIa ratio differed widely among the various LMW heparin products, and continues to do so.

Because of all these problems it became clear that the UFH Standard was unsuitable for measurement of the anticoagulant activities of LMW heparins. It was therefore decided to establish a separate standard for LMW heparin, on the basis that "like vs. like" would give better reproducibility. It was recognized that LMW heparins as a group were not identical to each other, and so the appropriate material for a standard had to be carefully chosen to be "in the middle" of the group with regard to its molecular weight and anticoagulant properties.

Following a preliminary study, two of eight LMW heparins were identified as giving the least interlaboratory variability when used as a standard for assay of the other preparations, with CVs in the range of 4–14%.[15] These two preparations were then subjected to a large international collaborative study, and one of the materials was established by WHO as the first International Standard for LMW heparin in 1986.[16] Although WHO Standards are traditionally assigned a single potency, this would have been inappropriate in the case of LMW heparin, because of the large difference between potencies by anti-Xa and anti-IIa assays (around 2.5-fold). Accordingly, the LMW heparin Standard was assigned two values: one for anti-Xa assays and another for anti-IIa assays (including activated partial thromboplastin time [aPTT]).

The first International Standard has been used by manufacturers of all LMW heparins to calibrate their products, and was recently replaced by the second International Standard, following an extensive international collaborative study.[17]

Thromboplastins

The prothrombin time (PT), first described in 1938, remains the most widely performed of all coagulation tests. Despite its simplicity, standardization of the measurements on a global basis has proved surprisingly difficult, and efforts are still continuing. One of the main uses of the PT is for monitoring anticoagulant therapy, and a detailed account of this is given in Chapter 18.

Two major steps forward in standardization of the PT were the establishment of International Reference Preparations (IRP) by WHO, and the development of a method of conversion of locally measured PTs to a standardized value, the International Normalized Ratio (INR).[18,19] The first IRP for thromboplastin was a human brain combined preparation, chosen because human brain preparations were widely used at that time, and were the most sensitive to the reduced levels of vitamin K dependent clotting factors induced by oral anticoagulants. In the absence of a previously defined "unitage" for thromboplastin reagents, the first IRP was arbitrarily assigned an "International

Sensitivity Index" (ISI) of 1.0.[3] The system of measurement described originally by Kirkwood[19] was for batches of thromboplastin reagents to be given an ISI value by calibration against the IRP, or against a substandard calibrated against the IRP. The INR could then be calculated from the local PT ratio (PTR – patient's PT ÷ normal PT) as follows:

$$INR = local\ PTR^{ISI}.$$

On the whole, this system has worked well, but discrepancies between results with different reagents can still occur, as indicated in Chapters 6 and 18. At the time of establishment of the first IRP, reagents prepared from rabbit and bovine brains were in common use, and IRPs were also established for rabbit and bovine thromboplastin. These were intended for calibration of reagents of the appropriate species, in an endorsement of the "like vs. like" principle. The original IRPs, which were established in the 1970s, have been replaced, and the currently available IRPs are:
- Human – third IRP, established 1996;
- Bovine – second IRP, established 1983;
- Rabbit – fourth International Standard, established 2005 (WHO recently discontinued the IRP nomenclature).

Recently, it has been recognized that calibration of the ISI of thromboplastin reagents may vary depending on the instrumentation used, and plasmas with defined INRs have been developed to overcome this. The ISTH/SSC has developed guidelines on the calibration and use of such plasmas,[20] but as yet no International Standards have been established for plasmas with defined INRs (see also Chapter 18).

Coagulation factors and inhibitors

This is the largest group of International Standards in the hemostasis field and, as indicated in Tables 3.1 and 3.2, standards for most factors are available in both plasma and concentrate forms.

Factor VIII

The first International Standard for FVIII, established in 1971,[4] was a concentrate of low purity, typical of the relatively few products available at that time; it was calibrated against pools of fresh normal plasma in the 20 participating laboratories. The variability among laboratories in this first international collaborative study was extremely high, with potencies covering a 10-fold range. Variability was somewhat lower in assays of a lyophilized plasma, but this was not stable enough to qualify as an International Standard. The first International Standard for FVIII was used successfully to calibrate manufacturers' concentrate standards, but its use to calibrate plasma standards such as the British Plasma Standards for FVIII was less satisfactory because of high inter-laboratory variability and a 20% difference between the results of one-stage and two-stage assays.[21] This is another example of the "like vs. like" principle, and it became clear that a separate International Plasma Standard for FVIII would be desirable to calibrate local and commercial plasma standards. Changes in the method of collection and handling of plasma, and in freeze-drying techniques, led to improved stability of FVIII in lyophilized plasma, and eventually the first International Standard for FVIII Plasma was established in 1981,[22] by assay against normal plasma pools in participants' laboratories; it was calibrated also for FVIII clotting antigen (FVIII:Ag), and for von Willebrand factor (VWF) antigen and activity.

Both of these standards have been replaced at fairly frequent intervals because of high usage, and there have been three main issues in the last 25 years of FVIII standardization.

Different types of FVIII concentrate
Continuing developments of plasma-derived concentrates, resulting from requirements of viral inactivation and improved purification methods, as well as the introduction of recombinant products, have considerably broadened the range of FVIII products available. This makes the choice of material for the International Standard important, because it has been shown that some concentrates give discrepancies between one-stage and chromogenic or two-stage methods.[23]

Early attempts to measure FVIII:C in full-length recombinant FVIII concentrates, relative to the WHO third International Standard FVIII concentrate (plasma-derived), were associated with extremely large inter-laboratory variability, with geometric coefficients of variation (GCVs) ranging from 39 to 137% depending on method.[23,24] Initially, it was considered that a separate International Standard recombinant FVIII concentrate might be necessary to improve agreement between laboratories. However, subsequent studies revealed that the high variability could be overcome by the following specifications of assay methodology:

1 *FVIII deficient plasma.* The use of hemophilic plasma, or deficient plasma with a normal VWF level, was found to be essential to give full potency in one-stage assays.

2 *Assay buffers.* It was found that albumin at a concentration of 1% w/v was necessary in all assay buffers in order to obtain reproducible results.

3 *Predilution.* Predilution of both test and standard with hemophilic plasma, or its equivalent, was necessary for assay of all recombinant and high-purity plasma-derived products, whichever assay method was used.

These specifications precluded the need for a dedicated recombinant standard and were published as recommendations by ISTH/SSC[25] and also incorporated into the EP monograph for the assay of FVIII.[26]

The sixth International Standard was composed of recombinant FVIII, in recognition of the widespread use of recombinant products, and in anticipation that plasma-derived concentrates would suffer a rapid decline in production and use. However, in the event most manufacturers have continued to produce plasma-derived products, and because there are still more plasma-derived products than recombinant ones, the current (seventh) International Standard reverted to a plasma-derived product. In the calibration of both of these standards there has been good agreement between laboratories, and discrepancies between one-stage and chromogenic or two-stage methods have been less than 10%.[27,28] However, this is not always the case – several concentrates have shown larger discrepancies when assayed against the International Standard, including the EP standard and the Mega 2 Standard;[29] in the latter case the difference between one-stage and chromogenic potencies was over 30% and it was decided to label this standard with a different potency for each method. The B-domain deleted recombinant concentrate also has a large discrepancy between methods, and even between different types of chromogenic or one-stage method.[30] These differences appear to be an inherent property of the materials and as far as possible it is best not to use such materials for standards – fortunately, the majority of FVIII concentrates do not give discrepancies between methods when assayed against the International Standard using the ISTH/SSC recommendations.

International Unit vs. normal plasma
After establishment of the first International Standard against the existing unit, i.e. normal plasma pools, subsequent International Standards have been calibrated against the previous one. However, although FVIII has been found to be very stable in these plasma standards, there is a slight risk that the International Units could drift from "normal plasma" over several calibrations during a long period of time. Hence, in each collaborative study, normal plasma pools have been included to check the relationship between the International Unit and normal plasma.

For the first two replacements (second and third International Standard) the values against the previous standard were very similar to those against the mean of the plasma pools. However, for the calibration of the fourth vs. the third Standard, there was a discrepancy of about 15% between the two values, and it was decided to take the mean value as the potency of the fourth International Standard, in order to minimize the gap between the International Unit and normal plasma. The stability of FVIII in the plasma standards has been confirmed by real-time studies,[31] and it seems likely that the apparent drift in the ratio of the International Unit to normal plasma is because of differences in donor population, and in methods of collection of the blood. When the first International Standard was established most blood was collected by syringes, whereas more recently Vacutainers are almost universally used – there is some evidence that these can lead to higher FVIII values in the plasma.

For the most recent (fifth) International Standard, there was still a discrepancy of around 10% between the values against the fourth International Standard and against the mean of the plasma pools.[32] However, it was decided not to make a further adjustment to the International Unit, in view of the good stability data, and also because too frequent changes in the International Unit cause difficulties for manufacturers of secondary standards.

Plasma and concentrate units and in vivo *recovery*
The assay of FVIII concentrates against plasma standards has been a long-standing problem because of wide variability among laboratories and a basic dif-

ference between assay methods, and for this reason two separate WHO standards for plasma and concentrates were developed. However, although such comparisons are avoided in routine assays, they are relevant to manufacturers of plasma-derived concentrates, and especially to clinicians measuring *in vivo* recovery. In the latter situation, patients' post-infusion samples, which essentially consist of concentrates "diluted" in the patient's hemophilic plasma, are assayed against a plasma standard.

It was first found in 1978[33] that when concentrates were assayed against plasma the potencies were higher by the two-stage method than by one-stage assays – the average discrepancy from a number of collaborative studies at this time was 20%. Since then, the same trend has been found in almost every collaborative study, although the size of the discrepancy varies from study to study, and possibly with different types of concentrates.

In recent years the chromogenic method has largely replaced the two-stage clotting method for assay of concentrates, and not surprisingly it also gives higher results than the one-stage method, being based on the same principles as the two-stage. Despite considerable investigation the basic causes of this discrepancy remain unknown, although it is thought that the extensive processing applied to both plasma-derived and recombinant concentrates could lead to differences in their rates of activation and inactivation in the two method types from the FVIII in normal plasma, and there is some evidence for this from recent studies.[34] For largely historical reasons, when the WHO concentrate and plasma FVIII standards are compared against each other, the values are approximately equivalent by one-stage assays but not by two-stage or chromogenic methods.

There is some evidence that the discrepancy is greater for recombinant concentrates than for plasma-derived products. In the collaborative study to calibrate the fifth International Standard FVIII concentrate, which included both the WHO plasma standard and a recombinant concentrate, the ratio of chromogenic to one-stage potencies was 1.48, and in the sixth International Standard study[27] it was 1.26. These figures help to explain the large discrepancies between chromogenic and one-stage potencies found in patients' samples after infusion of recombinant concentrates.[35] It appears that after infusion the recombinant products behave in an essentially similar

manner in these assays to samples produced by diluting them *in vitro* in hemophilic plasma.

The situation with plasma-derived products is variable, dependent on the nature of the product and the test systems used. For instance, in a study by Lee *et al.*[36] Hemofil M was found to give a 20% discrepancy in post-infusion plasmas between one-stage and chromogenic methods, whereas in a study of a similar product performed at Sanquin, there was no difference between the methods (K. Mertens, personal communication). Equivalence between the methods was also found in a UK NEQAS study on a post-infusion sample from a different type of plasma-derived concentrate.

A resolution of this problem is only possible when the exact causes of the discrepancy are discovered; it may then be possible to adjust one or both of the methods to give similar values. In the meantime, a practical solution which has been discussed by the FVIII/FIX Subcommittee of ISTH/SSC is to regard the post-infusion samples as concentrates, "diluted" in a patient's plasma, which is essentially what they are, and use a concentrate standard, diluted in hemophilic plasma, instead of a plasma standard, to construct the standard curve. Considering the close agreement between assay methods on recombinant concentrates when concentrate standards are used (see p. 25), this should provide good agreement on *in vivo* recoveries of recombinant concentrates when measured by chromogenic and one-stage methods. However, the nature of the concentrate standard needs to be carefully considered, it should be as similar as possible to the injected product. Thus, whereas either of the full-length recombinant concentrates could serve as a standard for the other, plasma samples following infusion of the B-domain deleted product, ReFacto, would need a ReFacto concentrate standard.

This approach has recently been tested in *in vivo* recovery studies, in which patients' samples after infusion of Recombinate, Kogenate and Alphanate were assayed against both a plasma standard and a concentrate standard. As shown in Table 3.5, for Recombinate and Kogenate the discrepancy between one-stage and chromogenic methods using the plasma standard was completely abolished with the appropriate concentrate standard. However, in the case of Alphanate the use of a concentrate standard, in this case not the same as the product infused, made the situation worse. Therefore, the use of concentrate

Table 3.5 Comparison of plasma and concentrate standards on post-infusion samples.

| Concentrate infused | Ratio chromogenic : 1-stage | | |
	Plasma standard	Concentrate standard	Concentrate standard
Recombinate	1.24	1.02	Recombinate
Kogenate	1.20	0.99	Kogenate
Alphanate	1.00	0.86	Kogenate

standards needs to be product specific, and should probably be restricted to recombinant and very high-purity plasma-derived products.

Factor IX

Standardization of FIX assays has presented fewer problems than that of FVIII. This is because there is only a single assay method, the one-stage clotting assay, used for both plasma and concentrates. As for FVIII, a concentrate standard was the first to be established by WHO, for therapeutic materials, and this consisted of a prothrombin complex concentrate (PCC).[37] During the late 1990s there was a switch to high-purity single FIX concentrates as the mainstay of therapy. This did not appear to cause any problems in assay standardization; it was found that PCCs and single FIX concentrates could be assayed satisfactorily against each other. The current (third) WHO standard is a single FIX concentrate; as FIX is extremely stable it was feasible to produce a large batch in rubber stoppered vials, and stocks of this were shared among WHO, FDA/CBER and the EP/EDQM. Thus, the need for calibration of separate working standards by the later two organizations was avoided, and the labeling of FIX concentrates was harmonized on a worldwide basis.

As for FVIII, it was found that predilution of concentrates in FIX-deficient plasma was necessary to obtain optimum and reproducible potency when assaying concentrates against a concentrate standard, and also when comparing concentrates against plasma.[38] An international plasma standard for FIX, together with the other vitamin K dependent factors II, VII and X, was established by WHO in 1987,[39] and most local and commercial plasma standards are now calibrated in International Units. However, UK NEQAS surveys continue to show wide variability among laboratories, probably as a result of the multiplicity of aPTT reagents and deficient plasmas used (Chapter 9). As with FVIII, artificially depleted plasmas have become the main type of FIX-deficient reagent used, but there has been no systematic study of their performance compared with hemophilia B plasma.

Von Willebrand factor

Development of the VWF standard differed from FVIII and FIX, in that a plasma standard was established first – this was the same plasma as that calibrated for FVIII. The first International Standard was calibrated for both VWF antigen and ristocetin cofactor activity, against the mean of the plasma pools, comprising over 200 donors.[22] As in established WHO practice, subsequent standards were calibrated against the previous one but, as for FVIII, comparisons were also made against normal pools. In the collaborative study to calibrate the fourth International Standard there were significant differences between the values against the third International Standard and against the mean of the normal pools – 14% for VWF:Ag and 20% for VWF:RCo, and as for FVIII it was decided to take the mean of the two values as the potency of the fourth International Standard. In the calibration of the most recent (fifth) International Standard there was no significant difference in the values against the previous (fourth) International Standard and against the mean of the plasma pools. Following the introduction of the collagen binding assay as an alternative to the ristocetin cofactor method the fifth International Standard was calibrated also for this parameter.

The increasing use of concentrates containing VWF for treatment of von Willebrand's disease led to the need for a VWF concentrate standard – as is generally the case, assays of VWF concentrates against the plasma standard were found to be highly variable. Following an international collaborative study the first International Standard for VWF concentrate was established with assigned values for VWF antigen and VWF:RCo. However, despite the "like vs. like" principle, assays of collagen binding activity were too variable to allow an assignment of mean potency, with major differences in potency according to the different collagen reagents used.[40]

Fibrinogen

Fibrinogen is the only coagulation factor to be assigned a potency in milligrams rather than units of activity. This relates back to early methods of measurement when, because of its unique clottability, the amount of protein in a clot, which could be measured in milligrams, was assumed to be equivalent to the fibrinogen content of a plasma or purified sample. However, in practice this method proved difficult to standardize because of variable conditions of formation of the clot and different amounts of other proteins absorbed. Most clinical laboratories use the Clauss method, based on comparative measurement of thrombin clotting times of dilutions of plasma, against a plasma standard. Accordingly, a WHO standard for fibrinogen plasma was established in 1992,[41] and to maintain continuity with established clinical practice, this was calibrated in mg using clot weight methods. The second International Standard for fibrinogen was calibrated against the first International Standard, using mostly Clauss methods.

Although fibrinogen concentrates are rarely used as therapeutic materials in themselves, they are an essential component of fibrin sealant preparations, which have become increasingly widely used. The fibrinogen content of these preparations is measured as total protein and clotable protein and these measurements do not have an absolute requirement for a standard. However, in a collaborative study high variability was found for both these measurements and it was shown that variability could be considerably reduced by comparison against a fibrinogen standard. Accordingly, the first International Standard for fibrinogen concentrate was established by WHO in 1999, calibrated in milligrams for total and clottable protein.[42]

Thrombin

Thrombin was one of the earliest components of the coagulation system to be standardized; the unit of activity was originally defined by the National Institutes of Health (NIH) as the amount required to clot a fibrinogen preparation in 15 seconds, and a standard based on this unitage was established by the

NIH before the WHO Standard was prepared. When the first International Standard for thrombin was established by WHO in 1970, attempts were made to link the unitage to the NIH unit. However, it subsequently became apparent that there was a discrepancy between NIH units and International Units, the degree of difference depending on the assay methods used. This discrepancy was resolved a few years ago by establishment of a joint WHO/NIH Standard with a common unitage.[43]

Other coagulation factors and inhibitors

The establishment of International Standards for the other coagulation factors and inhibitors has followed the same pattern as for FVIII and FIX, with separate standards for plasma and concentrates where the latter exist (see Tables 3.1 and 3.2).

Prothrombin complex factors
The WHO Standard for FIX plasma was also calibrated for factors II, VII and X. However, following the switch to a single factor IX product for the International Standard for FIX concentrate, a separate International Standard was established for factors II and X concentrate, to be used by manufacturers of PCCs. A further separate International Standard was established for FVII concentrate, and because this was found to be unsuitable for assay of the recombinant FVIIa product, a different International Standard was established for the latter preparation.

Inhibitors
Antithrombin was the first plasma inhibitor to be standardized, with the establishment of an International Standard for plasma, followed by establishment of a separate standard for concentrate. In both these standards different values were assigned for activity and antigen, although the values are very similar. Plasma standards have been established for proteins C and S, and most recently an International Standard for protein C concentrate has been added.

Other plasma clotting factors
International Plasma Standards have been established for factors V, XI and XIII. Although therapeutic concentrates are available for factors XI and XIII, these are used rarely and the number of manufacturers is small; hence, the establishment of separate concen-

trate standards for these two factors has been of low priority.

Fibrinolysis standards

The absence of genetic deficiency states for fibrinolysis components in plasma has meant that assays of these components are carried out much less frequently in plasma samples than those of coagulation factors. As shown in Table 3.4, attention has focused on development of International Standards for therapeutic materials, for use by manufacturers of these products, as well as standards for some of the main components of the fibrinolytic system, i.e. plasmin and plasminogen activator inhibitor-1 (PAI-1). The first International Standard to be established in this area was streptokinase, in the 1960s, and this was followed by plasmin, urokinase and tissue plasminogen activator (tPA). Recently, the need for plasma standards for diagnostic purposes has been recognized, and work is in progress on development of International Plasma Standards for some of the fibrinolytic components. However, the most clinically useful measurement in this area, D-dimer, has proved difficult to standardize, as described in detail in Chapter 11.

References

1 Jeffcoate SL. From insulin to amylin: 75 years of biological standardisation in endocrinology. *Dev Biol Stand* 1999; **100**: 39–47.

2 Brozovic M, Bangham DR. Standards for heparin. *Adv Exp Med Biol* 1975; **52**: 163–179.

3 Biggs R, Bangham DR. Standardisation of the one-stage prothrombin time test for the control of anticoagulant therapy. The availability and use of thromboplastin reference preparations. *Thromb Diath Haemorrh* 1971; **26**: 203–204.

4 Bangham DR, Biggs R, Brozovic M, Denson KWE, Skegg JL. A biological standard for measurement of blood coagulation factor VIII activity. *Bull World Health Organ* 1971; **45**: 337–351.

5 Jaques LB. The heparins of various mammalian species and their relative anti-coagulant potency. *Science* 1940; **92**: 488–489.

6 Seegers WH, Brinkhous KM, Smith HP, Warner ED. The purification of thrombin. *J Biol Chem* 1938; **126**: 91–95.

7 Recommendations for the preparation, characterisation and establishment of international and other biological reference standards (revised 2004). World Health Organization (WHO) Technical Report Series 2007. Geneva, Switzerland: WHO 2007; **932**: 73–131.

8 Campbell PJ. International biological standards and reference preparations. I. Preparation and presentation of materials to serve as standards and reference preparations. *J Biol Stand* 1974; **2**: 249–258.

9 Campbell PJ. International biological standards and reference preparations. II. Procedures used for the production of biological standards and reference preparations. *J Biol Stand* 1974; **2**: 259–267.

10 Kirkwood TBL. Predicting the stability of biological standards and products. *Biometrics* 1977; **33**: 736–742.

11 Kirkwood TBL, Tydeman MS. Design and analysis of accelerated degradation tests for the stability of biological standards II. A flexible computer program for data analysis. *J Biol Stand* 1984; **12**: 207–214.

12 Barrowcliffe TW, Matthews KB. Standards and quality control in the blood coagulation laboratory. In *Haemophilia and Other Inherited Bleeding Disorders*. Rizza C, Lowe G, (eds.) Philadelphia, PA: WB Saunders, 1997: 115–149.

13 Gray E, Walker AD, Mulloy B, Barrowcliffe TW. A collaborative study to establish the 5th International Standard for Unfractionated Heparin. *Thromb Haemost* 2000; **84**: 1017–1022.

14 Barrowcliffe TW, Mulloy B, Johnson EA, Thomas DP. The anticoagulant activity of heparin: measurement and relationship to chemical structure. *J Pharm Biomed Anal* 1989; **7**: 217–226.

15 Barrowcliffe TW, Curtis AD, Tomlinson TP, Hubbard AR, Johnson EA, Thomas DP. Standardisation of low molecular weight heparins: a collaborative study. *Thromb Haemost* 1985; **54**: 675–679.

16 Barrowcliffe TW, Curtis AD, Johnson EA, Thomas DP. An international standard for low molecular weight heparin. *Thromb Haemost* 1988; **60**: 1–7.

17 Gray E, Rigsby P, Mulloy B. Establishment of the 2nd International Standard for low molecular weight heparin. NIBSC unpublished report, 2005.

18 Bangham DR, Biggs R, Brozović M, Denson KW. Calibration of five different thromboplastins, using fresh and freeze-dried plasma. *Thromb Diath Haemorrh* 1973; **29**: 228–239.

19 Kirkwood TB. Calibration of reference thromboplastins and standardisation of the prothrombin time ratio. *Thromb Haemost* 1983; **49**: 238–244.

20 van den Besselaar AM, Barrowcliffe TW, Houbouyan-Reveillard LL, Jespersen J, Johnston M, Poller L, *et al.* Subcommittee on Control of Anticoagulation of the

Scientific and Standardisation Committee of the ISTH. Guidelines on preparation, certification, and use of certified plasmas for ISI calibration and INR determination. *J Thromb Haemost* 2004; **2**: 1946–1953.

21 Barrowcliffe TW, Kirkwood TBL. Standardisation of factor VIII. I: Calibration of British Standards for factor VIII clotting activity. *Br J Haematol* 1980; **46**: 471–481.

22 Barrowcliffe TW, Tydeman MS, Kirkwood TBL, Thomas DP. Standardisation of factor VIII. III: Establishment of a stable reference plasma for factor VIII-related activities. *Thromb Haemost* 1983; **50**: 690–696.

23 Barrowcliffe TW, Raut S, Sands D, Hubbard AR. Coagulation and chromogenic assays of factor VIII activity: general aspects, standardization, and recommendations. *Semin Thromb Hemost* 2002; **28**: 247–256.

24 Barrowcliffe TW. Standardization of FVIII & FIX assays. *Haemophilia* 2003; **9**: 397–402.

25 Barrowcliffe TW. Recommendations for the assay of high-purity factor VIII concentrates. *Thromb Haemost* 1993; **70**: 876–877.

26 Assay of human coagulation factor VIII (2.7.4). In *European Pharmacopoeia*, 5th edn. Strasbourg, France: Council of Europe, 2005: 194–195.

27 Raut S, Heath AB, Barrowcliffe TW. A collaborative study to establish the 6th International Standard for factor VIII concentrate. *Thromb Haemost* 2001; **85**: 1071–1078.

28 Raut S, Bevan S, Hubbard AR, Sands D, Barrowcliffe TW. A collaborative study to establish the 7th International Standard for factor VIII concentrate. *J Thromb Haemost* 2005; **3**: 119–126.

29 Kirschbaum N, Wood L, Lachenbruch P, Weinstein M, Daas A, Rautmann G, *et al.* Calibration of the Ph. Eur. BRP Batch 3/Mega 2 (US/FDA) standard for human coagulation factor VIII concentrate for use in the potency assay. *Pharmeuropa Spec Issue Biol* 2002; **1**: 31–64.

30 Hubbard AR, Sands D, Sandberg E, Seitz R, Barrowcliffe TW. A multi-centre collaborative study on the potency estimation of ReFacto. *Thromb Haemost* 2003; **90**: 1088–1093.

31 Hubbard AR. International biological standards for coagulation factors and inhibitors. *Semin Thromb Haemost* 2007; **33**: 283–289.

32 Hubbard AR, Heath AB. Standardization of factor VIII and von Willebrand factor in plasma: calibration of the WHO 5th International Standard (02/150). *J Thromb Haemost* 2004; **2**: 1380–1384.

33 Kirkwood TBL, Barrowcliffe TW. Discrepancy between 1-stage and 2-stage assay for Factor VIII:C. *Br J Haematol* 1978; **40**: 333–338.

34 Hubbard AR, Weller LJ, Bevan SA. Activation profiles of FVIII in concentrates reflect one-stage/chromogenic potency discrepancies. *Br J Haematol* 2002; **117**: 957–960.

35 Lee CA, Owens D, Bray G, Giangrande P, Collins P, Hay C, *et al.* Pharmacokinetics of recombinant factor VIII (Recombinate) using one-stage clotting and chromogenic factor VIII assay. *Thromb Haemost* 1999; **82**: 1611–1647.

36 Lee C, Barrowcliffe T, Bray G, Gomperts E, Hubbard A, Kemball-Cook G, *et al.* Pharmacokinetic *in vivo* comparison using 1-stage and chromogenic substrate assays with two formulations of Hemofil-M. *Thromb Haemost* 1996; **76**: 950–956.

37 Brozovic M, Bangham DR. Study of a proposed International Standard for factor IX. *Thromb Haemost* 1976; **35**: 222–236.

38 Barrowcliffe TW, Tydeman MS, Kirkwood TBL. Major effect of prediluent in factor IX clotting assay. *Lancet* 1979; **2**: 192.

39 Barrowcliffe TW. Standardisation of factors II, VII, IX, and X in plasma and concentrates. *Thromb Haemost* 1987; **59**: 334.

40 Hubbard AR. Von Willebrand factor standards for plasma and concentrate testing. *Semin Thromb Hemost* 2006; **32**: 522–528.

41 Gaffney PJ, Wong MY. Collaborative study of a proposed international standard for plasma fibrinogen measurement. *Thromb Haemost* 1992; **68**: 428–432.

42 Whitton C, Sands D, Barrowcliffe TW. Establishment of the 1st International Standard for fibrinogen, concentrate. NIBSC unpublished report, 2003.

43 Whitton C, Sands D, Lee T, Chang A, Longstaff C. A reunification of the US ("NIH") and International Unit into a single standard for thrombin. *Thromb Haemost* 2005; **93**: 261–266.

4 Sample integrity and preanalytical variables

D. M. Adcock

Laboratory testing is an integral component of clinical decision-making as it aids in the determination of patient diagnosis and treatment. The ability to provide optimal clinical care is highly dependent on accurate and reliable laboratory results. Laboratory error leading to the reporting of an erroneous result can be introduced at any point of the testing process, from sample collection to result reporting. Because of the advances in instrument technology and informatics, analytical variability no longer represents the major cause of laboratory inaccuracy. Today the preanalytical phase of testing is the source of many, if not the majority, of inaccurate laboratory results.[1-3]

The preanalytical phase of testing refers specifically to the point of time beginning with patient identfication and continues to specimen analysis. Errors in the preanalytical phase are generally a reflection of improper specimen collection, processing or unsuitable conditions during sample transportation and/or storage. Samples for hemostasis testing are particularly susceptible to conditions that may impair sample integrity because of a number of factors including the *in vitro* lability of platelets and coagulation factors, the complex nature of the reactions commonly measured in the hemostasis laboratory and because clot formation is naturally initiated with sample collection and must be completely inhibited for analysis of many of the hemostatic factors. In the coagulation laboratory, knowledge of preanalytical variables and their impact on accurate test results is crucial. Patient-related conditions such as intravascular hemolysis, lipemia, icterus and certain medications may also interfere with accurate result reporting. Although these patient conditions must be recognized and acknowledged, they are largely out of the control of the laboratory and are not emphasized in this chapter.

In every step of this process, from sample procurement to analysis, the potential exists for sample integrity to be compromised. Improper sample collection, processing and/or handling can have a critical impact on both the platelets and plasma factors involved in hemostasis. The effect of improper preanalytical conditions can be to reduce some platelet-related and plasma factor activities and surprisingly elevate others. For example, activation of a sample as a result of exposure to cold may cause an elevation of factor VII activity and a drastic drop in factor VIII activity levels.[4,5] A spurious decrease in factor VIII activity because of improper sample storage may lead to an inappropriate diagnosis of hemophilia A or von Willebrand disease. Compromise of sample integrity leading to erroneous result reporting may lead not only to patient misdiagnosis, but also to improper medication dosing and overall patient mismanagement which may cause life-threatening therapeutic misadventures.

In order to assure the highest quality of laboratory testing results, it is imperative that sample integrity be preserved at every step of the process. Guidelines for sample handling should be strictly

Quality in Laboratory Hemostasis and Thrombosis, 1st edition. By Steve Kitchen, John D. Olson and F. Eric Preston. Published 2009 by Blackwell Publishing. ISBN: 978-1-4051-6803-8

followed and deviations avoided unless their impact, or lack thereof, on coagulation testing is known.

Sample acquisition (specimen collection)

The importance of positive patient identification cannot be overemphasized. The conscious patient should be asked to identify him or herself and asked for a form of identification. In the case of the hospitalized patient, the positive identification provided for patients by the institution must be verified. Positive identification of hospitalized patients using bedside electronic or bar-code methods reduce the risk of patient misidentification. The labels for the specimens to be collected must be prepared in advance, taken to the collection site or bedside and, after collection, the filled tubes labeled in the presence of the patient and before leaving the bedside. Each tube should be labeled with the patient's name and an additional identifier, e.g. date of birth or medical record number.

Venipuncture is the most common and preferred method of sample collection for coagulation testing. Ideally, the patient should be made comfortable and at ease during the procedure. In situations of stress, e.g. if a child is very tearful or upset at the time of the phlebotomy, certain hemostastic proteins such as von Willebrand factor (VWF), factor VIII and fibrinogen may increase, as these are acute phase reactant proteins. This may cause spurious shortening of the activated partial thromboplastin time (aPTT) or bring low levels of these factors into the normal range resulting in a missed diagnosis of hemophilia or von Willebrand disease.

Blood samples should be procured in a relatively atraumatic fashion, and during collection the blood should flow freely into the collection container. When obtaining plasma for coagulation testing, it is imperative that clotting of the sample be avoided. Samples in which the blood is slow to fill the collection container, where there is prolonged use of a tourniquet or considerable manipulation of the vein by the needle may develop a clot *in vitro*.[6] These situations must therefore be avoided. The presence of clot in the collection container is cause for specimen rejection. Clot development may result in *in vitro* consumption of clotting factors, activation of clotting factors, activation of platelets and platelet granule release, any of which may alter results of hemostasis assays. Integrity of the sample may be affected even if the clots are not visible to the naked eye.

Another important means to prevent *in vitro* clot formation is to adequately and promptly mix the sample following collection, to insure complete distribution of anticoagulant. When using evacuated collection tubes, 3–6 complete end-over-end inversions are recommended.[7] Vigorous shaking is to be avoided so as not to induce hemolysis or activate platelets.[6]

Specimen collection system

Each component of the specimen collection system may potentially impact the quality of the sample for coagulation testing. Knowledge regarding the impact of these various components, including needle gauge, composition of the specimen container, fill volume, and anticoagulant composition and concentration, on sample integrity is therefore imperative.

Needle gauge

In general, needle gauge of 19–22 is optimal for blood collection. Gauge refers to the measure of the diameter of the needle bore. The larger the gauge, the smaller the needle bore. For collection of plasma samples, 21 gauge needles are most commonly used although 22 gauge needles provide adequate blood flow, potentially with less discomfort.[8] Very small needles, such as those greater than 25 gauge, should be avoided, as the slower rate of blood flow through the small bore may induce clotting or activation of the sample.[2,8] Very large bore needles, such as those less than 16 gauge, may induce hemolysis of the sample because of turbulence of flow through the needle.[9]

Collection container

For hemostasis testing, the primary collection tube and all aliquot tubes must be composed of a non-activating material such as polypropylene plastic or silicon-coated glass, in order to avoid initiation of clotting resulting from contact activation in the collection container.[10] Blood for hemostasis testing can be collected in either evacuated tubes or syringes as long as the composition of the container is non-activating. Variations in normal range and assay results may occur, depending on whether the sample is collected in glass or plastic containers. Facilities should therefore standardize their collection containers to one composition or another. Plastic evacuated tubes may be preferred or required in certain regions as these carry a lower risk of breakage and therefore reduced potential for injury and exposure to infectious materials. If a syringe is used to collect the sample, a smaller size such as 20 mL or less is recommended to avoid *in vitro* clot formation. Anticoagulant should be added to the syringe within 30 seconds following the phlebotomy. In order to prevent clotting of the sample *in vitro*, all samples must be adequately and rapidly mixed (3–6 complete inversions) to ensure complete distribution of anticoagulant.

Anticoagulant
Samples for hemostasis testing should be anticoagulated with sodium citrate. Some evacuated tube manufacturers standardize the color of the evacuated tube stopper and, in this instance, sodium citrate is the type of anticoagulant found in a light blue stopper tube. The World Health Organization (WHO) and Clinical Laboratory Standards Institute (CLSI) recommend 105–109 mmol/L, 3.13–3.2% (commonly described as 3.2%) of the dihydrate form of trisodium citrate ($Na_3C_6H_5O_7 \cdot 2H_2O$), buffered or nonbuffered as the anticoagulant of choice for hemostasis

testing rather than 129 mmol/L, 3.8% (commonly described as 3.8%), although either is acceptable.[7,11]

In order to reduce result variability it is important to standardize to only one anticoagulant concentration within a laboratory system. This is because clotting times, such as aPTT and prothrombin time (PT) may vary among concentrations of sodium citrate, particularly if the clotting time is prolonged (Table 4.1).[12] Clotting times tend to be longer in 3.8% vs. 3.2% sodium citrate because the higher concentration of citrate binds more assay-added calcium, making less available to promote clot formation. Significant error can be introduced, in particular when determining the International Normalized Ratio (INR), if different concentrations of sodium citrate are used in the sample to be tested versus the concentration of anticoagulant used to determine mean normal PT and International Sensitivity Index (ISI).

Other anticoagulants such as ethylenediaminetetraacetic acid (EDTA) or heparin are not acceptable for hemostasis testing. Samples collected in EDTA or heparin anticoagulated tubes or the use of serum for testing will lead to aberrant results. In serum, factors VII and IX are activated resulting in supranormal values while factors V and VIII are low and PT and aPTT result in no clot. However, EDTA plasma demonstrates moderate prolongation of the PT and aPTT with significant reduction of factor VIII. *Importantly*, plasma collected in EDTA shows an **inhibitor effect** in mixing studies and may lead

Table 4.1 Comparison of prothrombin time (PT) and activated partial thromboplastin time (aPTT) between citrate concentrations.

Treatment	PT (Innovin*) Citrate concentration			aPTT (Actin FS*) Citrate concentration		
	3.2%	3.8%	P**	3.2%	3.8%	P**
No anticoaguant	11.2 ± 2.5	11.8 ± 2.3	<0.0004	28.2 ± 4.0	30.3 ± 3.5	0.0006
UFH	16.4 ± 8.3	17.8 ± 9.9	<0.0005	44.0 ± 11.0	48.6 ± 14.0	0.0001
UFH plus AVK	25.1 ± 28.0	26.3 ± 28.0	<0.2	65.5 ± 16.0	69.0 ± 14.0	0.0109
AVK	27.6 ± 13.0	34.3 ± 17.0	<0.0001	40.2 ± 9.7	44.1 ± 13.0	0.0001

AVK, anti-vitamin K therapy; UFH, unfractionated heparin.
*Dade Behring, Marburg, Germany.
**All show statistical significance.

Table 4.2 Effect of collection tube on commonly performed hemostasis assays. From Valcour A, Marshall T. 2007 Laboratory Corporation of America, Inc., unpublished data.

Assay	Tube type			
	3.2% Citrate (Mean/range)	EDTA (Mean/range)	Sodium heparin (Mean/range)	Serum (Mean/range)
aPTT (sec)	29/25–33	68/45–92	>180	>180
PT (sec)	12.4/11.5–13.2	23/19–27	>60	>60
dRVVT (sec)	34.6/27–43	55/45–64	>150	>150
FV Act (%)	113/84–142	71/39–103	81/59–103	23/13–33
FVII Act (%)	115/50–180	116/51–182	77/43–107	308/80–437
FVIII Act (%)	141/80–202	7.5/2–19	<1	4.5/1.3–7.7
FIX Act (%)	122/97–148	115/63–168	<1	350/135–565
VWF:Ag (%)	122/50–194	143/59–228	70/42–98	101/32–169
VWF:RCo (%)	114/41–188	131/46–215	37/13–60	74/25–124
PC Ag	97/60–134	115/97–159	125/94–156	120/71–169
PC Act (%)	111/66–155	152/100–205	<1	21.6/0–70
PS Act (%)	96/73–119	30/17–42	<1	15.3/0–39.5
Free PS Ag (%)	108/72–144	131/91–171	126/94–159	131/97–164
AT Act (%)	102/86–118	121/105–138	126/108–143	47/30–65
AT Ag (%)	110/832–138	121/92–150	100/83–118	114/79–148

Act, activity; aPTT, activated partial thromboplastin time; Ag, antigen; AT, antithrombin; dRVVT, dilute Russel viper venom time; EDTA, ethylenediaminetetraacetic acid; F, factor; PC, protein C; PS, protein S; PT, prothrombin time; VWF, von Willebrand factor.

to spurious identification of a factor V or VIII inhibitor (see Table 4.2 for the effect of incorrect sample type on common hemostasis assays).[13] The receipt of serum or plasma other than that collected in sodium citrate for the performance of clot-based assays must result in specimen rejection. Reference laboratories that receive frozen plasma aliquot tubes rather than the primary collection tubes must be especially keen to the possibility that the sample is other than citrated plasma, as the appearance of these samples is the same once they have been aliquoted into a secondary tube.

Special sodium citrate collection tubes
Sodium citrate collection tubes may contain special additives that are necessary or preferable in order to ensure optimum sample integrity for certain hemostasis assays. These tubes can be categorized as those that: (i) Prevent platelet activation; (ii) Are highly acidified to stabilize factors of the fibrinolytic system; (iii) Contain protease inhibitors.

Citrate, theophylline, adenosine and dypyridamole (CTAD) is a cocktail of additives that prevents *in vitro* platelet activation. CTAD tubes, which are often difficult to obtain in North America, must be stored at cold temperature and shielded from light. These tubes afford more reliable measure of unfractionated heparin (UFH) levels because of diminished effect of platelet factor 4 (PF4),[14] a potent neutralizer of UFH which is released from platelets. Whole blood samples containing UFH show significant PF4 neutralization of heparin with time, within 4 hours; UFH levels, measured by an anti-FXa assay, may be diminished by up to 50%.[15] For this reason, whole blood samples containing UFH must be processed within 1 hour of collection. If samples are collected into CTAD and stored at room temperature, 4 hour stability has been reported.[14] In general, CTAD tubes are recommended for measure of markers of platelet activation such as β-thromboglobulin or PF4. These tubes may also be useful when determining plasma levels of analytes that have significant platelet stores such as plasminogen activator inhibitor-1 (PAI-1). In this situation, CTAD prevents release of the analyte from the platelet store during collection and processing and allows more accurate measure of the plasma concentration.

Additionally, the use of sodium citrate with added protease inhibitor(s) such as D-phenylalanine-proline-arginine-chloromethylketone (PPACK) can protect the integrity of the plasma sample from protease activity prior to performing non-routine coagulation assays.[16] The special evacuated tube package insert should be referenced to determine for which assays these different anticoagulant tubes are recommended. If these special collection tubes are used for routine hemostasis assays, reference range must be determined based on samples collected in the same type of special collection tube in order to avoid matrix effect.

Blood to anticoagulant ratio (fill volume)

Sodium citrate is provided as a liquid anticoagulant and the recommended ratio of blood to sodium citrate anticoagulant in blood collection containers is 9:1. Anticoagulant effect of sodium citrate is attributed to its ability to bind calcium in the plasma, making the calcium unavailable to promote clot formation. Collection containers that are underfilled contain proportionally more sodium citrate, which binds a greater amount of calcium, potentially leading to longer clotting times.[17] Dilutional effect of the plasma resulting from the liquid anticoagulant in underfilled tubes may also contribute to prolonged clotting times. The degree to which fill volume affects clotting time depends, in addition, on citrate concentration used, the size of the evacuated tube, assay to be measured and reagent used in testing. Samples drawn into 3.8% sodium citrate are more prone to prolongation of clotting time in underfilled tubes than those drawn into 3.2% sodium citrate. Underfilling the blue stopper tube causes greater prolongation of the aPTT than the PT. Small volume or "pediatric" tubes, such as those that draw in the range of 2 mL or less, may show statistically significant elevations in INR when sample tube fill volumes are less than 90%.[18] Unless local studies have been performed to demonstrate acceptability of reduced fill volumes, or package inserts state differently, blue stopper evacuated tubes that are less than 90% filled are considered unacceptable for testing. Overfilling of evacuated tubes may occur if the rubber stopper is removed and additional sample added. This should be avoided as it may lead to inadequate volume of anticoagulant and limited sample mixing potential with resultant *in vitro* clot formation.

Combining samples from different evacuated collection tubes into a sodium citrate tube is *prohibited*, even if contents of two underfilled sodium citrate tubes are combined. Adding specimen from one blue stopper tube to another alters the blood to anticoagulant ratio, potentially prolonging the clotting time. The addition of blood from a red stopper tube to an incompletely filled blue stopper tube causes activation of the plasma sample and may spuriously shorten the plasma clotting time. This could bring an prolonged result spuriously into the normal range.

Hematocrit

Samples from patients with hematocrits greater than 55% may demonstrate spuriously prolonged PT and aPTT results, particularly if the sample is drawn into 3.8% rather than 3.2% sodium citrate.[19,20] Samples with elevated hematocrits mimic the effect of an underfilled tube because the volume of packed cells is increased and the volume of plasma is reduced. This may cause spurious prolongation of the aPTT and PT. Prolongation of clotting times is caused by the dilutional effect of the liquid anticoagulant and the excess citrate concentration.[20] Samples with hematocrits above 55% should have the volume of sodium citrate adjusted (decreased) using the following formula:

$$C = (1.85 \times 10^{-3}) (100 - Hct) (V_{Blood})$$

where C is the volume of citrate remaining in the tube; Hct is the hematocrit of the patient; V is the volume of blood to be added and (1.85×10^{-3}) is a constant.[7]

A simplified method to overcome citrate effect in most samples with elevated hematocrit is to remove 0.1 mL sodium citrate from the evacuated tube. Removing this constant volume of anticoagulant is generally sufficient, because most samples with an elevated hematocrit have values that fall between 0.55 (55%) and 0.65 (65%).[7] It is not necessary to adjust the volume of sodium citrate concentration for anemic samples, as low hematocrit values do not affect aPTT and PT test results.[21]

Tourniquet use

Tourniquets are often used during phlebotomy to assist in localization of the vein. Application should be tight enough such that venous but not arterial flow is obstructed. The tourniquet should be applied for the minimum period of time necessary to identify the vein and should be removed when the needle is safely in the vein.[22] In general, tourniquets should not remain in place for more than 1 minute. Tourniquets are often incorrectly left in place, not just to localize the vein but until sample collection is complete. This may not only promote *in vitro* clot formation but also cause a spurious change in test results as venous stasis induced by the tourniquet causes local hemoconcentration.[23] This can cause clinically significant variations in a variety of assays such as the aPTT, PT, fibrinogen, D-dimer and select factor activities. While an effect on assay parameters may be evident after as little as 1 minute of tourniquet use, application of a tourniquet for 3 minutes may cause significant variation in results. Comparing application of a tourniquet for 3 vs. 1 minute, Lippi *et al.*[23] demonstrated a 3.1% shortening of the PT, 10.1% increase in fibrinogen, 13.4% increase in D-dimer, 10.6% increase in factor VII activity and 10.2% increase in factor VIII activity.

Certain special coagulation assays, such as those that measure thrombin generation markers (e.g. thrombin antithrombin complex [TAT] and prothrombin fragment 1.2 [PF 1.2]), should be drawn without the use of a tourniquet. Tourniquet application during sample procurement may lead to spurious elevation of these markers, particularly if the tourniquet is left in place for more than 1 minute. To demonstrate the potential of improper specimen collection handling, three blue stopper tubes were collected from a healthy volunteer and tested in the author's laboratory. Sample designated "reference" was drawn according to proper technique, specifically with minimal use of a tourniquet and adequate mixing of the evacuated collection tube. The sample designated "inadequate mix" was collected without use of a tourniquet and was subjected to only one inversion of the evacuated tube post collection versus the recommended 3–6 inversions of the sample. The sample designated "tourniquet 3 minutes" was collected following the application of a tourniquet for 3 minutes and was adequately mixed by five end-over-end inversions of the evacuated tube. Results are shown in Table 4.3. Although an effect of improper sample handling can be seen in both assays, TAT results demonstrate exquisite susceptibility to preanalytical variables.

Table 4.3 Effect of improper sample handing on TAT and PF1.2 results.

	TAT (ng/mL)	PF 1.2 (nmol/L)
Reference range	<5.1	0.4–0.8
Reference sample*	1.75	0.59
Inadequate mix	4.18	0.7
Tourniquet 3 minutes	47.4	1.5

PF, prothrombin fragment; TAT, thrombin antithrombin complex.
* Reference sample is a sample that has been properly handled.

Order of draw and use of a discard tube

For many years it was standard practice to draw a discard tube or non-additive tube before filling a coagulation tube, in order to minimize contamination by "tissue juice" (tissue thromboplastin).[24] In the 1940s, Armand Quick, the originator of the PT assay, cited "tissue juice" as the most important external substance that could influence the coagulation reaction, suggesting that it was of "utmost importance to exclude all traces from the specimen to be tested."[25] To avoid tissue thromboplastin contamination, a "two-syringe" technique was introduced and is still practiced in some laboratories. For the "two-syringe" technique, a needle and attached syringe containing no additive is used to draw (and discard) a small quantity of blood (e.g. 2–5 mL). With the needle left in place, the first syringe is removed and a second syringe attached and additional sample drawn. Following collection of blood into the second syringe, the appropriate volume of anticoagulant is added and the sample is properly mixed. Coagulation testing is performed on blood collected into the second syringe. This technique was extrapolated to an evacuated tube system, giving rise to the use of a discard tube.

A number of published studies have refuted the need for a discard tube and have consistently demonstrated no significant difference in the aPTT and PT results between the first and second tubes drawn.[26–28] For routine coagulation testing therefore, the use of a discard tube is no longer required. It is currently recommended that specimens for routine coagulation testing be the first tube drawn if a series of tubes are being collected.[29] Discontinuation of the use of a discard tube for routine coagulation testing not only minimizes the amount of blood withdrawn from a patient but also reduces the amount of medical waste, without compromising quality of results.

There is no published evidence to demonstrate the need, or lack thereof, of using a discard tube for special coagulation studies. If a discard tube is used *prior* to collecting blood for coagulation testing or if the blue stopper tube is collected with a series of tubes, the coagulation tube must be filled after a non-additive tube. This recommendation is based on potential contamination of the sample for coagulation testing by additive adherent to the plunger of the evacuated tube holder if the coagulation tube is drawn following an additive tube.[30] A red stopper serum collection tube containing clot activator is considered an additive tube and should not be used as a discard tube for coagulation studies.

A discard tube is recommended if citrated plasma is obtained using a winged (butterfly needle) collection system.[7] The volume of blood that is drawn and discarded should equal, at the minimum, the amount of blood that fills the tubing of the winged collection set.

The general recommendations for order of draw when collecting a sample for routine coagulation testing are as follows:
• If multiple evacuated tubes are to be collected, the coagulation tube should be the first tube drawn.
• If only one evacuated tube is to be collected, the blue stopper tube can be the only tube drawn and a discard tube is not necessary.
• There are no data to support the need for a discard tube for specialty coagulation testing.
• If using an evacuated tube collection system, the tube for hemostasis testing should not be collected following collection of an additive tube.
• When using a winged collection system, a discard tube is recommended to account for the volume of blood in the flexible tubing.

Collecting samples from a vascular access device

Blood for hemostasis testing should ideally be collected directly from a peripheral vein. It may be necessary, on occasion, to obtain blood from an existing vascular access device (VAD) such as an intravenous (IV) line, a central line or saline lock. When drawing a sample from a VAD, the potential exists for heparin contamination and sample dilution because of contamination of the specimen with IV fluids. In order to collect samples for coagulation testing, it is recommended that the line is flushed with saline and that six dead space volumes of the VAD discarded.[7,31] If the sample is drawn from a capped intravenous port such as a saline lock, two dead space volumes of the catheter extension set should be discarded.[32]

Transportation of whole blood specimens to the laboratory

Following collection, samples should be transported to the laboratory at room temperature in a manner consistent with the institutional policy to prevent infectious exposure. The practice of transporting samples on ice for coagulation testing is no longer recommended. This is because of the potential for cold activation of the sample (see p. 31).[4,5] In order to prevent sample deterioration, samples should preferable be transported to the laboratory and processed within 1 hour of collection. During transportation and storage, samples should remain capped; for both safety reasons and to maintain proper pH of the sample. Transportation using a pneumatic tube system is generally acceptable for hemostasis testing, as long as the pneumatic system does not induce excessive vibration and shock that may denature proteins and activate platelets.[33] Samples for platelet function testing should not be transported in a pneumatic tube as this method of transportation may activate platelets. During sample transportation, extremes of temperature must be avoided in order to maintain sample integrity.[34]

Refrigerated storage of whole blood – adverse effects

Cold storage of citrated whole blood prior to centrifugation, either by placing samples in an ice bath or in refrigerated (2–8°C) storage, may lead to platelet activation, activation of factor VII and significant time-dependent loss of both factor VIII and VWF. Bohm et al.[35] demonstrated that whole blood samples stored on crushed ice demonstrated significant loss of VWF antigen, VWF activity and factor VIII activity after 3 hours storage with up to 50% loss from baseline at 6 hours. The effect of cold storage is greater in the functional VWF assay (VWF activity) than with the antigen assay (VWF antigen).[5] Improper storage of whole blood at cold temperatures may cause VWF and factor VIII values to fall into the abnormal range and result in the misdiagnosis of hemophilia A or von Willebrand disease. As VWF activity tends to fall to a greater degree than VWF antigen, cold storage may simulate a type 2 pattern of von Willebrand disease.

Loss of VWF antigen and activity may be because of cold-induced activation of platelets, or release of VWF-cleaving proteases or reductases that degrade VWF in the sample.[35–37] Details regarding preanalytic issues and VWF are discussed in Chapter 13.

Specimen processing

To maintain the highest level of specimen integrity, all samples should be processed as quickly as possible – ideally within the first hour after collection. In order to maintain the highest integrity, samples should remain capped and at room temperature until centrifugation. Prior to processing, samples should be examined for the presence of a clot. This is often accomplished by observation with tilting of the tube or by inserting and removing two wooden applicator sticks. The identification of a clot demands specimen rejection.

Centrifugation

Plasma is generally prepared by centrifugation of the whole blood sample. Centrifugation should take place at room temperature in a centrifuge that has a rotor with swing out buckets to facilitate the separation of plasma from the cellular components.[38] It is generally recommended that the primary tube for coagulation testing be centrifuged at 1500 g for no less than 15 minutes.[7]

The generation of platelet-poor plasma is especially important if the sample is to be subjected to certain assays such as lupus anticoagulant testing, antiphospholipid antibody testing, monitoring of UFH therapy or if the sample is to be frozen prior to analysis. It has been demonstrated that platelet counts of at least 199×10^9/L or greater do not compromise results of PT and aPTT assays when the samples are tested fresh.[39] In general, centrifugation should occur at a determined g force to produce platelet-poor plasma such that the post centrifugation plasma platelet count is $\leq 10 \times 10^9$/L. Using relative centrifugal forces (RCFs) greater than 1500 g are not recommended as this may induce platelet activation and lysis of red blood cells.[40]

Lippi et al.[38] have demonstrated that centrifugation of samples at 1500 g for either 5 or 10 minutes yields PT, aPTT and fibrinogen results essentially identical to those samples centrifuged for 15 minutes. In this study, samples spun for 2 minutes or less demonstrated an increased bias in aPTT in seconds with no significant bias in PT. Nelson et al.[41] have reported that STAT centrifuges or those that spin at a greater speed over a shorter period of time are acceptable as long as the plasma is made platelet poor by the process.

Filtration of plasma to reduce platelet contamination

Micropore filters such as a 0.2 μm Millipore filter have been used to prepare platelet-poor plasma and therefore remove platelet phospholipid that may interfere with tests for antiphospholipid antibodies.[42] However, filtered plasmas may demonstrate falsely prolonged aPTT and PT results and plasma prepared in this manner should not be used for factor analysis and VWF testing. It has been shown that filtration of plasma through a micropore filter selectively removes a number of plasma factors including factors V, VIII, IX, XII and VWF. Loss of factor VIII and VWF through a micropore filter is especially striking and may lead to an erroneous diagnosis of hemophilia A or von Willebrand disease.[43]

Hemolyzed, lipemic and icteric samples

Plasmas that are lipemic or icteric may show interference with light transmission when a coagulation analyzer with an optical end point determination is used. Ultracentrifugation to clear lipemia is used in some centers; however, no published studies have been performed to validate this procedure. The concern is that ultracentrifugation may result in spuriously low fibrinogen values. Mechanical and/or electromechanical methods for clot detection should be utilized when possible for plasma samples that are icteric, lipemic or contain substances that interfere with light transmission. While hemolysis may interfere with light transmission, the greater concern is that lysis of the red cell membranes may lead to activation of the plasma sample altering coagulation parameters.[44] Lippi reported that hemolysis may lead to statistically significant increases in PT and D-dimer and significant decreases in aPTT and fibrinogen while others have reported that hemolysis has no significant effect on aPTT and PT.[44,45] Until further studies are published, it is recommended that hemolyzed samples are not analyzed. Samples that appear hemolyzed because of the presence of a hemoglobin substitute are not a cause of specimen rejection and these samples should be evaluated using a mechanical or electomechanical method for clot detection.

Stability and storage of plasma samples

Once the whole blood sample is centrifuged, plasma can remain on the cells until testing or it can be aliquoted and stored in a secondary tube. When aliquoting the plasma, care must be taken not to disturb the buffy coat (layer of cells between the red cells and plasma) or introduce this cellular component back into the plasma. During storage, samples should remain capped.

Stability of plasma samples depends on which assay(s) are to be performed as well as the temperature and conditions of storage. The following sample stabilities are provided as a guideline and generally represent the most conservative approach to specimen handling. Laboratories may choose to perform their own studies and validate sample stabilities that are different from those listed:
• Samples for platelet function testing should remain at room temperature and testing completed within 4 hours of collection.
• Samples for PT/INR evaluation are stable at room temperature for 24 hours.[15] Samples can be stored as whole blood or centrifuged.

• Samples for aPTT testing that *do no contain UFH* should be maintained at room temperature if testing will be complete within 4 hours.[15] Limited stability is caused largely by time-dependent degeneration or loss of labile factors, particularly factor VIII and possibly factor V.[46,47] Samples that cannot be tested within 4 hours should be centrifuged and the plasma aliquot frozen.
• Samples containing UFH must be processed within 1 hour of collection because of the release of PF4 from platelets *in vitro* and subsequent neutralization of heparin, resulting in a spuriously low heparin level as measured by an aPTT and/or anti-FXa assay. If the whole blood sample is centrifuged within 1 hour of collection, the plasma can be left at room temperature for up to 4 hours prior to testing.[15]
• Stability of plasma samples for special coagulation assays (except factor VIII, anti-FXa for UFH as described above) is largely unknown. Stability of the vitamin K dependent factors has been reported to be 24 hours at room temperature.[48] This is consistent with other studies that report 24-hour stability of PT/INR determination. Protein S activity is labile with statistically significant loss of activity demonstrated at 8 hours while fibrinogen, protein C and antithrombin activity remain relatively constant for up to 7 days.[47]

If samples for coagulation testing are stored frozen, they should not be maintained in a frost-free freezer (freezer that has an automatic defrost cycles). For long-term storage of plasma samples, samples should remain in at −20°C for no more than 2 weeks. Storage for longer periods of time can be accomplished by maintaining samples at −70°C or colder. Stability of many common plasma coagulation factors at ultracold (less than −70°C) temperatures has been published by Woodhams et al.[49]

Controlled thawing of frozen plasma samples

Prior to testing, previously frozen plasma samples should be thawed in a 37°C water bath for approximately 5 minutes or until completely thawed. Samples should be monitored closely to avoid inadequate or excessive incubation in the heated water bath. Plasma samples that are inadequately thawed may have spuriously low factor VIII, VWF and fibrinogen levels

Table 4.4 Common sources of error.

- Anticoagulant other than sodium citrate
- Incomplete filling of evacuated tube
- Inadequate mixing of evacuated tube
- Storage of the whole blood sample on ice or in a refrigerated setting

Table 4.5 Ideal sample for hemostasis testing.

- Atraumatic phlebotomy with minimal tourniquet use
- Draw 3.2% blue stopper tube first or only after a non-additive tube
- Fill tube adequately (no less than 90% fill)
- Adequately and thoroughly mix with anticoagulant
- Transport promptly at room temperature
- Centrifuged within 1 hour of phlebotomy to obtain platelet poor plasma
- Test plasma or aliquot into a non-activating secondary tube immediately following centrifugation

Table 4.6 Causes for specimen rejection.

- Specimen collected into tube containing other than sodium citrate anticoagulant
- Samples that contain a clot
- Samples with other than a 9 : 1 blood to anticoagulant ratio
  - Samples less than 90% filled
  - Samples that are overfilled
  - Samples with hematocrit >55%
- Samples that are hemolyzed

because of the presence of cryoprecipitate. Likewise, plasma that is subjected to prolonged heating or excessive temperature during thawing may be compromised. In our laboratory we demonstrated that VWF antigen levels can decrease by 50% and activity levels by 80% when samples are subjected to excessive temperatures (e.g. 60°C for 10 minutes). Once thawed, samples must be thoroughly mixed prior to testing.

Conclusions

In summary, Tables 4.4, 4.5 and 4.6 present the common sources of error, common causes of specimen rejection and important factors that determine an ideal sample for hemostasis testing.

Attention to the preanalytical phase of hemostasis testing is crucial in order to provide the highest quality of laboratory results. Deviations from published guidelines may significantly impact sample integrity leading to the potential for patient misdiagnosis and management. Unless local validation is performed, guidelines for proper sample collection, handling and transport should be made widely available and strictly followed.

References

1 Lippi G, Mattiuzzi C, Guidi GC. Laboratory quality improvement by implementation of phlebotomy guidelines. Letter to the Editor. *Med Lab Observ* 2006; January: 6–7.

2 Lippi G, Salvagno G, Montagnana M, Franchini M, Guidi GC. Phlebotomy issues and quality improvement in results of laboratory testing. *Clin Lab* 2006; **52**: 217–230.

3 Kalra J. Medical errors: impact on clinical laboratories and other critical areas. *Clin Biochem* 2004; **37**: 1052–1062.

4 Morrissey JH, Macik BG, Neuenschwander PF, Comp PC. Quantitation of activated factor VII levels in plasma using tissue factor mutant selectively deficient in promoting factor VII activation. *Blood* 1993; **81**: 734–744.

5 Favaloro EJ, Soltani S, McDonald J. Potential laboratory misdiagnosis of hemophilia and von Willebrand disorder owing to cold activation of blood samples for testing. *Am J Clin Pathol* 2004; **122**: 686–692.

6 Ernst DJ, Ernst C. Phlebotomy tools of the trade: Part 4. Proper handling and storage of blood samples. *Home Health Nurse* 2003; **21**: 266–270.

7 Clinical and Laboratory Standards Institute (2008) *Collection, Transport and Processing of Blood Specimens for Testing Plasma-based Coagulation Assays and Molecular Hemostasis Assays: Approved Guideline*, 5th edn. CLSI: H21-A5.

8 Ernst DJ, Ernst C. Phlebotomy tools of the trade. *Home Health Nurse* 2002; **20**: 151–153.

9 Sharp MK, Mohammad SF. Scaling of hemolysis in needles and catheters. *Ann Biomed Eng* 1998; **26**: 788–797.

10 Jaques LB, Fidlar E, Felsted ET, Macdonald AG. Silicones and blood coagulation. *CMAJ* 1946; **56**: 26–31.

11 WHO Expert Committee on Biological Standardization (1999) *Guidelines for Thromboplastins and Plasma used to Control Oral Anticoagulant Therapy*. WHO Techni-

cal Report series. No. 880, Geneva: World Health Organization.

12 Adcock DM, Kressin DC, Marlar RA. Effect of 3.2% vs. 3.8% sodium citrate concentration on routine coagulation testing. *Am J Clin Pathol* 1997; **107**: 105–110.

13 Favaloro EJ, Bonar R, Duncan E, Earl G, Low J, Aboud M, *et al.* (2006) Identification of factor inhibitors by diagnostic hemostasis laboratories: a large multi-centre evaluation. *Thromb Haemost* 2006; **96**: 73–78.

14 van den Besselaar AMHP, Meeuwisse-Braun J, Jansen-Gruter R, Bertina RM. Monitoring heparin by the activated partial thromboplastin time: the effect of pre-analytical conditions. *Thromb Haemost* 1987; **57**: 226–231.

15 Adcock DA, Kressin DC, Marlar RA. The effect of time and temperature variables on routine coagulation tests. *Blood Coagul Fibrinolysis* 1998; 9; 463–470.

16 Rahr HB, Sorenson JV, Danielsen D. Markers of coagulation and fibrinolysis in blood drawn into citrate with and without D-Phe-Pro-Arg-Chloromethylketone (PPACK). *Thromb Res* 1994; **73**: 279–284.

17 Adcock DM, Kressin DC, Marlar RA. Minimum specimen volume requirements for routine coagulation testing. Dependence on citrate concentration. *Am J Clin Pathol* 1998; **109**: 595–599.

18 Chuang J, Sadler MA, Witt DM. Impact of evacuated collection tube fill volume and mixing on routine coagulation testing using 2.5 mL (pediatric) tubes. *Chest* 2004; **126**: 1262–1266.

19 Koepke JA, Rodgers JL, Ollivier MJ. Pre-instrument variables in coagulation testing. *Am J Clin Pathol* 1975; **64**: 591–596.

20 Marlar RA, Potts RM, Marlar AA. Effect on routine and special coagulation testing values of citrate anticoagulant adjustment in patients with high hematocrit values. *Am J Clin Pathol* 2006; **126**: 400–405.

21 Siegel JE, Swami VK, Glenn P, *et al.* Effect (or lack of it) of severe anemia on PT and aPTT results. *Am J Clin Pathol* 1998; **110**: 106–110.

22 Kiechle FL, Adcock DM, Calam RR, Davis C, Schwartz JG. *So You're Going to Collect a Blood Specimen. An Introduction to Phlebotomy*, 12th edn. Northfield, IL: College of American Pathologists, 2007.

23 Lippi G, Savagno GL, Montagnana M, Guidi GC. Short-term stasis influences routine coagulation testing. *Blood Coagul Fibrinololysis* 2005; **16**: 453–458.

24 McPhedran P, Clyne LP, Ortoli NA, Gagnon PG, Sanders FJ. Prolongation of the activated partial thromboplastin time associated with poor venipuncture technic. *Am J Clin Pathol* 1974; **62**: 16–20.

25 Quick AJ, Honorato R, Stafanini M. The value and limitations of the coagulation time in the study of hemorrhagic diseases. *Blood* 1948; **3**: 1120–1129.

26 Brigden ML, Graydon C Mcleod B, Lesperance M. Prothrombin time determination: the lack of need for a discard tube and 24-hour stability. *Am J Clin Pathol* 1997; **108**: 422–426.

27 Yawn BP, Loge C, Dale J. Prothrombin time: one tube or two. *Am J Clin Pathol* 1996; **105**: 794–797.

28 Adcock DM, Kressin DC, Marlar RA. Are discard tubes necessary in coagulation studies? *Lab Med* 1997; **28**: 530–533.

29 *Procedures for the Collection of Diagnostic Blood Specimens by Venipuncture.* Approved Standard, 5th edn. Wayne PA: CLSI: 2003, H3-A5.

30 Calam RR, Cooper MH. Recommended "order of draw" for collecting blood specimens into additive-containing tubes. *Clin Chem* 1982; **28**: 1399.

31 Laxson CJ, Titler MG. Drawing coagulation studies from arterial lines: an integrative literature review. *Am J Critical Care* 1994; **1**: 16–24.

32 Powers JM. Obtaining blood samples for coagulation studies from a normal saline lock. *Am J Critical Care* 1999; **8**: 250–253.

33 Dyszkiewicz-Korpanty A, Quinton R, Jassine J, Sarode R. The effect of pneumatic tube transport on PFA-100™ closure time and whole blood aggregation. *J Thromb Haemost* 2004; **2**: 354–356.

34 van Geest-Daalderop JH, Mulder AB, Boonman-deWinter LJ, Hoekstra MM, van den Besselaar AM. Prenanlytical variables and off-site blood collection: influences on the results of the prothrombin time/international normalized ratio test and implications for monitoring oral anticoagulant therapy. *Clin Chem* 2005; **51**: 561–568.

35 Bohm M, Teaschner S, Kretzschmar E, Gerlach R, Favaloro EJ, Scharrer I. Cold storage of citrated whole blood induces drastic time-dependent losses of factor VIII and von Willebrand factor: potential for misdiagnosis of haemophilia and von Willebrand disease. *Blood Coagul Fibrinolysis* 2006; **17**: 39–45.

36 Favaloro E, Nair SC, Forsyth CJ. Collection and transport of samples for laboratory testing in von Willbrand's disease (VWD): time for a reappraisal? *Thromb Haemost* 2001; **86**: 1589–1590.

37 Refaii MA, van Cott EM, Lukoszyk M, Hughes J, Eby CS. Loss of factor VIII and von Willebrand activities during cold storage of whole blood is reversed by rewarming. *Lab Hematol* 2006; **12**: 99–102.

38 Lippi G, Salvagno GL, Montagnana M, Monzato F, Guidi GC. Influence of the centrifuge time of primary plasma tubes on routine coagulation testing. *Blood Coagul Fibrinolysis* 2007; **18**: 525–528.

39 Carroll WE, Wolitzer AO, Harris L, Ling MC, Whitaker ML, Jackson RD. The significance of platelet counts in coagulation studies. *J Med* 2001; **32**: 83–96.

40 Aursnes I, Vikholm V. On possible interaction between ADP and mechanical stimulation in platelet activation. *Thromb Haemost* 1984; **51**: 54–56.

41 Nelson S, Pratt A, Marlar RA. Rapid preparation of plasma for 'stat' coagulation testing. *Arch Pathol Lab Med* 1994; **118**: 175–176.

42 Sheppard CA, Channell C, Ritchie JC, Duncan A. Pre-analytical variables in coagulation testing. Letter to the editor. *Blood Coagul Fibrinolysis* 2006; **17**: 425–428.

43 Favaloro EJ. Preanalytical variables in coagulation testing. Letter to the editor. *Blood Coagul Fibrinolysis* 2007; **18**: 86–89.

44 Lippi G, Montagnana M, Salvagno L, Guidi GS. Interference of blood cell lysis in routine coagulation testing. *Arch Pathol Lab Med* 2006; **130**: 181–184.

45 Laga AC, Cheves TA, Sweeney JD. The effect of specimen hemolysis on coagulation test results. *Am J Clin Pathol* 2006; **126**: 748–755.

46 O'Neill EM, Rowley J, Hanson-Wicher H, McCarter S, Ragno G, Valeri CR. Effect of 24-hour whole-blood storage on plasma clotting factors. *Transfusion* 1999; **39**: 488–491.

47 Heil W, Grunewals R, Amnd M, Heins M. Influence of time and temperature on coagulation analysis in stored plasma. *Clin Chem Lab Med* 1998; **36**: 459–452.

48 Awad MA, Selim TE, Al-Sabbagh FA. Influence of storage time and temperature on International Normalized Ratio (INR) levels and plasma activities of vitamin K dependent clotting factors. *Hematology* 2004; **9**: 333–337.

49 Woodhams B, Giradot O, Blanco M, Collesse G, Gourmelin Y. Stability of coagulation proteins in frozen plasma. *Blood Coagul Fibrinolysis* 2001; **12**: 229–236.

5

Internal quality control in the hemostasis laboratory

S. Kitchen, F. E. Preston & J. D. Olson

Many tests performed in coagulation laboratories are vital for the accurate diagnosis and safe management of patients with familial and acquired bleeding and thrombotic disorders. There are many examples where an inaccurate result could have very serious consequences for patients. Safe use of dangerous drugs such as the anticoagulants used in the treatment of approximately 1% of the population in the industrialized world is only possible with well-controlled laboratory methods.

There are many other instances where treatment is highly dependent on the results of coagulation tests. In relation to diagnosis it is particularly important that results are accurate and reliable when investigations are undertaken to determine possible familial disorders of hemostasis. A laboratory error may lead to misdiagnosis, and if an error leads to a subject being misdiagnosed as having, or not having, a familial defect, there could be serious clinical consequences.

The scope and volume of testing in coagulation laboratories has continued to increase over recent years. Workload increases and major expansion in the regulatory requirements in terms of documentation have not always been fully matched by increases in staffing. Furthermore, automated analyzers in hemostasis laboratories are increasingly complex, requiring a higher level of understanding and vigi-

lance than might not have previously been the case. Taking all these factors together, the potential for error in hemostasis laboratories has increased substantially. The purpose of quality control is to provide the documentary evidence that test results are correct and safe to be released to clinicians for patient management.

The following text deals with all aspects of internal quality control (IQC) in relation to laboratory tests of hemostasis for the benefit of patient care. This is only one component of quality management (Chapter 1). Issues related to quality control of near-patient testing or point-of-care tests of hemostasis are dealt with elsewhere (Chapter 8).

Internal quality control materials

Materials used for IQC should be similar in properties to test samples. Wherever possible, quality control materials of human origin should closely resemble human test samples. Preparation of all vials or aliquots of the control material should be identical so that any variation in test results is not a consequence of vial-to-vial variation. The IQC material should also be stable for its intended period of use. In respect of hemostatic tests and assays, IQC materials are stable over a restricted time period, often dependent on the storage conditions. For IQC materials it is advantageous for the same batch or lot number of material to be used over a period of months. This limits the frequency with which the batch number is changed and facilitates detection of drift in the assay system under assessment (see p. 47). Stability of

Quality in Laboratory Hemostasis and Thrombosis, 1st edition. By Steve Kitchen, John D. Olson and F. Eric Preston. Published 2009 by Blackwell Publishing. ISBN: 978-1-4051-6803-8

plasma for many coagulation test measurements is restricted to several hours, although for some tests plasma is stable for 24 hours or more. In order to extend this stability IQC materials should be deep frozen (preferably at −35°C or lower) or lyophilized in order ensure adequate stability over time. If deep frozen QC material is used this should be thawed rapidly at 37°C for 5 minutes and the vial inverted several times to ensure full dissolution of any precipitated protein such as fibrinogen or von Willebrand factor (with associated FVIII:C). Frozen IQC material has the advantage that reconstitution is not required and therefore precludes the necessity of adding distilled water, a potential source of pipetting error. Use of contaminated or impure distilled water for reconstitution can also adversely affect the results of coagulation tests, and again this is avoided if frozen material is employed. The use of deep frozen material can result in some longer term instability leading to prolongation of screening tests and/or loss of activity. This can be avoided by rapid freezing of the IQC material during preparation and use of lower storage temperatures.

Domestic grade −20°C freezers are inadequate for storage of frozen plasma for coagulation tests, particularly where auto-defrosting cycles lead to temperatures fluctuating above −20°C where partial defrosting of stored material can occur. Such plasma samples are especially susceptible to cryoprecipitation and cold activation.

Poorly handled frozen material may suffer from gain of function through cold activation of factor VII (FVII) and FXII/FXI which, in addition to affecting assays of these two procoagulants, also causes shortening of activated partial thromboplastin times (aPTT) or prothrombin times (PT). Despite these potential disadvantages, the use of deep frozen material remains an attractive option. In this regard Woodhams et al.[1] have demonstrated that many tests of hemostasis, including PT, aPTT, thrombin time (TT), fibrinogen, factors II, V, VII, VIII, IX, X, XI, XII, D-dimer, protein C (PC), protein S (PS) and antithrombin (AT) activity are stable for up to 3 months in plasma frozen at −24°C and for at least 18 months at −74°C where stability was defined as <10% change from the baseline result immediately after freezing. Intermediate storage temperatures of around −35 to −40°C as used in many centers are suitable for storage of frozen IQC plasma for at least 3 months. It should

not be assumed that these findings are applicable to all test systems. Results may be reagent dependent, particularly for screening tests. The authors have seen minor shortening or lengthening of screening tests (PT and aPTT) with different measurement systems.

The majority of manufacturers of commercial IQC material prefer lyophilization as a means to extend the stability of plasma, mainly because such plasmas are normally stable for several weeks at ambient temperatures (at least in temperate climates) and this allows material to be transported inexpensively between sites without special measures. Lyophilized IQC plasma material normally requires buffering to ensure that the reconstituted plasma will be stable. Manufacturers of commercial materials may not state the nature of buffering used but will normally give an indication of the period of time over which the IQC will be stable. Lyophilization increases the pH of plasma as a consequence of loss of dissolved gasses. Buffering of plasma prior to lyophilization reduces this effect but does not abolish it completely. Unbuffered lyophilized plasma normally suffers more from post reconstitution instability with a gradual increase in pH. This may be accompanied by altered results in coagulation tests. This is particularly apparent for screening tests such as aPTT and changes in results may be less marked in tests where the reagents are well buffered, such as coagulation factor assays. If buffering is inadequate the aPTT may prolong by 10–20% within 1 hour of reconstitution, depending on the reagent. For reconstitution of lyophilized samples it is important to use distilled water with pH 6.8–7.2 and to allow at least 10 minutes for reconstitution. If commercial quality control (QC) material is used this should be reconstituted according to manufacturers' instructions using an accurate pipetting system.

It is extremely useful to test at least two QC samples with different levels of abnormality. The most suitable levels will depend on the nature of the test sample population. For screening tests, centers should analyze QC samples with normal levels and at least one further level where the result is outside the reference range. This means that within limits QC results can confirm that the method is under control for both normal and abnormal sample analysis. If control of oral anticoagulant (OAC, e.g. coumarin) therapy is an important component of the workload then the second level of IQC for the PT/International Normalized Ratio (INR) test system could have an INR in the mid therapeutic range. If a center is involved in the diagnosis of bleeding disorders, then an IQC with a level of FVIII:C, FIX and von Willebrand factor (VWF) in the range 30–50 IU/dL is particularly appropriate because this is a critical area for establishing a diagnosis or for monitoring response to therapy. For thrombophilia work, IQC samples with results around the interface between normal and abnormal are useful because once again this is a critical area where good evidence that the method is under control is helpful.

In the selection of QC material the risk of transmission of blood-borne viruses should be considered and high-risk material should not be used.

Frequency of IQC testing

There are number of issues to take into account when considering the frequency of IQC testing including the number of patient samples being analyzed and the way in which these samples are processed. For tests that are performed in discrete batches at least one level of QC material should be included with each batch. Where there is continuous processing, e.g. when using many types of modern auto-analyzer, then a QC sample should be included at regular intervals. There is some evidence that a combination of IQC testing at fixed time intervals with further IQC testing performed randomly at additional times may be better for detection of error conditions.[2]

When large numbers of samples are processed then QC testing can be fixed at timed intervals or after a certain number of test samples have been analyzed. Such decisions should also take account of the consequences of releasing incorrect results. The frequency should be set so that recall of erroneous patient results is avoided. For screening tests such as PT/INR or aPTT in departments processing more than 100 samples per day, testing every 2 hours does not represent too large a financial burden in relation to the cost, and is easily achieved.

There are published recommendations in relation to the frequency of testing IQC material for some coagulation tests. The Clinical Laboratory Standards Institute (CLSI – formerly NCCLS) have recently updated their guideline document dealing with PT and aPTT.[3] This recommends testing at least two levels of control material every 8 hours for all non-manual PT and aPTT coagulation test systems, but recognizes that if the volume of testing is high, more frequent QC testing should be performed. This document also recommends that when continuous sample processing occurs, as in many large laboratories in established centers, then at least one from the two or three levels of IQC should be alternately tested at least every 4 hours. In our experience, the frequency should be increased to every 2 hours during periods of testing when more than 20 samples per hour are being analyzed. This CLSI document also reminds us that the first test performed after reagent addition or important instrument change should be the QC sample. This is of particular importance after daily instrument maintenance. Some analyzers now allow several different positions to be occupied by the same reagent. The instrument is then programmed to switch automatically to a new vial of reagent when the first has been consumed. When this occurs it is important that an IQC sample is tested from each reagent reservoir before patient samples are analyzed. Only after an IQC result within the target range has been obtained is it safe to proceed with patient testing.

In relation to fibrinogen testing the inclusion of at least one abnormal control with a decreased fibrinogen level of 0.8–1.2 g/L with each batch of samples has been recommended,[4] although in practice any abnormal control with a level between 0.3 and 1.4 g/L is probably suitable. The same authors recommend testing normal and abnormal samples at a minimum of every 20 samples in laboratories where many fibrinogen determinations are performed. For current auto-analyzers, a single normal IQC every 20 samples is acceptable for routine purposes. The inclusion of an abnormal control at least daily gives additional confidence that the method is under control for measurement at a level where inaccurate results are of particular importance for patient management. When performing coagulation factor assays there is a recommendation to include both an abnormal and normal IQC with each batch of tests.[5] In contrast, the UK Haemophilia Centre Doctors Organisation (HCDO)[6] and the World Federation of Hemophilia (WFH) recommend a single level of IQC with each test batch.[7]

The extra information provided by testing two levels of IQC has to be balanced against the additional costs incurred. When tests are performed in batches of less than 10 then a single level of IQC is reasonable. This can be increased to two for larger test batches.

Acceptable limits for IQC

All analytic techniques are subject to variability. It is not possible to eliminate this totally but it is important to minimize variability by good laboratory practice. There are essentially two sources of variation in coagulation test analyses: random and systematic. Random error is described by the precision of the test. Systemic variation is a reflection of the accuracy of the test.

Because all tests suffer to a greater or lesser degree from variability, some authors prefer to use the term imprecision rather than precision. These describe the same effects in opposite ways, so low variability can be described either as high precision or low imprecision. Precision can be defined as the closeness of agreement between independent results of measurements obtained under a particular set of conditions. For practical purposes this is measured by a number of replicate measurements on the sample. The degree of precision will normally depend on the analytical conditions. The precision of replicate measurements by one operator using a single set of reagents in a short time period of time (within-run error) will normally be lower than a set of measurements made by different operators on different days using fresh reagent sets on each occasion (between-run error). This means that setting acceptable limits for analysis of an IQC material must take account of day-to-day variability. The most commonly used measure of precision is the coefficient of variation (CV% = SD/mean × 100). Thus, a high CV indicates poor reproducibility.

In the case of screening tests and occasionally assays, the results obtained will be dependent on the reagents and end point detection system used to perform the tests. The target range must take account of these effects. For commercial IQC samples, manufacturers often provide a target range of acceptable values; however, this should only be used as guide and the target range for any coagulation test should be established locally. The IQC material should be tested repeatedly (minimum 20 times) with testing spread over at least 10 sessions. When collecting

these data it is useful to have evidence that the method is under control and so any available IQC that has been used previously should be included and only if results on this previous material are within limits can the results on the material under evaluation be used. This may not always be possible, e.g. when establishing a method for a new analyte. In this case any outliers amongst the data should be excluded from the calculation of target values. Identification of outliers can be performed by statistical methods but visual inspection of the data may well be sufficient.

It is not recommended to use the observed range of results obtained to define the limits of the target range. Once the raw data are collected some form of data analysis is used to set the limits of the acceptable range The mean and standard deviation (SD) of the results are calculated. The SD is a measure of the spread of results: the larger the SD, the greater is the spread of results. Random variation follows a Gaussian distribution, i.e. the classic bell-shaped normal distribution. In this case the mean ± 2 SD encompasses 95.5% of the values. This is the most commonly used range so that intervention occurs if an IQC result is more than 2 SD above or below the mean. The mean ± 3 SD encompasses 99.7% of the values and could be considered as overtolerant in respect of the target range that has to be exceeded before suspension of patient sample testing and subsequent method investigation. The acceptable limits of variation for an IQC material are therefore statistically based and reflect the causes of error. These limits reflect how reproducible the process is and do not describe the accuracy of the test, accuracy being how close the measured test result is to the true value.

Storage and processing of IQC results

The most convenient way to record and visualize IQC results is by using a chart. The most widely used system is the Levey–Jennings chart. First reported more than 50 years ago,[8] its continued and widespread use in an essentially unchanged format is good evidence of its ease of use and fitness for purpose. A more recent perspective on this has been published,[9] which reminds the reader that Levey and Jennings in their original publication comment that review of

IQC results helps in the development of an appreciation of quality issues. This in turn helps improve patient care through increased pride amongst laboratory workers as a consequence of good IQC data and records.

Although originally designed for several biochemistry tests, Levey–Jennings charts are suitable for a wide range of analytes including coagulation tests. Control charts are useful to judge what has happened to an analytical process in the past, and are useful for ongoing evaluation of the process over time. Ongoing evaluation can be used to help document the improvement over time as a consequence of any interventions, actions or efforts to reduce the causes of variation. The Levey–Jennings chart is constructed to show the mean value of initial testing performed to define the acceptable limits. The chart should also have lines showing the upper and lower limits of acceptable results – these being 2 SD above and 2 SD below the mean. An example is shown in Fig. 5.1 which

illustrates the expected distribution of control values as well as examples where problems are occurring.

There are a number of changes that can be made to a test system with the potential to alter the bias between a measured IQC result and the target or true value. These include a change in the calibration of the method, a change in lot number of reagents or consumables or even a change in operator where there is potential for different operators to perform tasks differently. Many of these would be apparent as systematic shifts in the means of IQC results placed on a typical chart.

Out of limits IQC results

As soon as an out-of-limits IQC result is obtained all patient testing must be suspended pending identification and correction of the problem. When an indi-

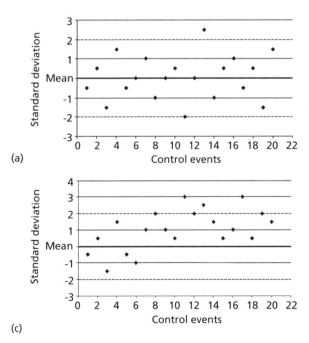

(a)

(c)

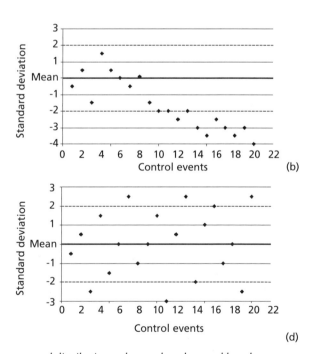

(b)

(d)

Fig. 5.1 Examples of Levey–Jennings charts recording control values. (a) Expected distribution of control values. (b) Control events demonstrating a trend. (c) Control events demonstrating a shift. (d) Control events demonstrating an increased random error. This shows the expected distribution and examples where problems have occurred indicating that a method is moving out of control. In each case the dotted lines show the 2 standard deviation limits of acceptable results.

vidual IQC test result falls outside limits then either there is a problem with the individual vial of IQC material, the entire batch of IQC has deteriorated or there is a problem with the analytical system. It is important to differentiate between these possibilities by sequential investigations so that appropriate action can be taken. Analysis of a second vial of the same batch of IQC with the same reagents/method should be the first action. If this is within limits then it is highly likely that the test system is under control but the IQC sample analyzed earlier had deteriorated or been contaminated and should be discarded. This should be confirmed by performing a third IQC test. If this is within limits then patient testing can be safely resumed.

However, if a second out-of-limits result is obtained on the replacement IQC vial of the same batch then the most likely explanation is that the test system is out of control. In this case, analysis of a second lot or batch of IQC material would also give out-of-limits results.

If further vials of the first batch give out-of-limits results but the second batch of material gives within-limits results, then the entire batch of the first IQC material may have deteriorated. This is a rare occurrence. Thus, having more than one level of IQC available can be very useful when investigating the cause of out-of-limits IQC results.

The most common cause of an out of control test system in hemostasis laboratories is reagent deterioration or contamination. All IQC results will be out-of-limits and in this case reagents should be discarded. Patient testing should only be safely resumed after the problem has been identified and rectified.

In many centers PT and aPTT methods are in operation on the same analyzer at the same time. In this case scrutiny of the whole pattern of IQC results for both methods may be informative. Table 5.1 illustrates how different patterns of IQC results can help identify the nature of the analytical problem.

In some instances there are compelling reasons to investigate a method with subsequent intervention, even though recent IQC results are within the target range. For an IQC sample with appropriate target limits, analyzed with a well-controlled method, the results obtained should fluctuate around the mean (Fig. 5.1). However, a series of 7–10 results on the

Table 5.1 Troubleshooting internal quality control (IQC) problems. How different patterns of IQC error for two levels of IQC material tested for prothrombin time (PT) and activated partial thromboplastin time (aPTT) can direct the sequence of investigations required to correct the problem.

PT Level 1 IQC	PT Level 2 IQC	aPTT Level 1 IQC	aPTT Level 2 IQC	Conclusion/check
Out	In	In	In	PT Level 1 IQC material
Out	Out	In	In	PT reagent
In	In	Out	In	aPTT Level 1 IQC material
In	In	Out	Out	aPTT reagent
Out	Out	Out	Out	Instrument

same material showing a progressive trend in one direction, i.e. gradually increasing or decreasing over time (Fig. 5.1), may be an indication of drift in the analytical process. A gradual deterioration of a particular reagent over time, or gradual change in an analyzer could be associated with such a pattern of IQC results. On other occasions there may be a series of individual IQC results all within limits but consistently lying above or consistently below the mean (Fig. 5.1). This may indicate that there has been a change in the method since the target range was established. In this case a new target range should be established and investigation of recent changes in the method as well as an assessment of the accuracy of the test is merited (e.g. through external quality assessment or analysis of reference samples/materials). Where a batch or lot number of IQC is used for more than 3–4 months a recalculation of mean and SD is useful to confirm that the original range remains appropriate.

When the cause of out-of-limits IQC results has been identified it is necessary to assess which patient results need to be repeated. If the problem relates to the deterioration of IQC material no retesting is required. If the problem relates to reagents then all patient results obtained since the last within-limits IQC result should be reviewed. One practical approach is to retest every 10th sample in reverse order to establish at which point the problem developed. Any patient samples from that point onwards require retesting.

The comments above involve use of a single rule for intervention – if a single result exceeds a particular threshold then intervention follows. There are more complex procedures for assessing a series of IQC results based on multiple rules. These have come into use because an IQC result may fall outside a target range by chance alone, without any problem being present in the analytical system. This is statistically inevitable from time to time and represents a false alarm. This is a limitation of using a single rule when assessing IQC results. The so-called Westgard rules[10] are one example that use a combination of decision criteria from five different control rules. These have the advantage of fewer false rejections while maintaining a high rate of error detection. These were originally described for use with clinical chemistry testing with 2–4 control measurements per run. Some centers make use of multiple rules in coagulation testing but these have not been widely adopted in hemostasis laboratories.

Accreditation and regulatory bodies

The program of IQC employed within the laboratory should comply with any local legislation, regulations, guidelines or standards issued by relevant bodies. In many countries there are local standards which are often constructed to be compatible with ISO 15189[11] Medical Laboratories – Particular requirements for quality and competence. For example, in the UK the accreditation process is undertaken by Clinical Pathology Accreditation (CPA) (www.cpa-uk.co.uk) who require written procedures to include: records of the date; source and storage of IQC materials; the process used to validate IQC material prior to use; details of the statistical procedures employed; acceptance criteria for results obtained on IQC material in use. This body also requires that all IQC results shall be recorded, regularly evaluated and subsequent corrective and/or preventative actions taken recorded.

We strongly recommend use of such an error log which can be extremely useful for informing the troubleshooting process. The above CPA standards further require that the period of retention for records should be defined. These recommendations and requirements should be followed in addition to any other local recommendations from relevant accreditation or professional bodies, or legislation.

Conclusions

Any out-of-limits IQC result should lead to an immediate investigation together with suspension of patient testing pending resolution of the problem. This whole process helps to establish well-controlled methods. Recognition of the causes of problems facilitates the process of minimizing errors in the future. All of this serves to improve the overall quality of the service but IQC testing and regular scrutiny of results obtained should be merely one component of the quality assurance and quality management program. Quality control is a continuous process and is the responsibility of all staff at all levels in the hemostasis laboratory. The wider issues around quality management are dealt with in Chapter 1.

References

1 Woodhams B, Girardot O, Blanco BJ, Colesse G, Gourmelin Y. Stability of coagulation proteins in frozen plasma. *Blood Coag Fibrinolysis* 2001; **12**: 229–236.

2 Parvin CA, Robbins S. Evaluation of the performance of pandomised versus fixed time schedules for quality control procedures. *Clin Chem* 2007: **53**; 575–580.

3 Marler KA, Cook J, Johnston M, Kitchen S, Machin SJ, Shafer D, *et al. One Stage Prothrombin Time and Activated Partial Thromboplastin Time Test: Approved Guideline*, 2nd edn. CLSI, 2007. H47-A2.

4 Day J, Arkin CF, Bovill EG, Bowie EJW, Carroll JJ, Joist JH, *et al. Procedure for the Determination of Fibrinogen in Plasma: Approved Guideline*. NCCLS, 1994. H30A.

5 Arkin CF, Bowie EJW, Carroll JJ, Day HJ, Joist JH, Lenahan JG, *et al. Determination of Factor Coagulant Activator: Approved Guideline* NCCLS/CLCI, 1997. H48-A.

6 Bolton-Maggs P, Perry DJ, Chalmers EA, Parapia LA, Wilde JT, Williams MD, *et al*. The rare coagulation disorders: review with guidelines for management. *Haemophilia* 2004; **10**: 1–36.

7 Kitchen S, McCraw A. *Diagnosis of Haemophilia and Other Bleeding Disorders*. World Federation of Haemophilia, 2001. (http://www.wfh.org/2/docs/Publications/Diagnosis_and_Treatment/Lab_manual_web.pdf)

8 Levey S, Jennings ER. The use of control charts in the clinical laboratory. *Am J Clin Pathol* 1950; **20**; 1059–1066.

9 Barger JD. Levey and Jennings revisited. *Arch Pathol Lab Med* 1992: **116**; 799–803.

10 Westgard JO, Barry PL, Hunt MR, Groth T. A multi-rule Shewart chart for quality control in clinical chemistry. *Clin Chem* 1981; **27**: 493–501.

11 International Organization for Standardization. ISO 15189. 2007: Medical Laboratories: Particular requirements for quality and competence. http://www.iso.org/iso/iso_catalogue/catalogue_tc/catalogue_detail.htm?csnumber=42641

6

External quality assessment in hemostasis: its importance and significance

F. E. Preston, S. Kitchen & A. Srivastava

The coagulation laboratory has a vital role in the diagnosis and management of patients with familial and acquired hemorrhagic and thrombotic disorders. Its involvement in oral anticoagulant control is of particular importance.

For all clinical laboratories, the results generated should be accurate, reliable and reproducible. This applies to all laboratory investigations and particularly to those performed to diagnose, or to exclude, a possible familial disorder. The workload and scope of the coagulation laboratory has increased substantially over recent years and this has been accompanied by the introduction of increasingly sophisticated automated equipment employing a variety of technologies. The potential for error is therefore considerable. Consequently, it is essential to monitor a laboratory's performance through its participation in an external quality assessment program.[1]

External quality assessment (EQA) provides a comparison of results obtained on the same sample among different laboratories. Consequently, it provides information in respect of the accuracy of results produced by the participating laboratories. Of equal importance is that the larger programs also provide comparisons of results obtained with different reagents and different instrument – reagent combinations on a single sample.

In hemostasis EQA programs, plasma samples, usually lyophilized, are distributed to participating laboratories and these are instructed to perform specific tests using their standard methods. It is important that the EQA samples are tested in the same way and by the same personnel as for patient samples. In most programs the laboratory is requested to return its results to the program organizer for detailed analysis.

It is important to stress that, for obvious reasons, the samples that are distributed to participating laboratories are not identical to routine patient samples. The plasma samples are usually obtained by single donor plasmapheresis but occasionally it is necessary to pool donations, e.g. for heparin dosage monitoring. In general, genuine patient samples such as these are preferable to samples that have been created by manipulation of normal plasma, e.g. by artificial depletion. Unless it is impossible to avoid, all distributed samples should be negative for human immunodeficiency virus (HIV), hepatitis C virus (HCV) and hepatitis B virus (HBV) infection. If this cannot be avoided then prior approval for the distribution of infected material should be obtained from the participant.

In most programs the distributed samples are lyophilized. Consequently, it is incumbent on the EQA providers to ensure that following reconstitution, the results obtained on their materials are similar to those obtained on the native plasma before lyophilization and also following reconstitution.[2,3] Very rarely, a matrix effect is responsible for differences in EQA results. This has been noted by UK National External Quality Assessment Scheme (NEQAS) with

Quality in Laboratory Hemostasis and Thrombosis, 1st edition. By Steve Kitchen, John D. Olson and F. Eric Preston. Published 2009 by Blackwell Publishing. ISBN: 978-1-4051-6803-8

respect to a particular thromboplastin for International Normalized Ratio (INR) testing (F.E. Preston & S. Kitchen 2006, personal communication). It is also important to establish the stability of the lyophilized samples over a range of different temperatures, especially where distributed materials may be exposed to higher temperatures for prolonged periods of time.

Target values

The most important component of any EQA program is the assignment of the target value, i.e. the "correct" result because this is the yardstick by which all laboratories are assessed. Target value assignment is difficult. Possible candidates include results obtained using an approved reference method results obtained by "expert laboratories" and overall consensus results.

Although target values derived from results obtained through reference methods are acceptable for EQA programs in clinical chemistry, this approach is not feasible for EQA programs in hemostasis and thrombosis. Although common principles are employed for all tests of hemostasis, the number of variables operating within most, if not all, laboratory procedures is extremely large and there is no consensus for specific reference methods.

Another possible approach to target value assignment is to deploy the results obtained by laboratories recognized for their expertise in the area. Although this sounds reasonable there is no unanimous agreement as to what constitutes an expert laboratory. There is no guarantee that because a laboratory has a long-standing reputation in hemostasis and thrombosis it is able to produce accurate and reliable results across a broad spectrum of investigations. Indeed, when we explored this possibility in an EQA program, it was soon apparent that the results obtained by internationally accepted expert laboratories were as diverse as those derived from smaller institutions. When using expert laboratories it is vital that the participating centers in any EQA program accept the validity of target results derived from these laboratories. In respect of this, difficulties may arise and the efficiency of the EQA program compromised when professional rivalries exist between different high profile centers.

The overall consensus value of the results obtained by all participants can also be adopted as the target value for EQA participants. This can be the mean, the median or, after the removal of statistical outliers, the truncated mean value of the overall results. However, even this approach is not without its problems. In any large EQA program the number of variables with respect to reagents, instruments and calibrants is extremely large and major differences may be observed in the results obtained with different combinations. For example, in the UK NEQAS program for INR testing, participants used at least 27 different thromboplastins and 35 different coagulometers in at least 110 different combinations during 2006. Although the INR system is designed to give identical results with different thromboplastins, this ideal situation is not always realized (see Chapter 18).[4] Consequently, if different results are obtained with different reagent–calibrant–instrument combinations then the overall consensus result will be influenced by the numbers of participants employing any single combination of these variables.

An example of this is provided by the results obtained by UK NEQAS participants in an exercise of unfractionated heparin monitoring by activated partial thromboplastin time (aPTT). In this exercise participants received a lyophilized plasma sample derived from patients receiving unfractionated heparin. They were asked to perform an aPTT test using their usual reagent. Results were expressed as a ratio of the sample aPTT divided by the mid-point of their reference range using the same reagent. Six reagents were used by 10 or more participants. These results are presented in Table 6.1.

Table 6.1 UK National External Quality Assessment Scheme (NEQAS) results: pooled *ex vivo* heparinized plasmas.

Reagent	n	Median aPTT ratio
A	143	1.93
B	10	1.93
C	47	1.63
D	37	1.55
E	62	1.45
F	35	1.30

It can be seen from Table 6.1 that there were major differences in the results obtained by users of the different reagents, ranging from 1.30 to 1.93. This means that the median aPTT ratio of users of reagent "F" was 1.3 compared with a median aPTT ratio of 1.93 for users of reagents "A" and "B." The overall median aPTT for all participants was 1.7. Thus, if a user of reagent "F" obtained a ratio of 1.3 and this was assessed against the overall median of 1.7 then this would constitute "poor performance" because the result is 23.5% lower than the overall median. However, the median aPTT ratio for "F" reagent users was 1.3 and therefore if this result (1.3) is assessed against the group reagent median then it clearly represents a good performance. Conversely, if the result of a reagent "F" user was 1.7 this would constitute a good performance if assessed against the overall median but a poor performance if assessed against the group median.

It is clear from this example that there are inherent flaws in assessing results against the overall median (or mean) result for tests such as the prothrombin time and aPTT. Whenever possible therefore it is more appropriate to assess results against the peer group median result. An assessment against the overall median, i.e. all-methods analysis, is appropriate only where the number of laboratories deploying a specific method with the same reagents is too small, i.e. less than 10, for an accurate statistical analysis or when all methods are known to give the same result for any given analyte. Separate peer group analyses is therefore appropriate for tests whenever there are 10 or more users of any given combination.

Evaluation of laboratory performance

The methods by which individual EQA providers evaluate performance are very variable. Commonly used examples include a fixed percentage on either side of the overall or peer group mean or median and the application of the so-called "z" score. This is calculated from the formula $z = (R - T)/\sigma$, where R is the participant's result, T is the target value and σ is the standard deviation for proficiency. Using the "z score" model, performance is evaluated as follows

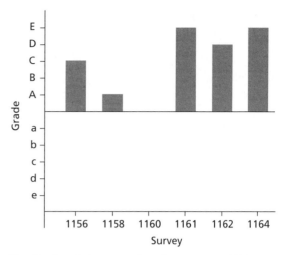

Fig. 6.1 Cumulative external quality assessment (EQA) results for antithrombin activity. In the final three surveys (1161, 1162 and 1163) the laboratory has obtained grades E, D and E for each of the test samples (see text for explanation of the grading system) indicating persistent poor performance over this period of time.

$0 < z < 2 =$ "acceptable",
$2 < z < 3 =$ "questionable"
and $3 < z =$ "unacceptable".

Some programs adopt a different approach in their assessment of performance analysis of simple tests such as the prothrombin time and the aPTT compared with that adopted for specific clotting factor assays such as FVIII:C or FIX:C. The UK NEQAS program, for example, employs a grading system of A–E for clotting factor assays (Fig. 6.1). This is based on the difference between the laboratory result and the overall median value. An "A" result covers all results that are either 25% above or below the overall median value. Conversely, an "E" grade is allocated to those laboratories that obtain the extreme 5% of results above and below the overall median result. The designation "persistently outwith consensus" is then based on the results of three consecutive surveys. For the simple tests such as the prothrombin time or aPTT, results are considered satisfactory if they fall within 15% above or below the peer group median result. Following statistical analysis the results are then forwarded to the participating laboratories. Most EQA providers also provide a corresponding performance analysis (see p. 54).

For those laboratories that participate in more than one EQA program the different approaches adopted by the providers may result in some ambiguity in that a satisfactory performance may be achieved in one program and an unsatisfactory performance in another. In our experience this often relates to differences between results assessed against the overall median compared with results analyzed against a method specific peer group median.

For some analytes different methods produce different results. For example, clotting and chromogenic-based protein C methods give different results when other abnormalities are present in the sample, e.g. factor V Leiden. In the case of von Willebrand factor (VWF) activity measurements we have shown that different results are produced by different methods, particularly in patients with type 2 VWD.[5] Where such differences occur, the assessment of individual laboratory performance should be determined by reference to results obtained by those laboratories that deploy the same technique.

In respect of the analysis of results and the evaluation of laboratory performance two quite distinct approaches are taken by EQA providers.[6] Some EQA providers set standards for satisfactory performance for individual analytes. The laboratory results are analyzed and the laboratory performance is graded according to the criteria established by the EQA program. The terms employed for performance analysis are extremely varied and include expressions such as "pass" or "fail," "desirable" or "undesirable," "within consensus" or "outwith consensus." Some of the programs do not perform a separate performance analysis for every analyte.

Other EQA providers adopt a different approach. These analyze the entire data set of results and report the statistics to the participating laboratory. The laboratory then assesses its own performance relative to the other results. Using this approach the laboratory thus assesses itself.

A questionnaire distributed by the recently formed External Quality Assurance in Thrombosis and Hemostasis (EQATH) has revealed that of the 11 EQA programs contacted, six were responsible for the analysis of performance of participating whereas the remaining five reported the overall statistics to the participating laboratories for their own evaluation.[6]

The criteria for the designation of poor performance by different EQA providers are extremely varied. In some programs, the method of performance analysis will always identify an apparent poor performer in each survey. For example, in the A–E system employed by UK NEQAS there will always be a number of laboratories that obtain results that are at the extreme 5% above and below the overall median result. However, contact is not made with participants until they are classified as being "persistently outwith consensus." As already indicated, the designation "persistently outwith consensus" is based on the results of three consecutive surveys. The overall probability of a laboratory obtaining three consecutive very low gradings by chance alone is 0.014.

Following their identification of persistently poor performance a very small number of EQA providers make direct contact with the laboratory, drawing attention to the problem and offering repeat samples and technical advice.

Irrespective of the manner in which an EQA program evaluates performance, this activity is of vital importance because it enables laboratories to recognize unsuspected analytical problems. Separate evaluation should be made for each analyte. There is no ambiguity when EQA programs adopt a pass/fail approach but some consider this to be somewhat too rigid. Some parameters are not easily assessed. In particular, the assessment of lupus anticoagulant detection has proved to be particularly difficult for EQA providers.[7,8]

In those instances where the interpretation of EQA results and corresponding performance analysis is performed by the participating laboratory rather than by the EQA provider, there appears to be an assumption that the laboratory will recognize its own unsatisfactory performance. In view of the many regulatory and fiscal pressures that are brought to bear on clinical laboratories we wonder whether absolute objectivity can always be maintained. This is clearly a controversial area.

In many countries, the grading of laboratory performance is an essential prerequisite for accreditation or licensure requirements. This has largely occurred because it was noted by regulatory authorities that laboratories were not voluntarily including EQA in their quality programs.[6] This enforcement of EQA has consequently resulted in increasing regulation and a corresponding reduction in its educational component and, possibly, limiting the program's ability to actually improve quality in the participant laboratory. Participation in EQA programs that are essential for accreditation is therefore mandatory and the professional relationship that exists between participants in these programs and the EQA provider will be quite different from that which exists between those involved in those EQA programs where these requirements do not operate. Understandably, the former group will view EQA as potentially punitive whereas the latter will be stimulated by the educational support of the latter. Stated another way, the former program will attempt to "drive" the laboratory to better quality while the latter will "lead" the program to better quality. Which approach provides better success in actually improving laboratory quality is not known, one hopes that it would be the latter, less punitive one; however, that may be wishful thinking.

Monitoring results: the role of the laboratory

EQA programs enable laboratories to assess their results against those obtained by other laboratories using the same reagents and the same methodology. This allows them to adjust their procedures and/or change their reagents in order to improve their quality of service. Poor performance, however defined, demands some response from the laboratory. A single poor result should be noted and consideration given to possible causes.

It is particularly important for a laboratory's performance to be monitored over time. Results that are consistently above or below the peer group median may indicate either a systematic or a calibration error and therefore provide information that is not apparent from single assessments. The limitations of a single assessment are supported by reports that in approximately 25% of cases it was not possible to identify the cause of a single poor performance.[9–11] A center with consistently poor performance should examine its internal quality control (IQC) records over the relevant time frame. This will help distinguish between imprecise and inaccurate results. Assay imprecision is likely when sequential EQA results fluctuate above and below the target values. In this case IQC results will usually be variable with low precision. EQA results that are consistently higher or lower than than those of its appropriate peer group indicate probable high precision in the assay. In this

case consistent IQC results indicate that the method is precise, which contrasts with the EQA results that demonstrate their inaccuracy. In these circumstances all of the components of the assay system should be investigated and, where necessary, replaced.

If a center obtains EQA results for a particular test that fluctuate above and below the median by a considerable degree then the method is poorly controlled and it is likely that the corresponding internal quality results will also show a high degree of imprecision. In this case the center needs to consider whether a particular analyzer is variable in its performance or whether there is instability in the reagents used. It is also necessary to ensure that staff performing the investigations are properly trained and competent. Serial monitoring of EQA results also allows laboratories to assess the impact of any method or reagent change or modification.

In general terms, an unsatisfactory laboratory performance may be caused by a clerical error, or else some problem in the laboratory or a problem with the EQA specimen. Unsatisfactory performance may reflect errors arising out of IQC, pipettes, instruments and inadequately trained or inexperienced laboratory staff. Most EQA samples are lyophilized and therefore require reconstitution prior to analysis. Occasionally, poor performance in EQA can be caused by inferior/contaminated distilled water, incorrect diluent volume or by failure to analyze the EQA sample within the stated period where sample stability is guaranteed. Some of these errors would not affect patient sample analysis because there is no requirement to reconstitute the plasma and in this case poor performance may not automatically confirm that patient results are unsafe.

In order to improve the quality of service it is clearly incumbent on the laboratory to reconcile the cause of its poor performance, particularly when this is recurrent. For some laboratories an additional, and arguably more pressing imperative, is the maintenance of its accreditation status. In some countries, clinical laboratories are required to provide documentary evidence of satisfactory participation in either an EQA program operated by the regulatory agency or else in a program that is approved by a government agency such as the College of American Pathology (CAP) in the USA. In the USA all laboratories must participate in proficiency testing and be inspected and accredited. This is undertaken by the government inspection program, run by the federal agency. The federal government does provide for EQA, this must come from an EQA provider that has been approved (i.e. has "deemed status"). There are 14 programs in the USA that have deemed status, one of which is the CAP. The CAP is, by far, the most comprehensive with about 6000 participants, mostly hospital or reference laboratories.

Of the 11 EQA programs participating in the EQATH initiative, seven have been granted "deemed" status by governmental agency that allows participating laboratories to cite their results for continued EQA accreditation.[6]

Educational role of EQA

EQA programs have an important educational role but this aspect may be minimal or even absent in those programs in which participation and success are essential for accreditation. Educational support is provided by printed or electronic commentaries and by regular participant meetings. A small number of EQA providers also offer technical support and repeat samples. Some of the EQA programs undertake supplementary exercises in which samples are distributed in order to address specific issues such as use of a common calibration plasma set for local calibration of INR, use of a common normal plasma for normalized ratios in detection of lupus anticoagulant or activated protein C (APC) resistance testing and so on.

Total confidentiality of results is usually maintained by those programs that are essentially educational in nature and the communication of EQA results and corresponding performance analysis is restricted to the individual nominated by the laboratory itself. The only exception to this approach is when a laboratory is financially sponsored by some agency such as the World Federation of Hemophilia (WFH).

Additional advantages of EQA programs

In addition to their role in identifying poor laboratory performance, the larger EQA programs have the important and added advantage of being able to identify problems relating to instruments, reagents and reference plasmas. This is achieved by comparing results obtained by peer group analysis. Persistent and significant differences of results between groups serves as an alert to the possibility of anomalies arising out of the method itself rather than unsatisfactory laboratory performance. Some years ago in the UK NEQAS program, the INR results obtained with a commonly used thromboplastin were significantly and consistently higher than those obtained by the users of a different thromboplastin.[12] In addition to determining the INRs, participants were provided with a clinical history and were asked, on the basis of their results, to state whether the patient was over, under or adequately anticoagulated. The differences in the INR results proved to be of considerable clinical importance because markedly differing conclusions were drawn by the two groups. For example, with one sample, 73% of the users of one of the thromboplastins concluded that the patient was over-anticoagulated whereas 71% of users of the other thromboplastin expressed the view that the patient was adequately anticoagulated. Following discussions with the program director, the matter was resolved by the manufacturers.

Discrepancies in clotting factor assays may also, on occasion, be attributed to anomalies relating to the use of commercial reference plasmas. In the UK NEQAS program this has been noted in respect of factors VIII:C and V:C assays. In a recent exercise the median factor VIII:C results obtained with six commonly used commercial reference plasmas varied from 72 to 86 IU/dL. All the other assay components were similar. Similar observations have also been noted in respect of factor V:C assays in that the use of different commercial reference plasmas was associated with markedly differing results.

The discrepant FV:C results focused attention on the need for an international standard for FV:C.[13] This has now been implemented through the auspices of the World Health Organization (WHO).[14]

It is clear that a comprehensive EQA program in hemostasis and thrombosis serves a number of important functions. By identifying, and assisting, those laboratories that fail to achieve satisfactory results it serves to improve laboratory performance and therefore patient care. Larger programs are able to identify unsatisfactory reagents, reference materials and methods and therefore are able to assist laboratories

Table 6.2 What does external quality assessment (EQA) not accomplish?

- EQA does not test the quality of the laboratory
- EQA does not test pre and postanalytical steps
- Limitations in evaluation of analytical steps (i.e. sample handled differently)
- EQA does not test staff competency

Table 6.3 What does external quality assessment (EQA) accomplish?

- Accesses current state of the art in laboratory medicine
- Provides information on reagents, calibrants and instruments
- Provides information to assist method selection
- Provides educational support
- Satisfies regulatory and accreditation requirements

in their choice of reagents and instrument–reagent combinations. EQA data also identifies poor methods and facilitates their elimination from laboratory practice.

It is important to appreciate the limitations of EQA programs (Tables 6.2 & 6.3).[15–17] EQA does not test the efficiency of participating laboratories.[6] Nor does it test the important pre and postanalytical steps of any analytical procedure.[18] There will always be some limitations in the actual analytical process because EQA samples are different from patient samples and are therefore handled differently. The concept of EQA is that the samples are tested alongside routine samples by the laboratory staff who routinely perform the tests. We are well aware that this does not always occur. Finally, EQA provides no information in respect of staff competency.

Recent developments

Within the last decade there has been a considerable increase in the number and complexity of tests performed by hemostasis laboratories.[19] These have included point-of-care testing for oral anticoagulant control, D-dimer assays for the exclusion of venous thrombovascular disease, lupus anticoagulant testing, familial thrombophilia testing, molecular genetic analysis and thromboelastography. These have presented EQA providers with a number of difficult challenges to which they have responded with varying degrees of success.

In the industrialized world, EQA programs in hemostasis and thrombosis are widely available but their coverage of tests of hemostasis and thrombosis is extremely variable.[19–23] Some attempt to cover virtually all routine tests of coagulation whereas others are more narrowly focused. One important area that does not receive EQA support is platelet function testing. We are unaware of any programs that distribute samples for this purpose. This undoubtedly reflects not only problems relating to sample collection, preparation and transportation but also to the time-consuming tests of platelet function.[24] A recent initiative has been an evaluation of the performance characteristics of the Platelet Function Analyzer-100 (PFA-100; Dade Behring), introduced by the CAP program in 2006.[21]

Point-of-care (POC) testing for oral anticoagulant control represents a major growth area in hemostasis and thrombosis and worldwide there is an increase in the number of individuals who are using POC devices to monitor their oral anticoagulant control. Although most laboratory scientists recognized the necessity for an EQA program for these monitors, an important initial drawback was that most of the devices were calibrated for whole blood rather than anticoagulated lyophilized plasma which is distributed in most EQA surveys. This means that that participants were not testing "like for like" materials. However, different EQA programs have demonstrated that with these monitors INR results on whole blood are similar to results on the corresponding plasma.[25,26] They have also demonstrated that EQA is achievable for POC/INR testing.[26,27] Currently, UK NEQAS provides EQA support for the CoaguChek series (Roche Diagnostics) including the recent XS models and Hemochron Signature series (International Technodyne). In the USA many tests have been classed as "waived" by the federal agency that oversees laboratory testing. These waived tests, including some POC/INR instruments are not required to participate in EQA.

A wide variety of molecular genetic defects is now recognized in respect of both inherited hemorrhagic and thrombotic disorders. As a consequence of this, molecular genetic testing represents another important growth area in hemostasis and thrombosis. It is also clear that as a direct consequence of the improved technology and simplification of molecular genetic techniques more of these investigations are now being performed in the hemostasis laboratory.

The accuracy and reliability of molecular genetic testing is of particular importance because clinicians appear to place particular reliance on these investigations and, surprisingly, the results are rarely questioned. Also, the results of these tests have important clinical and social implications, not only for the index patient but also for other family members. With these considerations it is clear that those laboratories that provide a diagnostic service by genetic analysis have an even greater responsibility for accurate testing and reporting than "routine" coagulation laboratories.

A number of EQA providers now provide molecular genetic programs for the diagnosis of familial thrombophila.[27,28] Although the majority of laboratories report accurate results there should be no sense of complacency. In respect of this Preston et al.[27] reported that in the UK NEQAS program 3–6% of laboratories failed to identify correctly samples for DNA analysis for familial thrombophilia in three distributions to 47 laboratories. Two types of error were noted. Four laboratories failed to make the correct diagnosis through analytical errors and confirmed transcription errors occurred in four other laboratories. We do not share the view held by some that a transcription error is less serious than an analytical error. Similar concerns regarding the reliability of DNA testing have been expressed by Tripodi et al.[28]

An EQA program for the molecular genetics of hemophilia A was established by UK NEQAS in 2003. To date there have been five distributions involving whole blood or immortalized cell line DNA. The latter was satisfactorily introduced in 2005. The EQA exercises have focused on screening for intron 1 and intron 22 inversions and also sequence analysis.[29]

It is essential that participants in EQA programs should have total confidence in their efficiency and effectiveness. EQA surveys should be sufficiently frequent to make sequential performance analysis meaningful. Routine tests of hemostasis and thrombosis should be distributed at least quarterly and data processing must be as rapid as possible, with prompt returns to participants. Industry may provide a useful service by organizing a program for users of their equipment but it is our strongly held view that the financing of an independent EQA program should remain totally independent of industrial support.

Establishing EQA programs in developing countries

The challenges

Initiating an EQA program in a developing country has several challenges. The first of these is to sell the concept to the laboratories that should participate in it. This requires a local champion, a person and a center that can conceptualize the need for EQA and communicate it to colleagues in the country. It is important that this group also understands the technicalities of running such a program, even if they are not involved in the preparation of the samples. This person or center should have the trust and confidence of the participating laboratories and should have the logistic support to be able to coordinate such a program. It can greatly help the cause if such help can come from a government agency or a non-governmental organization.

The second issue is with regard to recruitment of laboratories. As participation is not mandatory in most developing countries, significant effort is required to persuade individual laboratories to participate in EQA programs. It is particularly important to educate people about EQA, particularly with respect to its importance in improving and maintaining laboratory performance. One has to emphasize that the aim is educational and supportive and not regulatory and explain how confidentiality will be maintained. Support of the local professional societies can be very useful in achieving this.

The next important aspect is with regard to the service itself. Most importantly, the cost has to be maintained at a level that the community will be able to bear. If this is borne by governmental agencies, then it can be a great help but such examples are uncommon. Therefore, the service has to be designed in a way that the costs are kept low. Samples need to be prepared and transported in a way that they reach all participants in time and are stable through this process. Special attention needs to be given when ambient temperatures are over 40°C in some months of the year.

Another challenge is to ensure that reports are received consistently and punctually from all participants, especially for factor assays. Reported reasons for unreliable responses include the inability of some laboratories to obtain reportable results with the volume of sample provided (even though other laboratories are able to with the same samples) or lack of reagents needed for the tests. Technical support and advice is needed to help laboratories with these problems.

Finally, reports of performance need to be provided on time and in a format that is easily understood by the participants. The service provider must appreciate that the knowledge of the theoretical aspects of the tests of hemostasis are not necessarily the same in all laboratories and that very basic issues may need emphasis and clarification for some participants.

Establishment of an EQA program in India: a successful model

When initiated in the year 2000, the program was limited to laboratories associated with the chapters of the Hemophilia Federation (India) (HFI). Samples were obtained from UK NEQAS in Sheffield, UK and distributed to 27 such laboratories in different parts of the country. Results were then collected and sent to UK NEQAS for analysis, which then provided a report for each laboratory.[30] At the request of the Indian Society of Haematology and Transfusion Medicine, the program was converted into a national one in 2003 and called the ISHTM – CMC EQAS for Haemostasis.[31] The program aims to provide external proficiency testing to all laboratories in India providing diagnostic services for hemostatic disorders.

Samples for EQA
From 2000 until 2003, lyophilized samples for this EQA program was provided through UK NEQAS,

a critical reason this program could sustain itself at that stage. The cost of distribution and data analysis was covered by a grant from a charitable trust. Local logistics were supported from the infrastructure available at the Christian Medical College, Vellore with some support from the HFI. The EQA program ran without any cost to the participant laboratories that were supporting people with hemophilia in India. However, when the scheme expanded in 2003 into a national program for all laboratories performing tests of hemostasis, this model was modified. The program needed to sustain itself, both in terms of technology and finances. The team at the Christian Medical College, Vellore was expanded to include technical and scientific personnel in addition to staff for data management and a statistician.

Local production of samples for the scheme started in India in 2004 because it was not financially viable to obtain samples from overseas. Appropriately derived plasma for lyophilization is now sent to a suitable facility in the industry. Following receipt of the lyophilized samples from this source, they are evaluated for their suitability for the EQA. Apart from assessment of their physical characteristics and stability at different temperatures and inter-vial variability, the coagulation parameters are also tested. These include prothrombin time (PT), INR, aPTT, FVIIIC and FIXC after storage under a variety of conditions. Samples are distributed three times in a year. Laboratories are asked to perform the tests listed above.

Assignment of target value
This is undertaken in a manner similar to the UK NEQAS program.

Profile of participants
The number of participating laboratories has increased from 35, in 2003, to more than 120 in 2008. However, only about two-thirds are active in responding to all surveys. The participants range in size and function, e.g. very small laboratories (less than 20 samples/day); medium laboratories (20–200 samples/day); large laboratories (more than 200 samples/day), serving as stand alone services or within major hospitals, both in the public and private health care systems. All laboratories perform the clotting times and correction studies but only

about one-third of them are able to do the factor assays.[32]

The program and its impact

Participation in an external quality assessment program is not currently mandatory in India. Awareness of its necessity and its significance in ensuring quality of results is also not widely understood. This is reflected in the small number of participants in a national EQA scheme for hemostasis. The numbers have shown a gradual increase to over 120 registered participants in 2007, of which about two-thirds consistently return results for all surveys. Information about this program needs to be further disseminated to increase participation. However, it is only with mandatory requirements for accreditation that the number of participants is likely to become significantly higher. The program is now completely self-sufficient and is in fact helping, at subsidized costs, other developing countries start their own efforts.

The initial data obtained from the surveys are significant for several reasons. They give an overview of the types of laboratories offering this service and the reagents and methodologies being used for tests of hemostasis within India. For PT and aPTT, 17 and 20 different reagents are in use, respectively. It also helps these laboratories to become aware of the deficiencies, if any, in their performance and to seek solutions if required. This has resulted in improved performance over time. For PT ratios, fewer laboratories were "outwith consensus" (OWC) when it was low (median <2.0) than when it was higher (median >2.0). However, in each category, the percentage of laboratories that are OWC has reduced over the last 2 years: 32–16% and 80–40%, respectively. Improved methods for calculating mean normal PT and use of reagents with lower International Sensitivity Index (ISI) have probably contributed to this improvement. For aPTT, the number of participants who were OWC were similar regardless of the range of ratios (median 1.67–2.50). This same pattern was also noticed among 23 participants for FVIII:C (median 13.0–33.5%) and FIX:C (median 15.5–36.3%) assays. Fibrinogen assays, which were introduced in 2006 and involve 46 participants, initially had large numbers of OWC (61%) but this has subsequently reduced to 29%. Many of the participants who were OWC shifted from the dry weight precipitation method to the von Clauss method. These data show that errors are not always caused by methodology or reagents but also by the way calculations are performed or interpretations made.

Extension to other developing countries

Based on specific requests received from different countries this program is beginning to help them develop their own local schemes. From 2006 EQA samples have been sent to the Philippines. In that country the number of participating laboratories has increased from 20 to 30. Results from these participants are sent back to India for analysis. Reports of the analysis of performance of each laboratory are then sent back to the coordinator of the program in the Philippines for local distribution. In 2008, a similar program is likely to be initiated in Egypt. Thailand has also requested for samples to be sent to them for distribution within their existing program. The overall aim is to help as many developing countries introduce locally managed EQA programs with samples and services that can be obtained at costs that they can afford and in a way that suits their requirements at the national level.

References

1 Woods TAL, Kitchen S, Preston FE. Quality assessment of haemostatic assays and external quality assessment schemes. In *Laboratory Techniques in Thrombosis*, 2nd edn. Jespersen J, Bertina RM, Haverkate F (eds.). Kluwer Academic, 1999: 29–36.

2 Thienpont LM, Stöckl D, Fridecký B, *et al*. Trueness, verification in European external quality assessment schemes: Time to care about the quality of the samples. *Scand J Clin Lab Invest* 2003; 63: 195–201.

3 Middle JG, Libeer JC, Malakhov V, *et al*. Characterisation and evaluation of external quality assessment scheme serum. Discussion paper from the European External Quality Assessment (EQA) Organizers Working Group C. *Clin Chem Lab Med* 1998; 36: 119–130.

4 Kitchen S, Walker ID, Woods TA, Preston FE. Thromboplastin related differences in the determination of international normalised ratio: A cause for concern? *Thromb Haemost* 1994; 72: 426–429.

5 Preston FE. Assays for von Willebrand factor functional

activity: A UK NEQAS survey. *Thromb Haemost* 1998; **80**: 863.

6 Olson JD, Preston FE, Nichols WL. External quality assurance in thrombosis and hemostasis: An international perspective. *Semin Thromb Hemost* 2007; **33**: 220–225.

7 Tripodi A, Biasiolo A, Chantarangkul V, *et al*. Lupus anticoagulant (LA) testing: Performance of clinical laboratories assessed by a national survey using lyophilised affinity-purified immunoglobulin with LA activity. *Clin Chem* 2003; **49**: 1608–1614.

8 Jennings I, Kitchen S, Woods TA, Preston FE, Greaves M. Potentially clinically important inaccuracies in testing for the lupus anticoagulant: An analysis of results from the three surveys of the UK National External Quality Assessment Scheme (NEQAS) for Blood Coagulation. *Thromb Haemost* 1997; **77**: 934–937.

9 Clinical and Laboratory Standards Institute. *Using Proficiency Testing to Improve the Clinical Laboratory: Approved Guideline*, 2nd edn. GP 27-A2: 2007; **27**: No. 8.

10 Hoeltgee GA, Duckworth JK. Review of proficiency testing performance of laboratories accredited by the College of American Pathologists. *Arch Pathol Lab Med* 1987; **111**: 1011–1014.

11 Steindel SJ, Howanitz PJ, Renner SW. Reasons for proficiency testing failures in clinical chemistry and blood gas analysis. *Arch Pathol Lab Med* 1996; **120**: 1094–1101.

12 Kitchen S, Walker ID, Woods TA, Preston FE. Thromboplastin related differences in the determination of international normalised ratio: A cause for concern. Steering Committee of the UK National External Quality Assessment Scheme in Blood Coagulation. *Thromb Haemost* 2002; **87**: 921–922.

13 Preston FE, Jennings I, Kitchen DP, Woods TA, Kitchen S. Variability for factor V:C assays in UK National External Quality Assessment Scheme surveys: There is a need for an international standard. *Blood Coagul Fibrinolysis* 2005; **16**: 529–531.

14 Hubbard AT, Weller LJ, Johnes S. Calibration of the WHO 1st International Standard for blood coagulation factor V. *J Thromb Haemost* 2007; **5**: 1318–1319.

15 Ehrmeyer SS, Laessig RH. Inter-laboratory proficiency-testing programs: A computer model to assess their capability to correctly characterise intra-laboratory performance. *Clin Chem* 1987; **33**: 784–787.

16 Gambino SR, O'Brien JE, Mallon P. More on proficiency testing. *Clin Chem* 1987; **33**: 2321.

17 Klee GG, Forsman RW. A user's classification of problems identified by proficiency testing surveys. *Arch Pathol Lab Med* 1988; **112**: 371–373.

18 Shahangian S. Proficiency testing in laboratory medicine. *Arch Pathol Lab Med* 1998; **122**: 15–30.

19 Favaloro EJ, Bonar R. Emerging technologies and quality assurance in haemostasis: A review of findings from the Royal College of Pathologists of Australasia Quality Assurance Program. *Semin Thromb Hemost* 2007; **33**: 235–242.

20 Jennings I, Kitchen DP, Woods TA, Kitchen S, Walker ID. Emerging technologies and quality assurance: The United Kingdom National External Quality Assessment Scheme perspective. *Semin Thromb Haemost* 2007; **33**: 243–249.

21 Cunningham MT, Brandt JT, Chandler WL, *et al*. Quality assurance in hemostasis: The perspective from the College of American Pathologist Proficiency Testing Program. *Semin Thromb Hemost* 2007; **33**: 250–258.

22 Spannagl M, Dick A, Reinauer H. External quality assessment schemes in coagulation in Germany: Between regulatory bodies and patient outcome. *Semin Thromb Hemost* 2007; **33**: 259–264.

23 Meijer P, Haverkate F. An external quality assessment program for von Willebrand factor laboratory analysis: An overview from the European Concerted Action on Thrombosis and Disabilities Foundation. *Semin Thromb Hemost* 2006; **32**: 485–491.

24 Hayward CPM, Eikelboom J. Platelet function testing: Quality assurance. *Semin Thromb Hemost* 2007; **33**: 273–282.

25 Kitchen S, Kitchen DP, Jennings I, Woods TA, Walker ID, Preston FE. Point of care International Normalised Ratios: UK NEQAS experience demonstrates necessity for proficiency testing of three different monitors. *Thromb Haemost* 2006; **96**: 590–596.

26 Tripodi A, Bressi C, Carpenedo M, *et al*. Quality assurance program for whole blood prothrombin time–International Normalised Ratio point-of-care monitors used for patient self-testing to control oral anticoagulation. *Thromb Res* 2004; **113**: 35–40.

27 Preston FE, Kitchen S, Jennings I, Woods TAL. A UK National External Quality Assessment Scheme (UK NEQAS) for molecular genetic testing for the diagnosis of familial thrombophilia. *Thromb Haemost* 1999; **82**: 1556–1557.

28 Tripodi A, Peyvandi F, Chantaranqkul V, *et al*. Relatively poor performance of clinical laboratories for DNA analyses in the detection of two thrombophilic mutations: A cause for concern. *Thromb Haemost* 2002; **88**: 690–691.

29 Perry DJ, Goodeve A, Hill M, *et al*. The UK National External Quality Assessment Scheme (UK NEQAS) for

molecular genetic testing in haemophilia. *Thromb Haemost* 2006; **96**: 597–601.

30 Jennings I, Kitchen S, Woods AL, Preston FE. Laboratory performance of haemophilia centers in developing countries: 3 years' experience of the World Federation of Hemophilia External Quality Assessment Scheme. *Haemophilia* 1998; **4**: 739–746.

31 Hertzberg MS, Mammen J, McCraw A, Nair SC, Srivastava A. Achieving and maintaining quality in the laboratory (Laboratory Aspects of Haemophilia Therapy). *Haemophilia* 2006; **12** (Suppl 3): 61–67.

32 Mammen J, Nair SC, Srivastava A. External quality assessment scheme for hemostasis in India. *Semin Thromb Hemost* 2007; **33**: 265–272.

7

Initial evaluation of hemostasis: reagent and method selection

W. L. Chandler

The initial evaluation of hemostasis occurs in several situations including evaluation of patients who are bleeding, prior to invasive procedures and prior to starting antithrombotic medications. In these situations the initial assays used to assess hemostasis are selected to determine whether the patient has any evidence of a clinically significant acquired or hereditary deficiency of coagulation factors or platelets. The initial evaluation often includes measurement of the prothrombin time (PT), activated partial thromboplastin time (aPTT), fibrinogen and platelet count. Thrombin time and other assays may be added depending on the nature of the clinical situation. This chapter focuses on the selection and evaluation of instruments and reagents for the PT, aPTT, fibrinogen and thrombin time. Platelet counts are typically performed on automated cell counters as part of the complete blood count. Selection of platelet count methodology is outside the scope of this chapter and will not be considered further.

A variety of different methods have been described for measuring the PT and aPTT utilizing fingerstick samples, citrate anticoagulated whole blood and citrate anticoagulated plasma. Different technologies are used to detect the PT endpoint including optical and mechanical clot endpoint detection and chromogenic substrate methods. In general, there are two classes of instruments for determining PT and aPTT:

Quality in Laboratory Hemostasis and Thrombosis, 1st edition. By Steve Kitchen, John D. Olson and F. Eric Preston. Published 2009 by Blackwell Publishing. ISBN: 978-1-4051-6803-8

manual analyzers for point of care or small laboratory use and automated or semi-automated analyzers for larger laboratories. Several different point-of-care analyzers are available for performing the PT, typically for oral anticoagulant monitoring. This chapter discusses the selection of assays based on citrate anticoagulated plasma using clot-endpoint methods, other types of methods are not discussed further.

Instrument selection

The first step in selecting a test methodology is determining what clinical questions the test will help answer and how the test will be utilized. Table 7.1 summarizes a number of questions related to hemostasis instrument selection. A test that is only run on day shift without the option for stat requests might use a batch analyzer methodology while a test that will run 24 hours per day with stat testing would be handled better on a sequential analyzer with stat interrupt capability. If more than one type of test is typically ordered at the same time an analyzer that can do all the testing on a single platform may be best. Some analyzers are designed primarily to perform routine tests such as the PT, aPTT and fibrinogen, while others can be used for routine and more specialized assays such as factor activity. Another important consideration is the types of assays that will be needed including clot-based assays, chromogenic assays and antigenic assays. Some instruments are capable of performing all three types simultaneously. The types of panels offered and the turn around times needed

Table 7.1 Considerations for new instrument selection.

- Will the test be offered 24 hours per day?
- What is the anticipated test volume?
- Will the test be offered stat? If so what is the anticipated stat volume?
- What is the minimum sample volume anticipated for pediatric or other patients?
- What is the most common panel of tests that will be ordered? Can they all be performed on the same instrument?
- What types of hemostasis testing are anticipated: clot-based, chromogenic, antigenic?
- How many samples and reagents will the instrument hold?
- Does the instrument utilize barcoded reagents?
- Sample preparation requirements
- How many samples are processed per hour, how many reaction cuvettes does the instrument hold, how may tests can be run prior to operator intervention?

will help determine the type of instrument required. For clot-based assays such as the PT and aPTT, it is important to understand the mechanism of clot detection on the instrument (optical, mechanical, other) and potential sample interference problems that may affect the results such as sample hemolysis, icterus or lipemia.

There are other parameters to consider prior to selecting an instrument. Many modern instruments require barcoding prior to running the sample, this can be carried out in the laboratory or on the ward if computerized order entry is available. After centrifugation, some instruments can directly pipette through the cap into the tube, other instruments require the cap be removed, while still others require the plasma be separated from the cells and put in another aliquot container which is put on the instrument. Will the instrument only be used for tests predefined by a commercial vendor or will user-defined tests be on the instrument as well? Can the instrument store different test protocols in its memory and, if so, how many? How many of these are predefined by the vendor versus how many are open protocols or user-defined protocols if desired? On some instruments each dilution of a factor assay may represent a separate test protocol. If the instrument

will be used for assays requiring calibration curves, how does the instrument store, analyze and display these curves? If quality control data will be stored on the instrument then storage, analysis and display of quality control data may be important in instrument selection.

Other useful parameters to investigate related to instrument selection include the speed of processing samples (number of assays per hour). This can be important in high volume situations or when the analyzer is expected to perform many different assays. Speed may vary with the assay type depending on the number of reagents needed for each assay. This in turn may depend on the number of sampling probes the instrument uses. Instruments with only a single probe used to pipette plasma and all reagents may be slower than instruments with multiple probes. Throughput on an analyzer may also depend on other factors including the number of reaction cuvettes the instrument can store on board, waste capacity, etc. This may determine the number of assays the instrument can perform prior to operator intervention.

Reagent parameters may be an important consideration including the number of different reagents and controls that can be stored on the instrument and the storage temperature and stability of the reagents, particularly for reagents such as PT and aPTT that may stay on the instrument 24 hours per day. When evaluating reagent usage it may be important to know the minimum reagent volume the instrument can use and dead volume the instrument cannot utilize. Many instruments can now read barcodes on the reagent vials with details of reagent type, lot number, expiration date and other parameters to reduce errors when placing new reagents on the instrument. This may only be available for reagents made by the same vendor as the instrument. Sample parameters may be equally important including the number of samples that can be stored on the instrument, storage temperature and stability, minimum sample volume needed and sample dead volume that cannot be utilized. Other questions include the use of direct tube sampling and cap piercing.

Physical constraints may also be important including space, power, water and waste needs, instrument tolerance for temperature and power, and the ability to interface an instrument to the laboratory information system.

Evaluation of the method

For PT, aPTT, fibrinogen and thrombin time assays most instruments are sold in combination with coagulation reagents intended for use on that instrument. When selecting a methodology, a specific instrument–reagent combination is typically evaluated. Some companies offer several different versions of PT and aPTT reagents for their instruments. Some may choose to use only reagents from the same vendor as the instrument while others may choose to use a reagent from one company on an instrument from another company. Some instrument–reagent combinations may have disadvantages including lack of support If there are problems, inability to read bar codes between companies.

A number of different organizations, including the Clinical and Laboratory Standards Institute (CLSI), provide protocols for evaluation of clinical laboratory tests.[1-3] In addition, there are a number of different regulatory organizations dedicated to maintaining high quality clinical testing through proficiency testing, on-site inspections, education programs and other efforts. The goal of the following sections is to provide overviews of method selection for initial assessment of hemostasis applicable to all clinical laboratories, but they are not intended to cover all the specific details found in evaluation or regulatory protocols from different countries. Each section is designed to provide a detailed review of method (instrument–reagent) selection for a given test followed at the end of the section by a summary of the minimum evaluation steps that are recommended.

Prothrombin time method selection

The principal uses for the PT assay include monitoring of oral anticoagulant (OAC) therapy, evaluation of liver function and the initial evaluation of hemostasis prior to surgery and in patients with active bleeding or a prior history of bleeding. Typically, the same PT reagent is used for all of these purposes. For OAC monitoring the PT result is typically converted to an International Normalized Ratio (INR). Details regarding monitoring of OAC can be found later in this book (see Chapter 18).

The PT assay consists of combining citrated plasma with tissue factor, phospholipids and calcium followed by detection of the clotting time using optical turbidity, optical light scattering, mechanical clot detection or other methods. The two most common sources of tissue factor are rabbit brain and human recombinant preparations. To reduce interference from heparin, PT reagents often contain a heparin neutralizing agent, e.g. polybrene. The major difference among PT reagents is their analytic sensitivity to deficiencies of coagulation factors II, V, VII, X and fibrinogen. Highly sensitive PT reagents prolong more for the same level of factor deficiency than low sensitivity reagents. This is quantified to some extent for PT reagents used to calculate the INR by the International Sensitivity Index (ISI). A low ISI near 1 indicates a PT reagent with high sensitivity to factor deficiency. In general, PT reagents with a high ISI value (2 and greater) show higher levels of imprecision for the INR. It is recommended to use a lower ISI reagent to improve INR reproducibility. The current recommendation is to use an ISI less than 1.7. An ISI of 1 or less can result in poor precision at INRs of 5 or above. The optimal ISI may be in the range of 1.3–1.6.

The initial evaluation of any new PT instrument–reagent combination should include assessment of within-run and between-run imprecision at normal and prolonged values, stability of the reagent on the instrument and stability of the sample at room temperature and 4°C with respect to the PT. Imprecision for the PT assay should meet or exceed the manufacturer's specifications for the instrument–reagent combination. Modern automated instruments should show a between-run coefficient of variation less than 5% for the PT assay.[1] It is useful to determine the shortest and longest PT values the instrument can produce and what the reportable range of the assay will be. Depending on the clinical setting, it is also important to determine whether a critical value or cut-off will be used to alert clinicians to dangerously prolonged PT results.

If a new PT assay is being selected or a new batch of reagent evaluated it should be compared with the current assay across a wide range of possible values and patient types including patients on OAC. Both the PT and INR values should be compared among methods. Because of differences in the sensitivity of different reagents (different ISI), it is possible that PT values may show a substantial bias between methods, but should still be highly correlated. In contrast, the

INR between methods should show high correlation and little or no bias.

In some laboratories the INR is calculated by the instrument, which passes the INR value on to the laboratory information system. Another option commonly used is for the instrument to pass the PT result to the laboratory information system which then calculates the INR. Most medical care systems now have some form of electronic medical record that captures information from the laboratory information system. Whenever the PT reagent or method is changed it is important to verify that the INR is being correctly calculated and displayed in the instrument, the laboratory information system and downstream electronic medical record systems. Sources of error include the equation used to calculate the INR and the values for the geometric mean normal PT and the ISI used in the calculation. It is critical to good patient care to trace an initial PT and INR result produced in the laboratory and see that it is faithfully reproduced in all downstream systems.

When evaluating possible coagulation factor deficiencies there are three common clinical situations: single factor deficiency (either acquired or hereditary), vitamin K dependent factor deficiency (loss of factors II, VII and X in the PT reaction) and all factor deficiency seen in bleeding patients. The more factors that are deficient, the faster the PT will prolong. For example, a PT reagent with an ISI of 1.3 gave a clotting time of 16 seconds when only factor VII was reduced to 0.3 IU/mL of normal while all other factors were normal, compared to 21 seconds when factors II, VII and X were at 0.3 IU/mL, versus 29 seconds when all factors were reduced to 0.3 IU/mL of normal (Fig. 7.1). Depending on the how the PT assay will be used in a particular institution may determine how important it is to know the sensitivity of the assay to different types of factor deficiency. If the PT is only being used for OAC monitoring then knowledge of sensitivity to individual factors may not be needed. If the test is being used as an initial assay for unknown factor deficiency, or to assess factor deficiency in massively bleeding patients, knowledge of sensitivity to different forms of factor deficiency may be useful. Some groups have suggested the INR should only be used for OAC monitoring, while many other groups use the INR as a cut-off for factor deficiency, fresh frozen plasma transfusion and other uses. How the INR is used clinically is still under discussion.

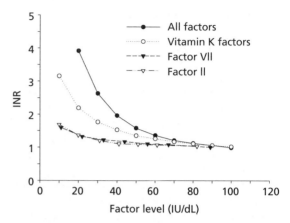

Fig. 7.1 Effect of single or multiple factor deficiency on the prothrombin time/International Normalized Ratio (PT/INR). The PT reagent used had an International Sensitivity Index (ISI) of 1.3. Plasma samples with varying degrees of factor II or VII deficiency were generated by mixing pooled normal plasma with plasma deficient in the appropriate individual factor. Plasma samples with varying degrees of vitamin K dependent factor deficiency were generated by mixing pooled normal plasma with aluminum hydroxide adsorbed plasma deficient in the vitamin K dependent factors. All other factors were near 100% normal (1 IU/mL). Plasma samples with varying degrees of deficiency for all factors including fibrinogen were generated by mixing pooled normal plasma with physiologic buffer.

Table 7.2 shows a list of factors that may potentially affect the PT result. Most PT reagents are relatively insensitive to unfractionated heparin because of the nature of the PT assay and inclusion of heparin neutralizing agents in many PT formulations. The PT assay is typically even less sensitive to low molecular weight heparin, heparinoids and pentasaccharides. While this is true, it is useful to know what heparin concentration prolongs the PT assay as this can occur if the assay is contaminated with concentrated heparin. Likewise, most PT reagents are relatively insensitive to lupus anticoagulants, but this varies with reagent. It is important to know how sensitive the PT reagent is to clotted or hemolyzed samples. Some instrument–reagent PT combinations are relatively insensitive to hemolysis[4] while others may be more sensitive.[5] Modest underfilling of the 3.2% citrate sample tubes may have little effect on some PT reagents, but this needs to be

Table 7.2 Factors potentially affecting the prothrombin time (PT) assay.

- Coagulation factors II, V, VII, X and fibrinogen deficiency
- Direct thrombin inhibitors, unfractionated heparin, low molecular weight heparin, heparinoids, pentasaccharides and other antithrombotic medications
- Clotted sample
- Hemolyzed sample
- Overfilled or underfilled sample tube
- Lupus anticoagulants
- Recombinant human factor VIIa
- Daptomycin therapy

---

carefully evaluated before any overfilled or underfilled tube is accepted.[6] A number of other medications may affect the PT including prolongations resulting from direct thrombin inhibitors such as lepirudin, argatroban or bivalirudin and shortened PT results resulting from recombinant human factor VIIa therapy.

Minimum evaluation, prothrombin time

Assuming an INR will be calculated with the PT result, the minimum assessment of a new PT instrument–reagent combination includes determination of the geometric mean normal PT for INR calculations, PT and INR comparison with the current method, determination or validation of the reference range, within-run and between-run imprecision at normal and prolonged values, sample and reagent stability.

Activated partial thromboplastin time method selection

Whereas the PT assay is primarily used to assess coagulation factor levels, the aPTT has many uses including assessing coagulation factor levels, monitoring antithrombotic agents such as heparin and direct thrombin inhibitors, and detecting lupus inhibitors. No standardization like the INR is available for the aPTT, so each aPTT instrument–reagent combination potentially has different abilities related to these different uses. The aPTT assay utilizes two

reagents. The first reagent is an activator composed of phospholipids (partial thromboplastin) and a negatively charged substance such as ground glass or kaolin to activate the contact system and form factor XIIa. The first reagent is added to citrate anticoagulated plasma and incubated for several minutes at 37°C, followed by addition of a calcium solution that allows coagulation system activation by factor XIIa to proceed.

The initial evaluation of any new aPTT instrument–reagent combination should include assessment of within-run and between-run imprecision at normal and prolonged values, stability of the reagent on the instrument and stability of the aPTT in the sample at room temperature and 4°C. An important consideration for the aPTT is the stability of heparinized aPTT samples. Activated platelets can release platelet factor 4 which reacts with and neutralizes heparin. If citrate anticoagulated plasma is not removed from the platelets, the heparin level in the sample can fall over time giving falsely reduced aPTT results. Imprecision for the aPTT assay should meet or exceed the manufacturer's specifications for the instrument–reagent combination. Modern automated instruments should show a between-run coefficient of variation less than 5% for the aPTT assay.[1] If a new aPTT assay is being selected or a new lot of reagent evaluated it should be compared with the current assay across a wide range of possible values and patient types, including patients with lupus inhibitors, patients on warfarin, heparin and other antithrombotic agents.

Depending on the composition of the aPTT reagent it may show different analytic sensitivity to deficiencies of coagulation factors II, V, VIII, IX, X, XI and fibrinogen. In particular, different reagents can show substantial differences in sensitivity to factors VIII and IX.[7-9] Like PT reagents, the more factors that are deficient, the faster the aPTT will prolong. For example, an aPTT reagent with a mean normal value of 30 seconds, gave a clotting time of 37 seconds when only factor VIII was reduced to 0.3 IU/mL of normal while all other factors were normal, compared to 48 seconds when factors II, IX and X were all at 0.3 IU/mL, versus 75 seconds when all factors were reduced to 0.3 IU/mL of normal (Fig. 7.2). Depending on the how the aPTT assay will be used in particular institution may determine how important it is to know the sensitivity of the assay to different types of factor deficiency. If the aPTT is only

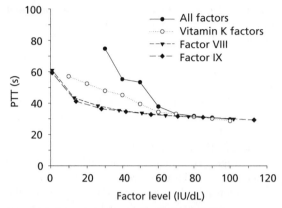

Fig. 7.2 Effect of single or multiple factor deficiency on the activated partial thromboplastin time (aPTT). Plasma samples with varying degrees of factor VIII or IX deficiency were generated by mixing pooled normal plasma with plasma deficient in the appropriate individual factor. Plasma samples with varying degrees of vitamin K dependent factor deficiency were generated by mixing pooled normal plasma with aluminum hydroxide adsorbed plasma deficient in the vitamin K dependent factors. All other factors were near 100% normal (1 IU/mL). Plasma samples with varying degrees of deficiency for all factors including fibrinogen were generated by mixing pooled normal plasma with physiologic buffer.

Table 7.3 Factors potentially affecting the activated partial thromboplastin time (aPTT) assay.

- Coagulation factor VIII, IX, XI deficiency. Also useful to know the sensitivity to factors II, V, X, XII, prekallikrein and high molecular weight kininogen and fibrinogen deficiency
- Lupus anticoagulants
- Direct thrombin inhibitors, unfractionated heparin, low molecular weight heparin, heparinoids, pentasaccharides and other antithrombotic medications
- Clotted sample
- Hemolyzed sample
- Overfilled or underfilled sample tube
- Elevated factor VIII levels

being used for heparin monitoring then knowledge of sensitivity to individual factors may not be needed. If the test is being used as an initial assay for unknown factor deficiency, or to assess factor deficiency in massively bleeding patients, knowledge of sensitivity to different forms of factor deficiency may be useful. In particular, aPTT reagents should produce abnormal prolonged results in plasmas that have less than 0.3 IU/mL factors VIII, IX or XI.[1] The reagent used for Fig. 7.2 shows similar factor VIII and IX sensitivity. Some aPTT reagents are less sensitive to factor IX. Care should be taken to determine the factor sensitivity of reagents if they will be used for factor deficiency detection. While factor deficiencies can prolong the aPTT, increases in factor VIII resulting from an acute phase response can shorten the aPTT making interpretation complex.

In addition to being sensitive to the coagulation factors, the aPTT is also sensitive to deficiencies of the contact system proteins including factor XII, prekallikrein and high molecular weight kininogen.

Patients with deficiencies of these factors do not have increased bleeding, but the aPTT will be variably prolonged depending on the degree of deficiency and the sensitivity of the particular reagent.

Table 7.3 shows a list of factors that may potentially affect the aPTT result. Different aPTT reagents show wide variations in their sensitivity to heparin.[10–12] When the aPTT is used to monitor unfractionated heparin therapy, care must be taken to determine the heparin therapeutic range accurately using one of several methods. The methods for doing this are discussed later in this book (Chapter 17).

If direct thrombin inhibitors are being used and if they will be monitored using the aPTT, then the sensitivity of aPTT to these medications will need to be determined. Several different direct thrombin inhibitors are available including argatroban, lepirudin and bivalirudin. APTT reagents may show different sensitivities depending on the direct thrombin inhibitor used.

Another common use for the aPTT is the initial detection of possible lupus anticoagulants. Most aPTT reagents show some sensitivity to lupus anticoagulants, but the degree of prolongation for a given lupus anticoagulant varies widely with different aPTT reagent preparations.[13,14] If the aPTT is to be used as an initial step in a lupus anticoagulant assay, then its sensitivity to lupus anticoagulants should be determined and compared with current reagents. It is important to know how sensitive the aPTT reagent is to clotted or hemolyzed samples. Some instrument–reagent aPTT combinations are relatively insensitive to hemolysis[4] while others may be more sensitive.[5] Modest underfilling of the citrate sample tubes may have little effect on some aPTT reagents,[6] but this needs to be carefully evaluated before any overfilled or underfilled tube is accepted. Greater detail on evaluation of lupus anticoagulants can be found later in this book (Chapter 16).

Minimum evaluation, activated partial thromboplastin time assay

Assuming the aPTT is used to monitor unfractionated heparin therapy, the minimum assessment of a new aPTT instrument–reagent combination includes determination of the heparin therapeutic range, comparison with current method, determination or validation of the reference range, within-run and between-run imprecision at normal and prolonged values, sample and reagent stability.

Fibrinogen method selection

Fibrinogen assays are most often used during the evaluation of hemostasis in patients with active bleeding or a prior history of bleeding. Low fibrinogen levels may occur as a result of blood loss, excessive intravascular coagulation activation and consumption or reduced production of fibrinogen as a result of hereditary fibrinogen abnormalities or liver damage resulting from cirrhosis or other causes. Fibrinogen may appear low using kinetic or activity assays in some patients with fibrinogen abnormalities that slow cleavage by thrombin. Fibrinogen is an acute phase reactant, its concentration rises during a variety of clinical syndromes including inflammation, infection and cancer. Elevated fibrinogen has been associated with an increased risk of thrombosis, although the assay is seldom used to assess this risk clinically.

Fibrinogen concentration in plasma can be measured in several ways including immunoassays for antigenic concentration, total clottable assays and activity or functional assays. Antigenic and total clottable fibrinogen assays are typically used only for research or the evaluation of dysfibrinogens as they are too slow and expensive for routine clinical use. Most clinical laboratories measure fibrinogen using a functional assay, either the kinetic method of Clauss[15]

or a turbity or light scattering method derived from the PT assay.

For the kinetic fibrinogen method, citrated plasma is diluted in buffer then clotted using a relatively high concentration of thrombin. The time required for the clot to form is inversely proportional to the fibrinogen concentration. Several international standard procedures for the kinetic (Clauss) fibrinogen have been published.[2,3]

For the PT-derived fibrinogen, a standard prothrombin time is run on the sample. In addition to determining the clotting time, the change in total light scattering or absorbance in the sample is determined which is proportional to the fibrinogen concentration.[16]

The initial evaluation of any new fibrinogen instrument–reagent combination should include calibration of the fibrinogen assay using a reference plasma calibrated against a standard plasma of known fibrinogen concentration. At least five points should be used to determine the fibrinogen calibration curve and the upper and lower limits of the reportable range determined for the standard dilution of plasma. If the fibrinogen falls outside this range, lower or higher dilutions of plasma can be used. New reference curves should be prepared with each change of reagent lot, any change in instrument, or with any deviation from quality control or proficiency testing limits. Next, the assay should be evaluated for within-run and between-run imprecision at normal and reduced fibrinogen values, stability of the reagent on the instrument and stability of fibrinogen in the sample at room temperature and 4°C. In most clinical settings the fibrinogen assay is used to assess low fibrinogen as a cause of bleeding. Ability to accurately and precisely measure fibrinogen levels below 1 g/L is important. At least one control for the fibrinogen assay should be a low control near or below 1 g/L in concentration. If a new fibrinogen assay is being selected or a new batch of reagent evaluated it should be compared with the current assay across a wide range of possible values and patient types, including patients on heparin and other antithrombotic agents.[2]

A number of things can affect the fibrinogen result. Underfilled tubes can result in falsely low fibrinogen because of dilution of the plasma by citrate. Clotted samples may show falsely low fibrinogen because of consumption of fibrinogen in the *in vitro* clot. The effect of hemolysis, icterus and lipemia should be evaluated; it can be method-dependent. Some fibrinogen assays based on optical clot detection or total light scattering can be affected by plasma interference more than methods using mechanical clot detection. Because of the dilution of the plasma and relatively high concentrations of thrombin used, kinetic fibrinogen assays are relatively insensitive to heparin contamination. However, it is important to know what level of heparin does interfere in the fibrinogen assay. High levels of direct thrombin inhibitors may interfere in fibrinogen assays.

Several studies have reported problems with PT-derived fibrinogen assays. Variable results, depending on the type of thromboplastin used for the PT assay and the patient group studied, have been reported, potentially producing clinically unreliable results in some situations.[17,18] How the fibrinogen assay will be used clinically and in which patient populations should be considered prior to selecting an assay.

Minimum evaluation, fibrinogen assay

The minimum assessment of a new fibrinogen assay includes calibration of the standard curve, comparison with the current method, determination or validation of the reference range, within-run and between-run imprecision at normal and reduced values, sample and reagent stability. If a PT-derived fibrinogen is selected, it should be evaluated in different patient groups to assure accuracy.

Thrombin time method selection

The principal uses of the thrombin time in the initial evaluation of hemostasis include detection of anticoagulants in the sample including antithrombin antibodies, heparin and direct thrombin inhibitors, acquired and hereditary abnormalities of fibrin formation or polymerization including higher levels of fibrin degradation products, paraproteinemias and dysfibrinogens. The sensitivity of the thrombin time in different clinical situations depends on the amount of thrombin used in the assay. If higher thrombin concentrations are used the thrombin time has a reference range of 12–16 seconds, is less sensitive to heparin and other anticoagulants. This

concentration range has been used to monitor heparin therapy. If lower concentrations of thrombin are used in the thrombin time the assay becomes more sensitive to heparin and other anticoagulants and is better able to detect low level heparin contamination, but is too sensitive for heparin monitoring.

The thrombin time assay consists of adding a dilute solution of thrombin to undiluted citrate anticoagulated plasma. The thrombin used in the assay may come from human or animal sources (often bovine thrombin). The thrombin time assay is not sensitive to deficiency of any coagulation factor except fibrinogen. Low fibrinogen levels prolong the thrombin time while high fibrinogen levels shorten it modestly.

The initial evaluation of any new thrombin time instrument–reagent combination should include assessment of within-run and between-run imprecision at normal and prolonged values, stability of the reagent on the instrument, stability of fibrinogen in the sample at room temperature and 4°C, and if applicable, comparison of the new instrument–reagent combination with the existing method across a wide range of possible values and patient types. Most thrombin time assays are sensitive to heparin in the sample, including many low molecular weight heparins. It is important to know the specific heparin sensitivity of the thrombin time being evaluated if it will be used to detect unexpected heparin contamination as occurs in samples drawn through intravascular lines or heparin locks. It is important to know how sensitive the thrombin time reagent is to clotted or hemolyzed samples. Some thrombin time assays are relatively insensitive to modest overfilling or underfilling of the sample tube, as citrate and calcium concentration are not important in the thrombin time assay, but this needs to be carefully evaluated before any overfilled or underfilled tube is accepted.

Minimum evaluation, thrombin time

The minimum assessment of a new thrombin time instrument–reagent combination includes comparison with the existing method, determination or validation of the reference range, within-run and between-run imprecision at normal and prolonged values, sample and reagent stability.

References

1 Arkin CF, Bowie EJW, Carroll JJ, Day HJ, Joist JH, Lenahan JG *et al. One-Stage Prothrombin Time (PT) Test and Activated Partial Thromboplastin Time (aPTT) Test; Approved Guideline.* NCCLS: 1996; **12**: 1–26.

2 Arkin CF, Adcock DM, Day HJ, Carroll JJ, Joist JH, Lenahan JG *et al. Procedure for the Determination of Fibrinogen in Plasma; Approved Guideline,* 2nd edn. NCCLS: 2001; **21**: 1–35.

3 DIN 58906–1, Ausgabe: 2000–03. Hämostaseologie – Bestimmung der Fibrinogenkonzentration – Teil 1: Referenzmeßverfahren für die Bestimmung des gerinnbaren Fibrinogens nach Clauss.

4 Laga AC, Cheves TA, Sweeney JD. The effect of specimen hemolysis on coagulation test results. *Am J Clin Pathol* 2006; **126**: 748–755.

5 Lippi G, Montagnana M, Salvagno GL, Guidi GC. Interference of blood cell lysis on routine coagulation testing. *Arch Pathol Lab Med* 2006; **130**: 181–184.

6 Adcock DM, Kressin DC, Marlar RA. Minimum specimen volume requirements for routine coagulation testing: dependence on citrate concentration. *Am J Clin Pathol* 1998; **109**: 595–599.

7 Sibley C, Singer JW, Wood RJ. Comparison of activated partial thromboplastin reagents. *Am J Clin Pathol* 1973; **59**: 581–586.

8 Hathaway WE, Assmus SL, Montgomery RR, Dubansky AS. Activated partial thromboplastin time and minor coagulopathies. *Am J Clin Pathol* 1979; **71**: 22–25.

9 Barrowcliffe TW, Gray E. Studies of phospholipid reagents used in coagulation. I. Some general properties and their sensitivity to factor VIII. *Thromb Haemost* 1981; **46**: 629–633.

10 Triplett DA, Harms CS, Koepke JA. The effect of heparin on the activated partial thromboplastin time. *Am J Clin Pathol* 1978; **70** (Suppl): 556–559.

11 Barrowcliffe TW, Gray E. Studies of phospholipid reagents used in coagulation. II. Factors influencing their sensitivity to heparin. *Thromb Haemost* 1981; **46**: 634–637.

12 Brandt JT, Triplett DA. Laboratory monitoring of heparin. Effect of reagents and instruments on the activated partial thromboplastin time. *Am J Clin Pathol* 1981; **76** (Suppl): 530–537.

13 Hirsh J, Raschke R. Heparin and low-molecular-weight heparin: the Seventh ACCP Conference on Antithrombotic and Thrombolytic Therapy. *Chest* 2004; **126** (Suppl): 188S–203S.

14 Mannucci PM, Canciani MT, Mari D, Meucci P. The varied sensitivity of partial thromboplastin and prothrombin time reagents in the demonstration of the lupus-like anticoagulant. *Scand J Haematol* 1979; **22**: 423–432.

15 Clauss A. Gerinnungsphysiologische Schnellmethode zu Bestimmung des Fibrinogens. *Acta Haematol* 1957; **17**: 237–245.

16 De Cristofaro R, Landolfi R. Measurement of plasma fibrinogen concentration by the prothrombin-time-derived method: applicability and limitations. *Blood Coagul Fibrinolysis* 1998; **9**: 251–259.

17 Mackie J, Lawrie AS, Kitchen S, Gaffney PJ, Howarth D, Lowe GD, *et al.* A performance evaluation of commercial fibrinogen reference preparations and assays for Clauss and PT-derived fibrinogen. *Thromb Haemost* 2002; **87**: 997–1005.

18 Lawrie AS, McDonald SJ, Purdy G, Mackie IJ, Machin SJ. Prothrombin time derived fibrinogen determination on Sysmex CA-6000. *J Clin Pathol* 1998; **51**: 462–466.

Point-of-care testing in hemostasis

C. Gardiner, S. Machin & I. Mackie

Point-of-care testing (POCT) and near-patient testing (NPT) are used synonymously to describe analytical testing undertaken by a healthcare professional or a non-medical person in a setting distinct from a conventional hospital laboratory. In principle, locating test equipment near to the patient provides a more rapid service than that which may be achieved in the hospital laboratory. This may be useful in a life-threatening situation, where the test may indicate an urgent therapeutic choice, in the management of long-term conditions, where the results can inform the consultation, influence a procedure, or where the patient may have heightened concern about the outcome of the test.

At present, the main applications of POCT in hemostasis are:
• Oral anticoagulant control (prothrombin time/ International Normalized Ratio [PT/INR]).
• High dose heparin management (activated clotting time [aCT], whole blood thrombin time).
• Global assessment of hemostasis during major surgery or in the intensive care unit (thrombelastography, thromboelastometry).
• Monitoring of therapy with certain coagulation factor concentrates in hemophilia.
• Platelet function testing.
• D-dimer testing in the negative exclusion of venous thromboembolism.

Quality in Laboratory Hemostasis and Thrombosis, 1st edition. By Steve Kitchen, John D. Olson and F. Eric Preston. Published 2009 by Blackwell Publishing. ISBN: 978-1-4051-6803-8

The devices differ in complexity from small, hand-held coagulation monitors intended for patient self-testing (PST), to small desk-top analysers designed for use by healthcare professionals in a clinic or hospital environment. They are mostly used with whole blood samples, sometimes making it difficult to compare the results with those from hospital laboratories using plasma. There is a wide range of platelet function POCT devices,[1] but these are mostly used for research purposes and there is little clinical validation. Quality control of these devices is difficult as platelet function is lost on storage and affected by any fixation process, therefore many users run a blood sample from a healthy normal control with each batch of tests. Platelet POCT devices will not be discussed further in this review.

Monitoring of oral anticoagulation

Oral anticoagulant therapy (OAT) using vitamin K antagonists is commonly used in the treatment and long-term prevention of thromboembolic events, with an estimated 0.95 million patients using warfarin in the UK and 3 million in the USA.[2,3] These patients require regular PT/INR determination. An aging population and the continuing expansion of clinical indications for OAT are likely to increase demand further still.[4] Consequently, several new models of patient care, involving various degrees of decentralization and POCT of PT/INR, have been implemented.[5–8] Since the introduction of POCT PT/ INR monitors in the 1990s,[9] the volume of blood required for testing has gradually decreased (now

10–50 μL), as well as the size and cost of devices (Table 8.1). The initial instruments were unreliable, particularly at higher INR values, showing considerable variability of the INR. However, with the development of new technologies and quality control procedures, their reliability has considerably improved.

There are several POC devices available for coagulation testing, which fall broadly into one of two types: devices for professional use; and devices for

Table 8.1 Point-of-care testing (POCT) devices for oral anticoagulant control (available in UK).

Device	Manufacturer	Blood sample	Sample volume (μL)	Available for self-testing	Calibration method	QC material	Data handling
CoaguChek S	Roche Diagnostics, Burgess Hill, UK	Venous or capillary blood	10	Yes	Code chip, automatic	Liquid QC	No data handling
CoaguChek XS	Roche Diagnostics, Burgess Hill, UK	Capillary or venous blood, non-citrated	10	Yes	Code chip; user must check	Strip integrity check	No data handling
CoaguChek XS Plus	Roche Diagnostics, Burgess Hill, UK	Capillary or venous blood, non-citrated	10	No	Code chip, automatic	Liquid QC; strip integrity check	Alphanumeric input; bi-directional interface
Hemochron Jr Signature+	ITC, Edison, NJ, USA	Venous or capillary blood	50	No	Barcode on cuvette, automatic	Internal QC and liquid QC	Numerical input; bi-directional interface
INRatio	Hemosense Inc, San Jose, CA, USA	Capillary blood	10	Yes	Manual entry of five digit code	Internal QC only	No data handling; RS232 interface
Protime 3	ITC, Edison, NJ, USA	Capillary or venous blood, non-citrated	27	Yes	Barcode on cuvette, automatic	Internal QC and liquid QC	No data handling; RS232 interface
Thrombi-Stat CD501WB	Hart Biologicals Hartlepool, UK	Capillary or venous blood, non-citrated	25	No	Manual entry of calibration details	Liquid QC	Numerical input; RS232 interface to RAID™ available

QC, quality control.

use by the patients themselves. The high cost of professional devices effectively rules out their use for PST.

Coagulation monitors intended for PST should satisfy certain requirements:
• There is a consensus of opinion, backed by proficiency testing data, that low International Sensitivity Index (ISI) thromboplastins (between 0.9 and 1.7 and ideally close to 1.0) should be used for INR determination. The higher ISI reagents are associated with a high degree of imprecision and may give less dependable INR values during the induction period of OAT and in poorly stabilized patients.[10–12]
• The INR result must be accurate and reproducible. Ideally, when compared to a reference method, >85% of samples within the therapeutic range should give an INR value within 0.5 INR units.[13]
• The result should be clearly and simply displayed.
• A suitable quality control (QC) system must exist to ensure the validity of results.
• Operation should be simple, with minimal user-definable steps, and should not require a high degree of dexterity.
• It must be small enough to be easily portable, ideally hand-held and low weight.
• Stored patient and QC results should be readily distinguishable.
• The sample volume requirement should be <30 μL with no requirement for accurate blood volume measurement.
• The sample application point must be easily accessible for patients with poor dexterity.
• The displayed INR value should be of large character size and be easily read.

Quality assurance of point-of-care INR monitors

As with any other diagnostic test, quality assurance of POCT devices is required to ensure that the results are reliable. All POCT monitors have a system verification procedure that is performed automatically when the instrument is switched on. Some instruments also have an electronic QC cartridge that simulates a test endpoint. However, electronic QC does not assess the performance of the test strip/cuvette and does not represent a valid

alternative to conventional QC procedures. Some devices have an internal QC system built into each test strip/cuvette and this helps to ensure the validity of each test, although a QC system independent from the manufacturer is preferred, because both device and internal QC could be miscalibrated. POCT coagulometers for professional use, which perform tests on citrated plasma, can use the same quality assurance programs as laboratory analyzers (with lyophilized plasmas) and will not be discussed further. Whole blood POCT coagulation monitors operate on several different measurement principles and it is these that dictate the type of QC that can be used.

The iron oxide particle/photo-reflection method detects clot by means of thromboplastin impregnated iron particles, mixed with the sample, which move within a magnetic field. This particle movement, detected by reflectance photometry, starts when the sample is introduced into the test strip and is halted by clot formation. Monitors that utilize this method (e.g. CoaguChek S, Roche Diagnostics) use liquid QC samples (reconstituted lyophilized plasma) provided by the manufacturer or external quality assessment (EQA) schemes.

Optical clot detection uses light-emitting diode (LED) optical detectors to measure the motion of a blood sample as it is pumped back and forth within a cuvette containing freeze-dried thromboplastin. As clot formation begins, the movement decreases below a predetermined rate and the endpoint is detected. These instruments (Protime III and Hemochron Jr. II series, International Technidyne Corporation) cannot detect clot formation in plasma samples and require the presence of red cells. Lyophilized whole blood controls, containing dried fixed red cells with buffered plasma are reconstituted in a diluent containing calcium ions. This is usually achieved by crushing a glass ampoule containing the diluent, within a plastic vial and mixing the contents by inversion. The reconstituted blood is then tested in the same way as a patient sample.

Some monitors use the amperometric (electrochemical) measurement of thrombin activity as a surrogate measure of clot detection (CoaguChek XS/XS Plus, Roche Diagnostics). In principle, lyophilized plasma QC materials may be used with this system, but at present the manufacturer using this technique does not offer a QC preparation for use with all of their instruments. However, in the UK, EQA schemes using lyophilized controls are available for all such instruments.

The electrical impedance method measures the change in electrical current flow that occurs when fibrinogen is converted to fibrin. These test strips contain thromboplastin reagent and electrodes within layered plastic. The only instrument currently using this detection method (INRatio, Hemosense Inc.) has an onboard QC but no commercial or external liquid QC material is available.

Integral onboard controls, contained within the test strip/cuvette are available for some POCT coagulation monitors. Some test strips (CoaguChek XS/XS Plus) have an incorporated QC control function which assesses integrity in the measuring channel after sample application. Resazurin is incorporated and this chemical is sensitive to ambient factors such as light, humidity and temperature and is transformed into Resorufin. The concentration of Resorufin is measured electrochemically and can be considered as a measure of strip damage.

Other POCT monitors (Protime, Hemochron Jr II series and INRatio) use cuvettes where one or more channels contain lyophilized plasma plus other additives, which become activated when mixed with the test sample. Typically, the controls are formulated to clot at a normal (low) and a therapeutic (high) clotting range. Onboard controls are designed primarily to detect test strip degradation and do not always display numerical values but do state whether the control meets the criteria set by the manufacturer as acceptable.

In the USA, the Food and Drug Administration (FDA) states that a QC should be run with each test. Consequently, POCT monitors that use onboard controls are widely used. In Europe, the preference is for liquid QC and this is reflected by the type of POCT monitors in common use. An alternative approach is to assess the POCT monitor normally used by the patient in a center that participates satisfactorily in an accredited EQA program. In this case the patient should test their blood on their monitor and the monitor belonging to the clinic; INR results between 2.0 and 4.5 should be within 0.5 INR units of each other. A paired venous sample may also be collected at the same time as the capillary blood sample for the POCT INR; the venous sample is then analyzed in an appropriate hospital laboratory. INR results of stabilized patients should be within 0.5 INR units of each other. If this "split sample" approach is used, the procedure must be repeated at least once every 6 months. One published study which used a single reference laboratory reported that satisfactory quality assurance could be achieved using this method.[14] However, there are difficulties with this approach because the quality of hospital laboratory INR results is variable and sometimes discrepant. Consequently, differences between the laboratory and the POCT method may not be a result of problems with the POCT device. Discrepancies between INR methods are known to be increased when OAT is unstable, especially at INR values >4.5. It is seldom feasible to use a single reference laboratory, especially if the postal service is poor, the distances involved are large or if the ambient temperature is high, as these factors could all adversely affect sample stability. Another study (performed in the UK) reported a high degree of discrepancy between POCT and laboratory INR values, which were largely a result of systematic errors in laboratory methods.[15]

Patient self-monitoring of oral anticoagulation

Several studies have shown that patient self-monitoring of oral anticoagulation is a reliable and effective alternative to hospital-based anticoagulant clinics. Patients who self-monitor their anticoagulation therapy have fewer thromboembolic events, major hemorrhages and lower mortality rates than those attending anticoagulant clinics. The potential benefit of self-monitoring depends very much on the existing quality of anticoagulation. Where patients are managed by dedicated anticoagulation clinics, and the time in target therapeutic range is ≥60%, an improvement in the quality of anticoagulation may not always be discernable.[16] However, where anticoagulation management is conducted in the physician's office, the time in target therapeutic range may be considerably less than 60% and, in this setting, substantial improvements in the quality of anticoagulation may be achieved. However, this is not feasible for all patients, and requires identification and education of suitable candidates.[17] Both the British Committee for Standards in Haematology[18] and the International Self-Management Association for Oral Anticoagulation[19] have produced guidelines for patient self-monitoring based on the available evidence. The main recommendations are summarized below:

• Under normal circumstances, only patients with long-term indications for OAT should be considered for self-monitoring.
• Previous stability of INR is not a prerequisite to self-monitoring as patients with poor control may benefit from increased independence and increased frequency of testing.
• Patients (or carers) must give informed consent to undertake self-monitoring. This should include agreement to record results accurately.
• Education and training on the theoretical and practical aspects of INR testing and anticoagulation is essential for all patients undergoing self-monitoring.
• Competence to perform a POCT INR must be assessed by a trained healthcare professional prior to allowing home testing.
• Competence to correctly interpret an INR result must be assessed by a healthcare professional prior to allowing self-management.
• Patients being considered for self-monitoring must have a documented INR target in line with accepted guidelines and clinical practice.
• Contraindications for self-monitoring include previous non-compliance in relation to clinic attendance or taking warfarin as instructed.
• Patients undertaking self-monitoring must retain contact with a named healthcare professional and be reviewed at least every 6 months by the responsible clinician.
• QC should be performed on a regular basis. The type of QC will be dependent on the type of monitor used and the institution.
• Self-monitoring patients should participate in some form of external QC/proficiency testing.
• Any INR result between 4.0 and 8.0 should be repeated with the POCT device to ensure that the prolonged result is not a consequence of poor sample quality.
• If an INR of >8.0 or sample error is obtained a venous sample should be collected the same day and analyzed in an appropriate hospital laboratory.

Activated partial thromboplastin time testing

POCT for aPTT is not widely used in the UK and many methods have been withdrawn worldwide, although methods are still available for the Hemochron Jr device. Several semi-automated coagulometers are suitable for use in hospital clinics and intensive care units, but require sample and reagent preparation as well as a certain degree of skill in pipetting technique and so are only suitable for experienced trained users. POCT aPTT only has clinical utility for heparin monitoring and is not advised for use in screening for inherited or acquired coagulation defects. As with all aPTT methods, the reagents and devices vary in their sensitivity to heparin, coagulation factors and lupus anticoagulant. Studies comparing POCT aPTT tests with traditional hospital laboratory tests have shown poor agreement in surgical patients, although the correlation was better for healthy volunteers.[20,21] Liquid QC plasmas are available for the semi-automated and Hemochron methods and these should be run daily or with every batch of tests.

Activated clotting time

The aCT is widely used for monitoring heparin anticoagulation during cardiopulmonary bypass (CPB) procedures.[22] The aCT is most frequently used to demonstrate that there is sufficient heparin anticoagulation to avoid blockage of the extracorporeal circuit. The required accuracy and precision of the test does not therefore have to be particularly high, i.e. it is sufficient to demonstrate that the clotting time is prolonged to within a relatively wide therapeutic range. ACT tests are sometimes performed at the end of cardiac bypass to ensure that suitable amounts of protamine have been used to reverse the heparin anticoagulation.

The sensitivity of the aCT to aprotinin (which is often given in difficult CPB procedures or during further cardiac surgery) appears to differ depending on the analyzer used and the formulation of the activator. Some reports have suggested that kaolin aCT is less affected by aprotinin than the celite aCT,[23] which probably reflects the weaker contact activation activity of celite.

The two best known manufacturers of aCT devices are Hemochron (Edison, NJ, USA) and Medtronic (Minneapolis, MN, USA), although methods are also available for the i-STAT (Abbott). The Hemochron Response is a two-channel analyzer that can measure aCT as well as a variety of other clotting times (aPTT, PT, thrombin time, fibrinogen assay). The reagents are preloaded in the reaction tubes, with color-coded tops for different types of test. Blood is placed in the tube, which also contains a plastic paddle which rotates when the tube is inserted into the analyzer. Clot detection is by a mechanical principle. The aCT tubes are generally designed to take 2 mL blood and the thrombin time tubes 1 mL. The Hemochron Junior Signature analyzer can measure aCT, aPTT and PT. Reagents are contained in test cuvettes, which require addition of approximately 15 µL blood. Clot detection is by an optical method, monitoring cessation of movement of blood along a capillary. The Medtronic ACT Plus analyzer can measure aCT only, although a similar instrument (ACT II) can measure a variety of clotting times. Reagents are preloaded in plastic cuvettes and contain plastic paddles, which facilitate mechanical clot end point detection. Less than 1 mL blood is required for each test.

Liquid QC samples are available for aCT methods and should be performed on each day that the method is used. No EQA schemes currently exist for aCT testing because the test is only performed on whole blood.

Thrombin time

The thrombin clotting time can be performed on citrated plasma or whole blood. The latter may be used during surgery for detecting the presence of heparin, investigating fibrinogen function in the presence and absence of heparin, and for monitoring heparin anticoagulation. The test is not affected by aprotinin. Various modifications of the test exist, using different concentrations of thrombin and with the addition of protamine sulfate to neutralize heparin.

The Hemochron Response analyzer may be used with three reagent tubes:

1 TT tubes (product A301) – containing low concentrations of human thrombin (manufacturer's predicted normal range 39–53 s), intended for the investigation of fibrinogen function and presence of heparin. 1 mL blood required.

2 HNTT tubes (Product A401) – containing human thrombi and protamine sulfate (manufacturer's predicted normal range 33–58 s), intended for the investigation of abnormal fibrinogen function and presence of heparin (in combination with the TT tubes). 1 mL blood required.

3 HiTT tubes (A501) – containing high concentrations of human thrombin, protamine and snake venom. Intended for monitoring high levels of heparin anticoagulation during CPB surgery. 1.5 mL blood required.

The thrombin time is not affected by aprotinin and therefore offers a potential means of assessing anticoagulation during CPB when this agent is used. The HiTT tubes can be used during CPB to ensure that the clotting time is prolonged and sufficient heparin has been given. If required, TT and HNTT tubes can be used to assess fibrinogen function in patients who are bleeding and to investigate whether prolonged clotting times are caused by heparin. The varying sensitivity to heparin of each tube type allows each situation to be covered. Liquid QC samples are available from the manufacturer.

Low molecular weight heparin monitoring

At present, there is only one POCT device intended for monitoring low molecular weight heparin (LMWH). The clot-based test (HEMONOX, ITC) measures the anticoagulant effect of LMWH in non-citrated fresh blood and is a modified dilute thromboplastin time. The manufacturers provide a lyophilized whole blood control but currently no EQA schemes are available. One study demonstrated sensitivity to therapeutic levels of intravenous enoxaparin,[24] but the test currently has limited clinical application.

D-dimer

There are a variety of POCT D-dimer tests available for use in the exclusion of venous thromboembolism (VTE). The earliest widely used test was a red cell agglutination assay (SimpliRED, Agen), and because of the principle of the method, independent EQA is difficult. Most of the other assays are based on enzyme-linked or turbidometric immunoassays. The Minquant (Biopool, Trinity Biotech Ltd.), Nycocard (Axis Shield POC, Oslo, Norway) and Cobas H 232 (Roche) methods all have liquid QC products available and these should be used daily. The CARDIAC D-dimer assay (Roche Diagnostics) has an instrument QC strip which checks the optical performance of the analyzer. A lyophilized plasma control is also supplied and EQA schemes are available. The sensitivity of POCT D-dimer assays to VTE is variable and some may not be as sensitive as the best laboratory tests.[25]

Thrombelastography

Thrombelastography was first described by Hartet in 1948.[26] The technology has been incorporated into two types of hemostasis analyzer: the thrombelastograph (TEG, Hemoscope, IL, USA) and the rotation thromboelastometer (ROTEM, Diagnostica Stago, Asnieres, France). These devices measure viscoelastic changes during coagulation, and provide information on the time taken for initiation of clot formation, the rate of clot formation, the tensile strength of the clot and its rate of dissolution. Thus, the test is influenced by the levels and activity of clotting factors, rate of fibrin polymerization, fibrinogen level, presence of inhibitors, platelet function and fibrinolysis.[27,28] Although the system may be used with plasma, it is more commonly used with whole blood and a variety of activators and reagents are available depending on the clinical application.

The most common applications of TEG/ROTEM are during cardiac surgery and liver transplant procedures, in order to detect excess heparin and coagulopathies. Data are rapidly obtained and indicate the type of therapeutic intervention required (protamine, plasma, cryoprecipitate, platelets, aprotinin). The analyzers have also been used in the assessment of hypercoagulability and in the evaluation of new hemostatic agents (e.g. recombinant factor VIIa) and platelet inhibitor compounds, but these are mainly research applications.

The TEG and ROTEM provide similar hemostatic information, but use slightly different technologies

to achieve this and so the results are not directly interchangeable and require separate reference ranges. Differences in measurement variables also occur depending on whether non-anticoagulated or citrated blood is used and depending on the time from blood collection (some authors recommend that citrated blood is not tested in the first 30 minutes from collection). During major surgery, results are often required rapidly and non-anticoagulated blood is usually tested immediately. Citrated blood should certainly be tested within 4 hours from collection, but standardization of the time is recommended. Before use each day, the analyzer set-up software should be run and baseline determination/adjustment performed. This verifies and maintains the electronic function of the analyzer. Lyophilized QC plasmas are available from the manufacturers and should be used daily (when test are performed) and with each new batch of reagents.

Management of POCT services

There may often be several types of POCT instrument in different departments of the same institution with similar clinical applications. In some countries these issues are addressed by POCT committees, which may include: a hematologist, a physician, nursing staff, laboratory managers, quality assurance managers, pharmacy managers, and others who are needed to train and implement the service. A specific POCT coordinator is recommended for larger institutions. In the UK, guidance is available about setting up and managing a hematology POCT service.[29]

Before a POC coagulation test is introduced, it is first necessary to be clear about the purpose of the test, i.e., diagnosis, monitoring or treatment of disease. A quality manual should be prepared and requirements related to POCT reviewed (ISO 22870, 2004). Standard operating procedures (SOPs) must be written and regularly reviewed. They should include full details of how to use the POCT device and manage the service, what actions to take on generation of a result and what to do in the event of a fault on the instrument. Safety regulations recognizing potential hazards should also be documented. Training protocols must be established and all potential operators must achieve an adequate level of competence; a list of authorized users should be drawn up and approved by the service director. Staff must have a clear understanding that they must not allow others access to tests without undergoing a formal training process. Some devices have security features that only allow accredited operators access, via a personal access code. Retraining intervals and a continuing education program should be established and POCT operator performance monitored as part of the quality assurance program.

Quality assurance requires the satisfactory recording of analytical data and it is essential that the POCT results are documented with operator identification. Ideally, results and patient/sample identification details should be transferred electronically from the POCT device to a computer, to avoid potential transcription errors, but this is not available on all devices (Table 8.1). In the absence of appropriate computer systems, results must be documented in a logbook, which also identifies reagent batch Lot numbers and the name of the operator; as well as the Lot numbers of any calibrants and IQC materials. The POCT results should be permanently stored in the medical record for the patient. When computers are available, the record should distinguish between POCT results and those from the central laboratory (ISO 22870, 2004). All computerized results should be password protected. Unfortunately, these standards are often not achieved and potentially significant clinical errors may occur. Regular effective QC procedures, as outlined above, are essential to allow POCT to become widely accepted, proven clinical practice.

Conclusions

POCT has the advantage of decentralization and reduced turn around times, because no transport of blood samples or return of results is required. The type of analysis (e.g. thrombelastography) will in some cases provide a different type of information to that available from traditional hemostasis laboratory tests, leading to improved health outcomes.

However, POCT methods have historically suffered from poor quality assurance procedures and a lack of standardization of methods. It is not uncommon for untrained operators to perform POCT, particularly in the operating theater. Devolving POCT to the community has been expected by many to reduce the overall costs of service delivery, but the higher costs per test in reagents, external QC and consumables actually tend (at least in the UK) to lead to increased costs.

References

1 Harrison P. Platelet function analysis. *Blood Rev* 2005; **19**: 111–123.

2 Baglin TP, Cousins D, Keeling DM, *et al*. Recommendations from the British Committee for Standards In Haematology and National Patient Safety Agency. *Br J Haematol* 2006; **136**: 26–29.

3 Gregoratos G. Perspectives. Oral anticoagulant therapy: current issues. *Prev Cardiol* 2000; **3**: 178–182.

4 Fitzmaurice DA. Oral anticoagulation control: the European perspective *J Thromb Thrombolysis* 2006; **21**: 95–100.

5 Cromheecke ME, Levi M, Colly LP, *et al*. Oral anticoagulation self-management and management by a specialist anticoagulation clinic: a randomised cross-over comparison. *Lancet* 2000; **356**: 97–102.

6 Gardiner C, Williams K, Mackie IJ, *et al*. Can oral anticoagulation be managed using telemedicine and patient self-testing? A pilot study. *Clin Lab Haematol* 2006; **28**: 122–125.

7 Fitzmaurice DA, Murray ET, McCahon D, *et al*. Self management of oral anticoagulation: randomised trial. *BMJ* 2005; **331**: 1057.

8 Beyth RJ, Quinn L, Landefeld CS. A multicomponent intervention to prevent major bleeding complications in older patients receiving warfarin: a randomized, controlled trial. *Ann Intern Med* 2000; **133**: 687–695.

9 Machin SJ, Mackie IJ, Chitolie A, *et al*. Near patient testing (NPT) in haemostasis: a synoptic review. *Clin Lab Haematol* 1996; **18**: 69–74.

10 Moriarty HT, Lam-Po-Tang PR, Anastas N. Comparison of thromboplastins using the ISI and INR system. *Pathology* 1990; **22**: 71–76.

11 British Committee for Standards in Haematology. Guidelines on oral anticoagulation, third edition. *Br J Haematol* 1998; **101**: 374–387.

12 Baglin TP, Keeling DM, Watson HG, for the British Committee for Standards in Haematology. Guidelines on oral anticoagulation (warfarin): third edition – 2005 update. *Br J Haematol* 2005; **132**: 277–285.

13 Gardiner C, Adcock DM, Carrington LR, *et al*. *Protocol for the Evaluation, Validation and Implementation of Coagulometers; Proposed Guideline*. CLSI: 2007. H57-P.

14 Solvik UO, Stavelin A, Christensen NG, *et al*. External quality assessment of prothrombin time: the split-sample model compared with external quality assessment with

commercial control material. *Scand J Clin Lab Invest* 2006; **66**: 337–349.

15 Kitchen DP, Murray ET, Jennings I, *et al.* Comparison of Coaguchek S INRs with hospital laboratory citrated plasma INRs. What is the truth? *Br J Haematol* 2005; **129** (Suppl. 1): 18.

16 Gardiner C, Williams K, Longair I, *et al.* A randomised control trial of patient self-management of oral anticoagulation compared with patient self-testing. *Br J Haematol* 2005; **132**: 598–603.

17 Heneghan C, Alonso-Coello P, Garcia-Alamino JM, *et al.* Self-monitoring of oral anticoagulation: a systematic review and meta-analysis. *Lancet* 2006; **367**: 404–411.

18 Fitzmaurice DA, Gardiner C, Kitchen S, *et al.* An evidence-based review and guidelines for patient self-testing and management of oral anticoagulation. *Br J Haematol* 2005; **131**: 156–165.

19 Ansell J, Jacobson A, Levy J, *et al.* Guidelines for implementation of patient self-testing and patient self-management of oral anticoagulation. International consensus guidelines prepared by International Self-Monitoring Association for Oral Anticoagulation. *Int J Cardiol* 2005; **99**: 37–45.

20 Ferring M, Reber G, de Moerloose P, *et al.* Point of care and central laboratory determinations of the aPTT are not interchangeable in surgical intensive care patients. *Can J Anaesth* 2001; **48**: 1155–1160.

21 Choi TS, Greilich PE, Shi C, *et al.* Point-of-care testing for prothrombin time, but not activated partial thromboplastin time, correlates with laboratory methods in patients receiving aprotinin or epsilon-aminocaproic acid while undergoing cardiac surgery. *Am J Clin Pathol* 2002; **117**: 74–78.

22 Despotis GJ, Gravlee G, Filos K, *et al.* Anticoagulation monitoring during cardiac surgery: a review of current and emerging techniques. *Anesthesiology* 1999; **91**: 1122–1151.

23 Despotis GJ, Filos KS, Levine V, *et al.* Aprotinin prolongs activated and nonactivated whole blood clotting time and potentiates the effect of heparin *in vitro*. *Anesth Analg* 1996; **82**: 1126–1131.

24 El Rouby S, Cohen M, Gonzales A, *et al.* The use of a HEMOCHRON JR. HEMONOX point of care test in monitoring the anticoagulant effects of enoxaparin during interventional coronary procedures. *J Thromb Thrombolysis* 2006; **21**: 137–145.

25 Heim SW, Schectman JM, Siadaty MS, *et al.* D-dimer testing for deep venous thrombosis: a metaanalysis. *Clin Chem* 2004; **50**: 1136–1147.

26 Hartert H. Blutgerrinnungsstudien mit der thrombelastographie, einem neuen untersuchungsverfahren. *Klin Wochenschr* 1948; **26**: 577–583.

27 Mallett SV, Cox DJ. Thrombelastography. *Br J Anaesth* 1992; **69**: 307–313.

28 Luddington RJ. Thrombelastography/thrombelastometry. *Clin Lab Haematol* 2005; **27**: 81–90.

29 Briggs C, Guthrie D, Hyde K, *et al. Guidelines for Point of Care Testing: Hematology*. British Committee for Standards in Haematology (BCSH) General Haematology Task Force: 2007. http://www.bcshguidelines.com/pdf/POCT_guidelines_310707.pdf QC, quality control.

9

Assay of factor VIII and other clotting factors

S. Kitchen & F. E. Preston

This chapter deals with issues relating to the assay of clotting factors in plasma, with particular emphasis on factor VIII:C. This will include assays of plasma from patients treated with concentrates but will not address the assignment of potencies to concentrates which is addressed elsewhere in this book (Chapter 3).

Pretest variables

The recommended anticoagulant for collection of blood samples for assays of clotting factors, including FVIII:C and FIX:C is normally tri-sodium citrate[1] at a concentration of 0.105–0.109 mol/L (3.2%).[2] It is likely that the use of 3.8% citrate has less impact on factor assays results than on the activated partial thromboplastin time (aPTT; Chapter 4) because the test plasma is diluted in buffer before testing. For the same reason factor assays may be more tolerant of tube underfilling or extremely low hematocrits, although there are few data to confirm this.

For factor assays it is essential that blood is collected as rapidly as possible by clean venepuncture. Any delay in mixing blood with the anticoagulant may affect the results. Before assaying, the blood samples should be inspected for the presence of clots by gentle inversion or by sweeping the tube with a wooden stick. Samples containing clots or exhibiting marked hemolysis should be discarded. Tests performed on partially clotted or activated samples can lead to overestimation of the activity present and activated clotting factors may be associated with non-parallelism in the assay graphs.

Samples should be stored at room temperature (20–25°C) prior to testing. If assays are not performed within 2–3 hours of collection plasma can be stored deep frozen for longer periods at −70°C, because clotting factors including FVIII:C and FIX:C have been shown to be stable for at least 18 months.[3] Frozen plasma should be transferred immediately to a 37°C waterbath, thawed for 4–5 minutes at 37°C and mixed by gentle inversion prior to analysis. A slow thaw at lower temperature must be avoided to prevent the formation of cryoprecipitate which reduces the FVIII concentration in the supernatant plasma.

Factor VIII is an acute phase reactant[4] and is also increased in pregnancy and by exercise. Caution is therefore required when interpreting FVIII assays when investigating for possible hemophilia A or von Willebrand disease (VWD) and these diagnoses should not be confirmed or excluded on the basis of a single result.

For a general discussion of preanalytical variables in relation to coagulation tests see Chapter 4.

One-stage assay of factors VIII:C or IX:C

The most commonly performed assay for FVIII:C worldwide for many years has been the one-stage

Quality in Laboratory Hemostasis and Thrombosis, 1st edition. By Steve Kitchen, John D. Olson and F. Eric Preston. Published 2009 by Blackwell Publishing. ISBN: 978-1-4051-6803-8

assay.[5,6] The following observations, relating to FVIII:C assays, can also be applied to assays of FIX:C or FXI:C. The one-stage assay is based on the aPTT and depends upon the ability of a sample containing FVIII to correct or shorten the delayed clotting of a plasma that has a complete lack of FVIII (FVIII-deficient plasma). It is important that the concentration of FVIII in this mixture is rate-limiting in its influence on the clotting time, as measured by the aPTT.

The assay requires a reference or standard plasma of known FVIII concentration. The preparation of several different dilutions of the reference plasma allows the construction of a calibration curve in which the clotting time response depends on the concentration (dose) of FVIII:C. If plasma is not sufficiently diluted then the other clotting factors in the test plasma will influence the clotting time and the assay is no longer specific for FVIII and is therefore invalid. For this reason most assays operate with a minimum dilution of 1 in 5. At very low concentrations of FVIII the clotting time may not be influenced by FVIII and the aPTT is similar to the aPTT of the FVIII-deficient plasma. If doubling dilutions of 1/5, 1/10, 1/20, 1/40, 1/80, 1/160 and 1/320 are selected then this may occur when dilutions of 1 in 160 or 1in 320 are analyzed (depending on the reagent).

In order to obtain a linear relationship, the data normally require transformation. Linearity of the reference or calibration curve is required for a valid assay. The most appropriate data transformation is that which gives the closest fit to a straight line relationship as indicated by an r value (relating clotting times to concentration) that is close to 1.0. This is most commonly achieved using log transformation so that the log of concentration is plotted against the log of the clotting times. For some assay systems the use of non-transformed data (linear scale) for the clotting times with log transformed concentrations may be suitable. Correlation coefficients of $r > 0.99$ are easily achievable and calibration curves with r values of <0.98 should be rejected.

Guidelines recommend that test plasmas are analyzed using at least three dilutions.[7–9] This is essential to confirm that two critical criteria for a valid assay have been met: that there is a straight line relationship through clotting times at different dilutions and

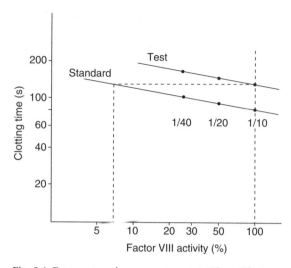

Fig. 9.1 Factor assay dose–response curve. Three dilutions of standard and test plasma are plotted with concentration (dose) on the horizontal axis and clotting time (response) on the vertical. In the example above the concentration of FVIII:C in the test sample is 7% of the activity in the standard plasma.

that the line through patient times is parallel to the calibration line. An example is shown in Fig. 9.1. If a test and standard line are parallel this indicates that the two materials have behaved in a similar way under the test conditions. Comparing unlike materials such as concentrate with a plasma standard or comparing plasmas containing animal clotting factors with a human plasma standard often leads to non-parallel lines, indicating that the criteria for a valid assay have not been met. Identifying parallelism is only possible if several test dilutions are analyzed. Non-parallel one-stage assays can also occur in the presence of heparin or thrombin inhibitors such as lepirudin.[10]

A second important reason to include multiple test dilutions is to improve the precision of the assay. In a UK National External Quality Assessment Scheme (NEQAS) exercise a test sample with FIX:C of 6 IU/dL was assayed in approximately 90 hemophilia centers. The CV of the FIX:C results in the 22 centers performing a single test dilution was 54%, compared with a CV of 22% for the 42 centers that performed the analysis using three test dilutions. The difference

Factor VIII MDA ID No 7004 29/9/97	[0004-04] 16:03	37.1°C

MDA ratio	Clot time	Activity %
1/1	99.0 sec	9.5 %
1/2	103.0 sec	15.3 %
1/4	106.0 sec	26.1 %
		Mean 17.0%
SCr = −1.000		Test r = −0.996

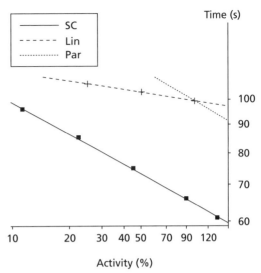

Fig. 9.2 This figure shows a printout from an autoanalyzer for an FVIII:C assay using a lupus-sensitive aPTT reagent in the assay. On the plot SC is the standard curve; Lin is the line of best fit through the three test dilutions; Par is a line drawn parallel to the SC through the first test dilution clotting time. In this example the Lin through patient dilution clotting times is not parallel to the SC. In the table, 1/1 represents the 1 in 10 dilution which in this case is the first test dilution and which suggests a FVIII test result of 9.5% of the standard. The next two dilutions, 1/2 and 1/4 (1 in 20 and 1 in 40, respectively) suggest test results of 15% and 26%, respectively. Two further test dilutions of 1/80 and 1/160 gave test results of 43% and 106% of standard (not shown in the figure). This patient has a normal level of FVIII:C and a strong lupus anticoagulant (LAC) which is causing the non-parallel assay effect and underestimation of activity in lower dilutions.

was statistically significant ($P < 0.05$). This indicates that the precision of assays is much improved by testing multiple dilutions.

If only one dilution is analyzed there can also be important errors in the accuracy of the assay, particularly if lupus inhibitors are present (see below)

Assays in the presence of strong lupus anticoagulant

Because lupus anticoagulant (LAC) can prolong phospholipid-dependent tests and in particular the aPTT, it is not surprising that in some cases these antibodies can compromise the quality of assay results by interfering in aPTT-based one-stage assays. In extreme cases such antibodies can completely block the reactions even when the test plasma has been diluted for analysis in a one-stage assay and in this case assay results of <1 IU/dL are obtained in both FVIII and FIX assays.[11] More typically, some clotting factor activity is detectable but the estimate of potency depends on the dilution of test plasma, with different results being obtained at different plasma dilutions.[12] The measured activity increases at higher dilutions. An example of LAC effect on a one-stage FVIII assay is shown in Fig. 9.2. LAC typically interferes to a similar extent in all one-stage PTT assays, so the non-parallel effects in Fig. 9.2 occur in assays of FIX:C, FXI:C and FXII:C in addition to FVIII:C. An accurate assay result can be obtained only if two different plasma dilutions give the same activity.

There are three possible solutions to this problem. One is to employ a chromogenic assay where the initial plasma dilution is high and the inhibitory effect of LA is diluted out.[10] In a report of 10 cases where LAC led to interference and underestimation of the FVIII:C, reliable estimates could be obtained in a chromogenic assay, including a case where the one-stage assay suggested that FVIII was completely absent even at a plasma dilution of 1 in 80.[12]

In respect of factor VIII:C a second way to obtain accurate assay results in the presence of LAC is to employ a two-stage clotting assay which is rarely affected by LAC despite the fact that phospholipid is required in the assay. The absence of LAC interference is related to the high initial test dilution (typically 1 in 50 or 1 in 100) used in two-stage clotting assays. Chromogenic assays are not widely used for FIX:C or FXI:C determinations.

The final option, which may be the favored choice for all one-stage aPTT-based assays, is to perform the assay in the presence of a high concentration of phospholipid so that there is an excess of phospholipid beyond the concentration that can be blocked by LAC. This can be carried out by addition of platelet-derived phospholipid[13] or more simply by using an aPTT reagent known to be insensitive to LAC as a consequence of higher phospholipid concentration. We have reported that Actin FS has approximately 20-fold more phospholipid than a number of other aPTT reagents[14] and one-stage assays performed with this reagent are only very rarely affected by the presence of LAC.

One-stage assay components

The quality of assay results is very much influenced by laboratory reagents currently in use. One-stage aPTT-based assays can be performed with any of the available aPTT reagents although it should be noted that they contain different types of activator including kaolin, cellite, silica particles and ellagic acid. Reagents employing ellagic acid as activator are unsuitable for assay of prekallikrein because activation by ellagic acid is largely independent of prekallikrein.

There is considerable variation in the concentration and composition of phospholipids in widely used reagents.[14] Because the phospholipids support the clotting reactions through bound clotting factors, different phospholipid preparations have the potential to give different assay results depending on the aPTT reagent used. One example we have reported is that in subjects with VWD Normandy higher one-stage FVIII:C results were obtained with the DAPTTIN aPTT reagent compared to the results obtained with other aPTT reagents.[15]

In general, differences between one-stage results of FVIII:C assays performed using different types of aPTT reagent are not sufficient to influence patient management.[16]

In the case of FIX:C assays differences between results obtained using different aPTT reagents are also minor.[17] The selection of aPTT reagent can influence the precision of both FVIII:C and FIX:C assays.[17,18] In both cases, precision is better for reagents where there is a greater increase in clotting time for a given change in concentration. Calibration curves of assays performed with such reagents have steeper slopes. While many different aPTT reagents are suitable for use in assays of FVIII:C and IX:C it remains important to select a reagent for which there is evidence (e.g. through proficiency testing surveys) that results are in agreement with those obtained with an alternative reagent.

For prothrombin time (PT) based assays the results may be influenced, albeit rarely, by the nature of the tissue factor present in the thromboplastin reagent. Some patients have normal levels of FVII:C (and normal PT) when the test is performed with a reagent containing human tissue factor, whereas reduced activity in both FVII:C assay and the PT is obtained with a thromboplastin of rabbit origin. Interestingly, in cases such as these bleeding symptoms normally correlate with the results obtained with reagents of human origin.[9]

One-stage assays require an appropriately deficient plasma. This should have a total lack of the factor being assayed, normal levels of other relevant clotting factors and no evidence of coagulation factor inhibitor. Even 1–2 IU/dL residual activity of the factor being assayed makes this unsuitable for use, leading to non-parallel assays and possible overestimation of the factor under analysis. Most commercially available factor-deficient plasmas are now prepared by immunodepletion of one factor from normal plasma. In general, this works well and in a study reported by Barrowcliffe et al.[19] no differences were observed between FVIII:C assay results obtained with a deficient plasma from severe hemophilia A patients and five different immunodepleted FVIII-deficient plasmas.

Some FVIII:C-deficient plasmas are prepared using an anti-von Willibrand factor (VWF) antibody. Such plasmas are deficient in both FVIII:C and VWF. This might influence the results of FVIII:C assays in some hemophilia patients. A normal level of VWF in the FVIII:C-deficient plasma is of particular importance when performing FVIII:C assays on concentrates.

It has been reported that the antibody against FVIII:C used to produce deficient plasma can leach off the column used for the depletion and then be present in the FVIII:C-deficient plasma. This can cause problems in FVIII:C inhibitor assays (Chapter 20)[20] and would therefore be unsuitable for use in one-stage FVIII:C assays of any kind.

The accuracy of all factor assays is dependent on the use of a reference or calibration plasma that has an accurately assigned potency. For commercial materials this is the responsibility of the manufacturer. Most often results in proficiency testing exercise confirm that results obtained by centers using different sources of reference plasma are in good agreement but this is not always the case. On rare occasions, results obtained using one reference plasma are consistently different from results obtained against all others.[6] This is normally caused by inaccurate assignment by the manufacturer and, in the UK at least, some manufacturers have issued revised potencies after correcting errors in the original assignment process. In an assessment by the Scientific and Standardization Committee (SSC) of International Society for Thrombosis and Haemostasis (ISTH) of six commercial reference plasmas, the observed potency as determined in nine expert centres differed from the labelled potency by as much as 17% for FVIII:C and 16% for FIX,[21] indicating that the problems above are not restricted to the UK.

Factor assays in the presence of severe deficiency

The SSC has defined severe hemophilia A and B as <0.01 IU/mL (<1% or <1 IU/dL), with levels of FVIII:C/FIX:C being 0.01–0.05 IU/mL (1–5%) defined as moderate and >0.05–0.40 IU/mL (5–40%) as mild.[22] The same publication points out that classification based on clinical symptoms has sometimes been used because some patients with reported levels of <0.01 IU/mL exhibit little or no spontaneous bleeding whereas some patients with reportedly moderate, or even mild disease, have frequent spontaneous bleeds and appear to be clinically severe. It may be that this discrepancy between laboratory assay and

clinical phenotype arises out of the difficulties in accurately assaying FVIII and FIX at very low levels. Following a proficiency testing survey we reported that approximately one-third of expert hemophilia centers wrongly classified two severe hemophilia A patients as mild or moderate.[23] There are particular difficulties in performing assays at levels below 0.03 IU/mL (3%).

One way to improve the accuracy of results in such samples is to extend the calibration curve and include reference plasma dilutions with activities of 1 or 2% as recommended by NCCLS.[7] If the patient results are more prolonged than the clotting time of the lowest dilution then the patient result can be reported as less than that activity.[7] It is also useful to perform a test using all the same reagents but with dilution buffer in place of the test plasma dilution. This is sometimes referred to as the blank time of the assays. Only patient dilutions with clotting times shorter than this blank can be properly interpreted. When the level of FVIII:C and FIX:C is genuinely <0.01 IU/mL then it is not usually possible to obtain clotting times on test plasma dilutions which are clearly shorter than this blank time. The comments in relation to FVIII:C assays above also apply to other factor assays.

For FVIII:C assays in the presence of severe deficiency there is also the option to use a modified chromogenic assay as described by Yatau et al.[24] who used the Coamatic chromogenic assay with a lower dilution of 1 in 30 (rather than the recommended 1 in 80) and prolonged the incubation time with chromogenic substrate to 30 minutes (rather than the recommended 10 minutes). The modified assay allowed precise and accurate determinations in the range 0.001–0.02 IU/mL (0.1–2%).

Assay of elevated FVIII:C

The recognition that elevated levels of FVIII:C are risk factors for thrombovascular disease has resulted in an increased demand, by clinicians, for FVIII:C determinations in individuals with both venous and arterial vascular disease. The same assay design used for investigation of bleeding disorders is generally suitable for assay of elevated levels of FVIII:C (and other factors) although the dilution of test plasma should be increased accordingly so that the clotting times of at least two of the three patient dilutions lie within the range covered by the calibration curve. The calibration curve should not be extended by testing dilutions lower than 1 in 5 because clotting factors in the test sample other than the one under assay may begin to influence the clotting time obtained and assay specificity is lost. For FVIII:C activities of 150 IU/dL or more chromogenic assays may be more precise than one-stage clotting methods.[10]

Two-stage clotting assay for FVIII:C

Mild hemophilia A is not excluded by the finding of a normal FVIII:C level by one-stage assay. Several groups have reported that a subgroup of mild hemophilia A patients have discrepant FVIII:C results, as determined using different types of assay.[25–27] More than 20% of mild hemophilia A patients are associated with assay discrepancy if a twofold difference between results obtained with different assay systems is used to define this.[25] In some cases the one-stage assay result may be five times higher than the two-stage clotting or chromogenic assay.[25] The most common manifestation of assay discrepancy is one-stage assay results that are more than twofold higher than those of two-stage clotting or chromogenic assays. In more than 75% of such patients all assay results are reduced below the lower limit of the reference range so that a diagnosis can be reliably made irrespective of which method is employed for analysis. However, a small proportion of patients have results by the one-stage assay which are well within the normal range with reduced levels by a two-stage clotting or chromogenic assays.[27,28] These patients have bleeding histories compatible with the lower levels obtained in two-stage clotting or chromogenic assay. In many cases the genetic defect has been identified so there is no doubt that these subjects do indeed have hemophilia.[28,29] In our experience about 5–10% of mild hemophilia A patients have a normal one-stage assay result. We screened 60 patients with mild hemophilia A and found seven patients from six families in whom the result by one-stage assay was within the normal range and was at least twice the level obtained by two-stage clotting assay. Results are shown in Table 9.1.

Because FVIII:C activity is normal in the one stage aPTT-based assay it is not surprising that the aPTT

Table 9.1 Comparison of factor VIIIc assays using three methods.

	One-stage assay (IU/dL)	Two-stage clotting assay (IU/dL)	Chromogenic assay case (IU/dL)*
A	101	34	13
B	88	15	28
C	63	30	40
D	55	24	40
E	58	21	33
F	72	21	36
G	84	19	45

* Chromogenic assay (Dade–Behring Ltd.)

is also normal in such patients. This means that patients with a clinical history compatible with hemophilia A should have a two-stage clotting or chromogenic assay even if the aPTT and one-stage assay are normal.

There are a small number of mild hemophilia A patients with the reverse pattern, i.e. reduced activity by one-stage but normal results by the two-stage assay.[30–32] In these cases the clinical phenotype once again correlates with the two-stage result in that there is no personal or family history of bleeding with no requirement for FVIII:C replacement therapy.[33]

The two-stage clotting assay was developed as a modification of the now rarely used thromboplastin generation test by Biggs *et al.* in Oxford and reported in the very first issue of the *British Journal of Haematology*.[34] It is a testament to the usefulness of this assay that after more than 50 years it continues to be used in some hemophilia reference centers largely unchanged except for a minor modification proposed by Denson[35] to facilitate automation of the test. Chromogenic FVIII assays were later developed from two-stage clotting assays using similar principles.

As the name implies, there are two distinct stages to the assay. The first stage involves creation of a reaction mixture that contains an excess of the components required for generation of the prothrombinase complex with the exception of FVIII: C. The initial reagent therefore needs to contain activated FIXa, FX, phospholipid, calcium ions and factor V. The FIXa and FX are provided by diluted activated human serum that has been fully clotted to remove all the FII, fibrinogen and FVIII, followed by incubation to allow antithrombin to neutralize thrombin and activated FX formed during the clotting process, and to allow activation of FIX to IXa via contact activation. This manipulated serum contains FX but not FXa and most of the FIX in the active form. For a full description of the reagent see Barrowcliffe.[36]

In the first stage of the assay the rate at which FIXa activates FX depends on the amount of FVIII that has been added. The FXa generated is bound through FV and calcium to phospholipid. This first stage must not contain FII and fibrinogen or the mixture will clot. Test and reference plasma are therefore mixed with alumina hydroxide to remove prothrombin, with other vitamin K clotting factors being removed as a side effect of this. Such adsorption also removes any trace quantities of thrombin or FXa. Barrowcliffe[36] provides a full description of the assay details.

Chromogenic assay for FVIII:C in plasma

The chromogenic assay method is based on the ability of FVIII to act as a cofactor in promoting the activation of FX:C by FIXa. The FXa generated in the assay is detected by the cleavage of a chromogenic substrate and the generation of color. The assay method ensures that the color development is dependent only on the concentration of FVIII:C in the test sample. The chromogenic method has some similarities to the two-stage clotting assay. In the first stage, the test sample containing FVIII:C is incubated in the presence of phospholipid, calcium and purified coagulation FIXa and FX. This mixture leads to the generation of FXa in amounts proportional to the concentration of FVIII:C in the test sample. The second stage of the assay involves the estimation of FXa by the cleavage of a chromogenic substrate and the generation of color by the release of *p*-nitroaniline (pNa) which is measured photometrically at 405 nm.

There are several different chromogenic assays available and there are important differences in the composition of the reagents so that results obtained using different chromogenic assays are not always interchangeable. Some chromogenic asays include added thrombin to fully activate FVIII:C, whereas in the original Chromogenix system thrombin is not added and must be generated in the first stage for FVIII:C activation.

For most (but not all) chromogenic assays the second stage includes a thrombin inhibitor in order to prevent cleavage of the chromogenic substrate by any thrombin that might be present. The generation of color may either be measured continuously or as an endpoint perhaps with an acid-stopped reaction. The generation of color in the second stage is directly proportional to the concentration of FVIII in the test sample. The data from calibration curves does not normally require transformation and can be plotted on a simple linear scale to give a straight line relationship.

The chromogenic method differs from the one-stage clotting method in that it is not sensitive to the presence of activated FVIII:C in the test plasma sample. A gross discrepancy between results of a one-stage and chromogenic assay may be caused by activation of FVIII:C during sample collection, although this can be a genuine finding in certain hemophilia A patients (see p. 86).

The chromogenic assay is currently recommended by the *European Pharmacopoeia*[37] and by SSC of ISTH for assignment of potency to FVIII:C concentrates.[38]

In addition to the lack of interference by LAC (see above), chromogenic FVIII:C assays may also be unaffected by the presence of heparin or lepirudin[10] making them the method of choice if assay is required in the presence of these kinds of anticoagulants.

Factor VIII:C and FIX:C assays following clotting factor infusions

In most cases the same factor assay design and reagents should be used for measuring samples from treated hemophiliacs as for other test samples. Issues related to the assay of such samples have been extensively reviewed.[39,40] There are particular issues related to the assay of samples containing recombinant FVIII:C. When measuring full-length recombinant FVIII:C in plasma, results of some chromogenic assays may be 40–50% higher than by one-stage clotting assays.[41]

A further issue relates to B domain depleted recombinant FVIII:C where results of one-stage assays were approximately 30% greater than results by chromogenic assay in plasma samples containing this material in an SSC/ISTH field study.[42] This discrepancy could be substantially reduced by calibrating the assay using B domain depleted material as calibrator. There is evidence that the higher result by one-stage assay (with the usual plasma standard) is a consequence of the artificial phospholipids present in the reagent.[43] The more appropriate result is considered to be the lower activity obtained either by chromogenic assay or one-stage clotting assay when calibrated against the B domain depleted standard. We have noted that there are differences between results of different chromogenic assays in samples from patients treated with this product. The SSC field study[42] concluded that the one-stage assay, when calibrated with the B domain depleted standard, provides an accurate and precise assessment of FVIII:C in plasma samples containing this material.

References

1 World Health Organization Report. *Use of Anticoagulants in Diagnostic Laboratory Investigations*. WHO/DIL/LAB/99, 1 Perl. 1999.

2 National Committee for Clinical Laboratory Standards (NCCLS, USA) (1998) *Collection, Transport and Processing of Blood Specimens for Coagulation Testing and General Performance of Coagulation Assays, Approved Guideline*, 3rd edn. NCCLS: 1998. H21-A3, UH 18, no. 20.

3 Woodhams B, Giradot O, Blanco MJ, Colesse G, Gourmelin Y. Stability of coagulation proteins in frozen plasma. *Blood Coagul Fibrinolysis* 2001; 12: 229–236.

4 Gallus AS, Hirsh J, Cade J. Relevance of pre-operative and post-operative blood tests in post-operative leg vein thrombosis. *Lancet* 1973; ii: 805–809.

5 Brandt JT. Measurement of factor VIII: A potential risk factor for vascular disease. *Arch Pathol Lab Med* 1992; 117: 48–51.

6 Preston FE, Kitchen S. Quality control and factor VIII assays. *Haemophilia* 1998; 4: 651–653.

7 National Committee for Clinical Laboratory Standards (NCCLS, USA). *Determination of Factor Coagulant Activities, Approved Guideline*. NCCLS: 1997. H48-A.

8 Kitchen S, McCraw A. *Diagnosis of Haemophilia and Other Bleeding Disorders: A Laboratory Manual*. Montreal, Canada: World Federation of Hemophilia, 2000.

9 Bolton-Maggs PH, Perry DJ, Chalmers EA, Parapia LA, Wilde JT, Williams MD, *et al*. The rare coagulation disorders: review with guidelines for management. *Haemophilia* 2004; 10: 1–36.

10 Chandler WL, Ferrell C, Lee J, Tun T, Kha H. Comparison of three methods for measuring FVIII levels in plasma. *Am J Clin Pathol* 2003; 120: 34–39.

11 Kazmi MA, Pickering W, Smith MP, Holland LJ, Savidge GF. Acquired haemophilia A: errors in the diagnosis. *Blood Coagul Fibrinolysis* 1998; 9: 623–628.

12 De Maistre E, Wahl D, Perret-Guillaume C, Regnault V, Clarac S, Briquel ME, *et al*. A chromogenic assay allows reliable measurement of FVIII levels in the presence of strong lupus anticoagulant. *Thromb Haemost* 1998; 79: 237–238.

13 Armitage J, Ashcraft J, Kim A, Kaplan HS. An approach to factor assays in patients with strong lupus anticoagulant. *Clin Appl Thromb Hemost* 1995; 1: 125–130.

14 Kitchen S, Cartwright I, Wood TAL, Jennings I, Preston FE. Lipid composition of seven aPTT reagents in relation to heparin sensitivity. *Br J Haematol* 1999; 106: 801–808.

15 Bowyer AE, Cartwright I, Kitchen S, Makris M. FVIII:C assay discrepancy in type 2N VWD is reagent dependent. *J Thromb Haemost* 2007; 5: Supplement 2.

16 Arkin CF, Bovill EG, Brandt JT, Rock WA, Triplett DA. Factors affecting the performance of factor VIII coagulant activity assays. Results of proficiency surveys of the College of American Pathologists. *Arch Pathol Lab Med* 1992; 116: 908–915.

17 Brandt JT, Atkin CF, Bovill EG, Rock WA, Triplett DA. Evaluation of aPTT reagent sensitivity to factor IX and factor IX assay performance. *Arch Pathol Lab Med* 1990; 114: 135–141.

18 Brandt JT, Triplett DA, Musgrave K, Atkins C, Bovill EG, Ljucas FV, *et al*. Factor VIII assays. Assessment of variables. *Arch Pathol Lab Med* 1988; 112: 7–12.

19 Barrowcliffe TW, Tubbs JE, Wong MY. Evaluation of FVIII deficient plasmas. *Thromb Haemost* 1993; 70: 433–437.

20 Verbruggen B, Giles A, Samis J, Verbeek K, Menisink E, Novakova I. The type of factor VIII deficient plasma used influences the performance of the Nijmegen modification of the Bethesda assay for factor VIII inhibitors. *Thromb Haemost* 2001; 86: 1435–1439.

21 Kasper C, Aronson DL, Davignon G, Foster P, Hillman-Wiseman C, Lusher J, *et al*. Comparison of six commercial reference plasma for FVII, Factor IX and von

Willebrand factor, on behalf of the Subcommittee for FVIII and IX of the SSC of the ISTH. *Thromb Haemost* 1995; **74**: 987–989.

22 White GC, Rosendaal F, Aledort LM, Lusher JM, Rothschild C, Ingerslev J. Definitions in hemophilia. Recommendations of the Scientific Subcommittee on FVIII and FIX of the SSC of ISTH. *Thromb Haemost* 2001; **85**: 560.

23 Preston FE, Kitchen S, Jennings I, Woods TAL, Makris M. SSC/ISTH classification of Hemophilia A: can hemophilia center laboratories achieve the new criteria? *J Thromb Haemost* 2004; **2**: 271–274.

24 Yatau R, Dayan I, Baru M. A modified chromogenic assay for the measurement of very low levels of factor VIII activity (FVIII:C). *Haemophilia* 2006; **12**: 253–257.

25 Parquet-Gernez A, Mazurier C, Goudemand M. Functional and immunological assays of FVIII in 133 haemophiliacs: characterisation of a subgroup of patients with mild haemophilia A and discrepancy in 1-stage and 2-stage assays. *Thromb Haemost* 1988; **59**: 202–206.

26 Duncan EM, Duncan BM, Tunbridge LJ, Lloyd JV. Familial discrepancy between one stage and two stage factor VIII assay methods in a subgroup of patients with haemophilia A. *Br J Haematol* 1994; **87**: 846–848.

27 Keeling DM, Sukhu K, Kemball-Cook G, Waseem N, Bagnall R, Lloyd JV. Diagnostic importance of the two stage FVIII:C assay demonstrated by a case of mild haemophilia associated with His[1954]-Leu substitution in the FVIII A3 domain. *Br J Haematol* 1999; **105**: 1123–1126.

28 Mazurier C, Gaucher C, Jorieux S, Parquet-Gernez A. Mutations in the FVIII gene in seven families with mild haemophilia A. *Br J Haematol* 1997; **96**: 426–427.

29 Rudzi Z, Duncan EM, Casey GJ, Neuman M, Favaloro RJ, Lloyd JV. Mutations in a subgroup of patients with mild haemophilia A and familial discrepancy between one-stage and two-stage factor VIII:C methods. *Br J Haematol* 1996; **94**: 400–406.

30 Goodeve AC, Hinks JL, Nesbitt IM, Sampson B, Burgess C, Khair K, *et al*. Unusual discrepant factor VIII:C assays in haemophilia A patients with Tyr346Cys and Glu-321Lys FVIII gene mutations. *Thromb Haemost* 2001; **86** (suppl. 1).

31 Mumford AD, Kemball-Cook G, O'Donnell J, Johnson DJD, Manning R, McVey JH, *et al*. A novel factor VIII variant Tyr346Cys in the acidic a1 domain is associated with an unusual one-stage/two-stage assay discrepancy and delayed thrombin activation. *Thromb Haemost* 2001; **86** (suppl 1).

32 Mumford AD, Laffan M, O'Donnell J, McVey JH, Johnson JD, Manning RA, *et al*. A Tyr346Cys in the interdomain acidic region a1 of FVIII in an individual with FVIII:C assay discrepancy. *Br J Haematol* 2002; **118**: 589–594.

33 Lyall H, Hill M, Westby J, Grimley C, Dolan G. Tyr346-Cys mutation results in factor VIII:C assay discrepancy and a normal bleeding phenotype: is this mild haemophilia A? *Hemophilia* 2008; **14**: 78–80.

34 Biggs R, Eveling J, Richards G. The assay of antihaemophilic globulin activity. *Br J Haematol* 1955; **1**: 20–34.

35 Denson KWE. Human blood coagulation. In *Haemostasis and Thrombosis*, Biggs R. (ed.). Blackwells, Oxford, 1976: 682–692.

36 Barrowcliffe TW. Methodology of the two stage assay of FVIII (FVIII:C). *Scand J Haematol Suppl* 1984; **41**: 25–38.

37 Council of Europe. Assay of blood coagulation factor VIII. *European Pharmacopoeia*, 3rd edn. Strasbourg: 1997: section 2.7.4, 111–114.

38 Barrowcliffe TW on behalf of the factor VIII and IX subcommittee of SSC of ISTH. Recommendations for the assay of high-purity FVIII concentrates. *Thromb Haemost* 1993; **70**: 876–877.

39 Lundblad RL, Kingdom HS, Mann KG, White GC. Issues with the assay of FVIII activity in plasma and FVIII concentrates. *Thromb Haemost* 2000; **84**: 942–948.

40 Barrowcliffe TW, Raut S, Sands D, Hubbard AR. Coagulation and chromogenic assays of FVIII activity: general aspects standardisation and recommendations. *Semin Thromb Haemost* 2002; **28**: 247–256.

41 Hubbard AR, Bevan SA, Weller LJ. Potency estimation of recombinant FVIII: effect of assay method and standard. *Br J Haematol* 2001; **113**: 533–536.

42 Ingerslev J, Jankowski MA, Weston SB, Charles LA. Colaborative field study on the utility of a BDD factor VIII concentrate standard in the estimation of BDDr Factor VIII:C activity in hemophilic plasma using the one-stage clotting assay. *J Thromb Haemost* 2004; **2**: 623–628.

43 Mikaelsson M, Oswaldson U, Sanderg H. Influence of phospholipids on the assessment of factor VIII activity. *Haemophilia* 1998; **4**: 646–650.

10 Application of molecular genetics to the investigation of inherited bleeding disorders

S. Lethagen, M. Schwartz & L.B. Nielsen

Hemophilia A and B

Hemophilia is an X-linked inherited bleeding disorder, with female carriers and affected males. There are two clinically indistinguishable forms. Hemophilia A is characterized by a deficiency of coagulation factor VIII and hemophilia B by a deficiency of FIX. The incidence of hemophilia A and B is 1 in 10,000 and 1 in 30,000 boys, respectively.

FVIII is synthesized as a single chain precursor glycoprotein with 2332 amino acids ($\approx$285,000 Da). It has a domain structure with three A domains, one B and two C domains and circulates as a dimer composed of one heavy chain (A1-A2-B domains) and one light chain (A3-C1-C2 domains) in a concentration of 150 ng/mL. In plasma (Fig. 10.1), FVIII is non-covalently bound to the von Willebrand factor (VWF), which protects FVIII from inactivation and clearance. VWF is required for normal release of FVIII and also targets FVIII to the site of vascular damage. FVIII is activated to FVIIIa initially by thrombin, which releases FVIII from VWF, and thereafter increasingly by FXa. FVIIIa is an unstable heterotrimer consisting of the A1, A2 and A3-C1-C2 chains. Inactivation is caused either by spontaneous dissociation of the A2 domain or cleavage of FVIIIa by activated protein C (aPC)[1] (Fig. 10.2).

Quality in Laboratory Hemostasis and Thrombosis, 1st edition. By Steve Kitchen, John D. Olson and F. Eric Preston. Published 2009 by Blackwell Publishing. ISBN: 978-1-4051-6803-8

FIX, a single chain glycoprotein with 415 amino acids ($\approx$55,000 Da), is one of the vitamin K dependent coagulation factors and contains 12 gamma-carboxyglutamate (gla) residues. The gla-domain, which requires vitamin K for normal synthesis, is essential for normal protein conformation, and for binding to phospholipid membrane surfaces via calcium. Other important functional regions are the catalytic and activation domains. FIX circulates as an inactive zymogen in a concentration of about 3–5 μg/mL. FXa or FVIIa in complex with tissue factor activates the zymogen FIX to FIXa by cleavage of two peptide bonds and release of an activation peptide.[2]

In the coagulation process, FVIIIa associates with FIXa on a phospholipid surface (physiologically the surface of the activated platelets) and forms the tenase complex, which activates FX to FXa.

Depending on the factor activity in plasma, hemophilia is divided into severe (factor levels <1%), moderate (factor levels of 1–4%) and mild (factor levels of 5–40%). The range of FVIII and FIX in plasma of normal healthy individuals is usually about 50–150% (0.50–1.50 kIU/L). One international unit (1 IU) is defined as the activity of the respective factor in 1 mL normal plasma and calibrated to an international standard.

Inhibitors to FVIII develop in about 20–30% of patients with severe hemophilia A[3] and in about 9–23% of those with severe hemophilia B.[4] Inhibitors are antibodies against FVIII or FIX that neutralize the coagulant activity of the respective factor, and which develop in response to exogenous administration of the factor. Exogenous FIX may even cause

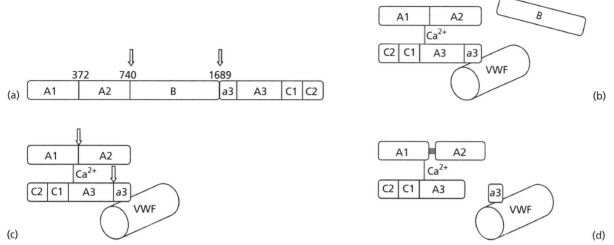

Fig. 10.1 Schematic cartoon of the activation steps of FVIII. (a) FVIII is synthesized as a single chain precursor glycoprotein with 2332 amino acids (≈285,000 Da), and consists of the main domains A1, A2, A3, B, C1 and C2. It is activated mainly by thrombin and FXa cleavage at positions 372, 740 and 1689. (b) FVIII circulates as a heterodimer consisting of a heavy chain (A1, A2 and B domains) and a light chain (A3, C1 and C2 domains) in complex with the von Willebrand factor (VWF). The *a3* region within the A3 domain contains the VWF binding site. During activation, the B domain is cleaved off. (c,d) The A2 domain is cleaved off at position 372, and stays loosely bound to the relatively stable A1/A3-C1-C3 dimer via weak electrostatic interaction. Activation of FVIII involves release from the VWF.

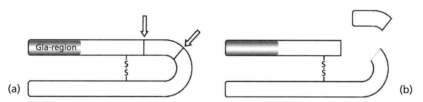

Fig. 10.2 Schematic cartoon of the activation steps of FIX. FIX is a single chain glycoprotein with 415 amino acids (≈55,000 Da) (a). It is activated by cleavage of two peptide bonds and release of an activation peptide (b).

anaphylactic reactions. About one-third to one-half of patients with inhibitors have low titers that may resolve spontaneously. High titer inhibitors (>5 Bethesda units, BU) preclude the effect of factor VIII or IX concentrates. Instead, bypassing agents, i.e. activated prothrombin complex concentrates (aPCC), or recombinant FVIIa (rFVIIa) are used to treat bleeding episodes. Different immune tolerance induction regimes are in use to eliminate the inhibitor, but are not always successful. Several risk factors for inhibi-tor development have been identified, including both genetic risk factors and non-inherited risk factors. The genetic factors include certain high-risk muta-tions in the *F8* or *F9* genes, inhibitors amongst first-degree relatives, variation in some immune response genes (IL-10, TNF-α) and Native American or African ethnicity.[3] Non-inherited risk factors are less well documented. Proposed risk factors are age at first exposure, immunologic challenge at the time of early factor substitution (e.g. infections or recent vaccinations), continuous infusion in mild hemophilia and type of factor concentrate.

Factor concentrates as a cause of inhibitor development has only been documented for two intermediate plasma-derived FVIII concentrates that had undergone a combined solvent–detergent and pasteurization process, which altered the antigenic presentation of the C2 domains in the FVIII molecule.[5] Apart from that, any proposed difference in risk of inhibitor development between plasma-derived and recombinant factor concentrates has not been proven in sufficiently powered controlled prospective trials.[6,7]

The genes and their mutations

Both the *F8* and *F9* genes are located on the long arm of the X chromosome at Xq28 and Xq27, respectively. *F8* spans 186 kb long and is comprised of 26 exons, ranging in size from exon 5 with 69 bp to the large exon 14 of approximately 3.1 kb.[8] The *F9* gene is much smaller with eight exons spanning 33.5 kb.[8,9]

Most common mutations

Hemophilia A
More than 800 different mutations have been described and can be found in the HAMSTeRS database (http://europium.csc.mrc.ac.uk) and in the Human Mutation database (http://archive.uwcm.ac.uk/uwcm/mg/hgmd0.html). The most common mutation is the inversion of exon 1 to exon 22 found in 45% of patients with severe hemophilia A.[9,10] The second most common mutation is the inversion in intron 1 found in 2–3% of patients with severe disease.[11,12] Except for these inversions the remaining mutations are point mutations, small insertions and deletions (Table 10.1). The most common insertion/deletion is a frameshift mutation in the tract of 9As (codons 1191–1194) in exon 14 (3637_3638insA/c.3637delA p.I1194fsX5).

Hemophilia B
More than 800 unique mutations have been described (Table 10.2) which are scattered all over the *F9* gene. There is no common mutation as found for hemophilia A, although some of the mutations have been

Table 10.1 Number of unique mutations in *F8* as of September 2007 (http://archive.uwcm.ac.uk/uwcm/mg/hgmd0.html).

Type	n
Missense/nonsense	544
Splicing errors	53
Regulatory	0
Small deletions	128
Small insertions	40
Small insertion/deletions	9
Gross deletions	95
Gross insertions	7
Complex rearrangements	9

Table 10.2 Number of unique mutations in *F9* as of September 2007 (http://archive.uwcm.ac.uk/uwcm/mg/hgmd0.html).

Type	n
Missense/nonsense	539
Splicing errors	76
Regulatory	16
Small deletions	110
Small insertions	29
Small insertion/deletions	8
Gross deletions	46
Gross insertions	7
Complex rearrangements	5

found several times in different families. Some of these relatively abundant mutations might be founder mutations, particularly mutations associated with a mild course of the disease. A list of the mutations can be found in the Haemophilia B Mutation database (http://www.kcl.ac.uk/ip/petergreen/haem Bdatabase.html) and in the Human Genome Mutation Database (HGMD; http://archive.uwcm.ac.uk/uwcm/mg/hgmd0.html).

Molecular diagnosis
Knowing the mutation in a patient with hemophilia A or B is now considered part of good practice in

larger clinics. However, a molecular genetic test is not necessary for the diagnosis or further treatment. In a few rare cases with mild symptoms, molecular genetic analyses can be used for establishing the diagnosis. For carrier diagnosis, genetic counseling, prenatal diagnosis and preimplantation diagnosis, it is important to know the disease causing mutation.

The molecular diagnosis of hemophilia A is not an easy task because of the size of the *F8* gene and the high number of different mutations that are distributed throughout the gene. The analysis of *F9* is much more straightforward. Several efficient *high throughput* mutation screening methods for both genes have been published and are now performed in many laboratories.[13,14] These methods will detect point mutations and small insertions and deletions. With the introduction of multiplex ligation-dependent probe amplification (MLPA) a very simple way to detect deletions is now available, which is also important for carrier analysis.[15] The overall mutation detection rate is high at >95%.

A diagnostic approach for mutation detection in a new hemophilia A patient (or obligate carrier) should start with a long range polymerase chain reaction (PCR) for detection of the very common intron 22 inversion[16,17] followed by detection of the intron 1 inversion.[14,15] If negative, amplification of all exons and their flanking intronic regions should be performed and the PCR products investigated using a screening method such as conformation sensitive gel electrophoresis (CSGE), denaturing high-performance liquid chromatography (dHPLC) and denaturing gradient gel electrophoresis (DGGE), or the recently developed high resolution melting (HRM), followed by direct sequencing of relevant exons.[13,14,18,19] However, all these methods analyze heteroduplexes. For X-linked diseases such as hemophilia, this means that the PCR product has to be mixed with a product from a control individual in order to create such heteroduplexes.

DNA sequencing is the gold standard for mutation detection. This could be the direct approach for the *F9* gene. Automated sequencing with the use of relevant software is very reliable for both males and heterozygous females. Detection of deletion in both patients and female carriers can reliably be investigated by MLPA or real-time PCR.

Genotypic–phenotypic relationship

The two common inversions in hemophilia A are always associated with a severe disease. This is also, with a few exceptions, the case for stop mutations, frameshift mutations and splicing errors in both *F8* and *F9*, because these are invariably predicted to result in a protein that is truncated if at all synthesized.

Depending of the type of the missense mutation these are associated with severe, moderate and mild form of the diseases, but the structure–function relationships of most mutations is not known. The role of novel mutations, especially missense mutations, may therefore be difficult to interpret as disease-causing and great care has to be taken before using this knowledge in genetic counseling and carrier diagnosis. When a novel missense mutation is found, the type of amino acid change (conservative/non-conservative) and the position in the protein should be taken into consideration. Furthermore, it should be checked if the involved amino acid is conserved across species. Several software tools are available for such evaluations (Con seq; http://conseq.bioinfo.tau.ac.il and SIFT; http://blocks.fhcrc.org/sift/SIFT.html).

The individual patient's FVIII or FIX gene defect is probably the single most important risk factor for inhibitor development. In hemophilia A, mutations that completely preclude the synthesis of FVIII, i.e. large deletions, stop mutations and nonsense mutations, are associated with a higher incidence of inhibitor formation. In such patients, infused FVIII will appear as a foreign protein. Gross deletions are less common in hemophilia B. About 75% of *F9* mutations are missense and only about 25% are major gene alterations. In severe hemophilia B, a much larger proportion of patients have detectable FIX antigen, and therefore immunologic tolerance to infused factor IX, than FVIII antigen in hemophilia A. This may, at least partly, explain the much lower inhibitor incidence in hemophilia B.

Genetic counseling, prenatal and preimplantation diagnosis

Hemophilia A and B are both X-linked recessive diseases. It is generally assumed that one-third of all isolated cases would arise by a *de novo* mutation. One-third of the remaining cases are caused by a new mutation in the grandparental generation. The mothers of severe hemophiliacs with the intron 22-inversion mutation are nearly all carriers.

Carrier diagnosis is a straightforward procedure if the mutation in the family is known. However, this is not always the case. In larger families with several known patients or obligate carriers, linkage analysis is still a rather powerful method, especially to determine female carrier status. Although such studies have been superseded by direct mutation analysis, linkage analysis protocols using intragenic linked markers should be considered when the mutation has not been identified. Linkage analysis is only useful in families where a *de novo* mutation has been ruled out. It always requires involving family members, which is not always possible.

Linkage analysis is highly reliable when intragenic polymorphisms are used, and is a cheap and easy approach for countries (clinics) with a low budget and without access to more expensive methods such as direct sequencing.[20]

Linkage analysis is highly dependent on informative intragenic markers. The mother of the index case must be heterozygous for the polymorphism and often several markers have to be tested in order to find a marker. Although several very useful polymorphisms are known for both *F8* and *F9*, the heterozygosity rates vary considerably among different ethnic groups, which has to be considered.[21]

Prenatal diagnosis is possible either as a direct mutation test, if the disease-causing mutation is known, or by marker analysis if informative linked markers have been identified.

Chorionic villus biopsy is performed at 11–13 weeks' gestation. Mutation analysis as well as sex determination is usually performed within 2–3 days. Because of the greatly improved treatment of the disease during the last 10–20 years, a fetal diagnosis of hemophilia does not always lead to termination of pregnancy.

Preimplantation diagnosis (PGD) is now feasible.[22,23] This method implies *in vitro* fertilization followed by an embryo biopsy at the 6–10 cell stage. There are two approaches in PGD:

1 A single blastomere is analyzed by fluorescence *in situ* hybridization (FISH) analysis to detect the sex of the embryo, and only female embryos are transferred to the uterus.

2 Direct mutation detection using single cell PCR and transfer of unaffected male or female embryos.

Other rare bleeding disorders

Hemophilia A and B, and von Willebrand disease are the most prevalent inherited bleeding disorders, together covering about 95–97% of all inherited deficiencies of coagulation factors. The remaining defects are generally recessively inherited to both sexes. They are rare, with prevalence ranging from approximately 1 in 2 million for FII (prothrombin) and FXIII deficiency to 1 in 500,000 for FVII deficiency. Prevalence may be higher in areas with a high frequency of consanguineous marriages, e.g. FXI deficiency in some Jewish communities, and also other deficiencies in the Middle East or Southern India. Being so rare, most centers have limited experience of their management. Some large international registries have enhanced our knowledge about these rare bleeding disorders.[24–26]

In contrast to hemophilia A, where approximately 50% of the patients have the same inversion of exon 1 to exon 22, the rare inherited bleeding disorders are often caused by mutations that are specific for each family, and mutations are scattered throughout the genes. The mutations can be missense, nonsense, or insertion/deletion types or mutations in non-coding regions affecting mRNA splicing. Gross deletions or large inversion have rarely been described, but this may to some extent reflect that such gene rearrangements will often escape detection with the conventional DNA sequencing strategies used in molecular diagnostics. Indeed, conventional DNA sequencing fails to identify specific mutations in approximately 10–20% of patients with rare coagulation factor deficiencies. The Institute of Medical Genetics, Cardiff maintains a large database of mutations in coagulation factors and a comprehensive summary of mutations described up to 2002 has been provided by Peyvandi *et al.*[27] Table 10.3 shows the occurrence of different mutation types in various types of rare bleeding disorders adapted from Mannucci *et al.*[25]

Severe deficiency of coagulation factors is mostly caused by large deletions. Null mutations may result in production of truncated proteins and very low or undetectable plasma factors, and may cause severe

Table 10.3 Mutations in genes causing rare bleeding disorders (adapted January 2008 from the human gene mutation database at the Institute of Medical Genetics, Cardiff).

Coagulation factor	Frequency of homozygous deficiency[$]	Gene	Type of mutation					
			Missense/ nonsense	Small insertion/ deletion	Splicing	Gross insertion/ deletion/ rearrangement	Regulatory	Total
Fibrinogen	1:1,000,000	FGA	29	20	3	4	1	57[†]
		FGB	27	1	4	1	2	35[†]
		FGG	51	2	5	0	1	59
Prothrombin	1:2,000,000	F2	36	5	3	0	3	47[†]
V	1:1,000,000	F5	30	17	6	1	0	54[†]
VII	1:500,000	F7	104	19	21	2	10	156[*†]
X	1:1,000,000	F10	64	6	4	3	0	77
XI	1:1,000,000	F11	69	10	10	1	0	90[†]
XIII	1:2,000,000	F13A1	41	18	8	1	0	68
		F13B	2	3	0	0	0	5
V + VIII	1:2,000,000	LMAN1	5	10	5	0	0	20
		MCFD2	2	3	2	0	0	7
Vitamin K dependent	1:2,000,000	GGCX	3	1	1	0	0	5[*‡]
		VKORC1	6	0	1	0	1	8[‡]

[*] Includes one repeat variation.

[†] Rarely mutations have been detected in individuals with increased plasma concentrations or a history of thrombosis.

[‡] Mutations have also been described in individuals with altered sensitivity to warfarin.

[$] Adapted from Manucci et al. (2004).[25]

bleeding symptoms. Missense mutations are less predictable and may lead to both mild and severe deficiencies.

Fibrinogen deficiency can present as afibrinogenemia, hypofibrinogenemia or dysfibrinogenemia, depending on the causing mutation. In contrast to other rare bleeding disorders, fibrinogen disorders are often inherited as autosomal dominant traits. Some patients have a bleeding tendency, others have thrombotic tendency and some may have both.[28]

Prothrombin deficiency is either characterized by a parallel decrease of activity and antigen levels or a dysfunctional protein with normal antigen levels. There are no reported cases of aprothrombinemia, which may not be compatible with life. FV deficiency, also called Owren's disease or parahemophilia is usually a type 1 deficiency. Only one case of type 2 FV deficiency has been described. FVII deficiency is the most common of the rare bleeding disorders. Two-thirds are missense mutations. One-third are null mutations that decrease or abolish the expression of FVII. Most mild cases have missense mutations. Most severe cases have null mutations (deletions, insertions, splicing, and promoter mutations). FVII deficiency may be combined with other coagulation factor deficiencies.[29] FX deficiency is caused by missense mutations in about 75% of cases, and most cases have measurable levels of FX. Complete absence of FX is probably not compatible with life. There are no reported nonsense mutations. FXI deficiency (hemophilia C) may be caused by a nonsense mutation in exon 5 (Glu117Stop), which is frequent in Ashkenazi and Iraqi Jews. The mutation causes very low or undetectable levels of FXI in plasma in homozygotes. Another mutation, frequent in Ashkenazi Jews, is a missense mutation in exon 9 (Phe283Leu) that leads to a defective secretion, with plasma levels of FXI low but detectable at approximately 10%. Compound heterozygosity for both mutations is the most common cause of FXI deficiency among Jews.[30] Other missense mutations have been described in some European non-Jewish populations. A dominant negative effect through heterodimer formation has been described for some missense mutations. In FXIII deficiency, most mutations are located in the gene that encodes the A subunit, and only a minority in the B subunit. The mutations are spread throughout the gene and most mutations are unique.

Patients with combined FV and FVIII deficiency have a type 1 deficiency, with levels of the respective factor usually between 5% and 20%. The disorder is caused by a dysfunction in a reciprocal intracellular transport mechanism. A lectin mannose-binding protein (LMAN1, also called ERGIC-53) binds both FV and FVIII in the endoplasmic reticulum/Golgi intermediate compartment (ERGIC) and functions as chaperone in their intracellular transport. Mutations in the *LMAN1* gene cause the combined deficiency in most cases. Some cases are caused by deficiency of a cofactor to *LMAN1*, encoded by a gene called multiple coagulation factor deficiency 2 gene (*MCFD2*).

Multiple deficiency of vitamin K-dependent coagulation factors can be caused by mutations that affect the gamma-glutamyl carboxylation of vitamin K-dependent proteins. This involves not only the coagulation factors II, VII, IX and X, but also the coagulation inhibitors proteins C and S, which are all vitamin K-dependent, and also some bone proteins. The molecular basis of the multiple deficiency are missense mutations in the gamma-glutamyl carboxylase gene (*GGCX*), or in the gene vitamin K epoxide reductase complex subunit 1 (*VKORC1*), which lead to the production of a dysfunctional enzyme.[25]

Genotypic diagnosis of rare bleeding disorders is not performed routinely. There are generally no high-frequency mutations. This implies that screening the whole gene is necessary in most cases.

Internal quality control

A water blank should be included with every PCR amplification to ensure that there is no contamination of PCR reagents by exogenous DNA. No amplified product should be visible in this tube. Whenever any product is seen, all simultaneously amplified PCR products should be discarded.

PCR primers should be designed using a software program such as Primer Design-Exon Primer (http://ihg.gsf.de/ihg/ExonPrimer.html) and checked for possible single nucleotide polymorphisms within the the primer annealing sequence (http://ngrl.man.ac.uk/SNPCheck/).

When setting up analyses for the two common inversions, positive controls should always be included. If possible, DNA from patients and female carriers should be included.

Always repeat the sequencing of an amplicon in which a candidate mutation has been identified, preferably by another method, e.g. restriction enzyme analysis. A second scientist should independently check sequences, nucleotide number and base change and its predicted effect on the protein. When analyzing family members for a previously identified mutation, include a familial positive control plus a normal control lacking the familial mutation.

When a sequence alteration is identified, use the relevant database to see if the mutation has been described before. If the mution is new, be sure to name it according to the Human Genome Variation Society (HGVS; http://www.genomic.unimelb.edu.au/mdi/mutnomen/). Nucleotide numbering should follow these rules that "A" in initiation codon ATG = +1. To convert to HGVS-type aminoacid numbering in FVIII (where initiator Met = +1) to the more common universal numbering add 20 to negative numbers below and 19 to positive numbers, e.g. Met–19 becomes Met+1 but Arg+3 becomes Arg+22. For FIX add 47 to the negative numbers and 46 to the positive numbers, e.g. Arg –4 becomes Arg43, but Gly+4 becomes Gly50.

If a sequence alteration is suspected to have an effect on mRNA splicing, a number of prediction tools are available and the use of the number of these tools in combination is recommended before suggesting that an effect on splicing is likely; these include Fruit Fly (http://www.fruitfly.org/seq_tools/splice.html), NetGene2 (http://www.cbs.dtu.dk/services/

NetGene2/) and Splice Site Finder (http://violin.genet.
sickkids.on.ca/~ali/splicesitefinder.html). Where an
effect on splicing is likely, follow-up by cDNA analysis can often confirm the prediction, but this usually
not possible in a routine setting up.

External quality assessment

Among the few external quality assessment (EQA)
schemes available for molecular testing in hemophilia,
the UK National External Quality Assessment Scheme
(NEQAS) for Blood Coagulation on Haemophilia
Genetics is one example. This scheme runs twice-
yearly exercises that alternate between hemophilia A,
hemophilia B and VWD. As with other molecular
genetic EQA schemes, the three areas of clerical accuracy, genotyping and interpretation are examined
(http://www.ukneqasbc.org/content/PageServer.asp?S
=932234149&C=1252&ID=32). Marks are lost for
errors in each of these three areas.

Reporting

Develop standard templates for commonly used
report types to avoid missing essential information.
Reports should be written so that they can follow the
patient and be interpreted by a number of different
healthcare professionals.

Nomenclature

Nucleotide and amino acid numbering, and nomenclature for sequence alterations should follow HGVS
recommendations (http://www.hgvs.org/mutnomen/).
GenBank reference sequences with version numbers
should be stated for both cDNA and protein (Ref.seq:
NM_000132 [*F8*] and ref.seq: NM_000133 [*F9*]).

References

1 Saenko EL, Ananyeva NM, Tuddenham EG, Kemball-
Cook G. Factor VIII: novel insights into form and function. *Br J Haematol* 2002; **119**: 323–331.

2 Schmidt AE, Bajaj SP. Structure–function relationships
in factor IX and factor IXa. *Trends Cardiovasc Med*
2003; **13**: 39–45.

3 Oldenburg J, Pavlova A. Genetic risk factors for inhibitors to factors VIII and IX. *Haemophilia* 2006; **12** (Suppl
6): 15–22.

4 DiMichele D. Inhibitor development in haemophilia B:
an orphan disease in need of attention. *Br J Haematol*
2007; **138**: 305–315.

5 Peerlinck K, Arnout J, Di Giambattista M, *et al*. Factor
VIII inhibitors in previously treated haemophilia A
patients with a double virus-inactivated plasma derived
factor VIII concentrate. *Thromb Haemost* 1997; **77**:
80–86.

6 Hoots WK. Urgent inhibitor issues: targets for expanded
research. *Haemophilia* 2006; **12** (Suppl 6): 107–113.

7 Hay CR. The epidemiology of factor VIII inhibitors.
Haemophilia 2006; **12** (Suppl 6): 23–28; discussion
28–29.

8 Gitschier J, Wood WI, Goralka TM, *et al*. Characterization of the human factor VIII gene. *Nature* 1984; **312**:
326–330.

9 Kurachi K, Davie EW. Isolation and characterization of
a cDNA coding for human factor IX. *Proc Natl Acad
Sci U S A* 1982; **79**: 6461–6464.

10 Antonarakis SE, Rossiter JP, Young M, *et al*. Factor VIII
gene inversions in severe hemophilia A: results of an
international consortium study. *Blood* 1995; **86**:
2206–2212.

11 Bagnall RD, Waseem N, Green PM, Giannelli F. Recurrent inversion breaking intron 1 of the factor VIII gene
is a frequent cause of severe hemophilia A. *Blood* 2002;
99: 168–174.

12 Cumming AM. The factor VIII gene intron 1 inversion
mutation: prevalence in severe hemophilia A patients in
the UK. *J Thromb Haemost* 2004; **2**: 205–206.

13 Jayandharan G, Shaji RV, Chandy M, Srivastava A.
Identification of factor IX gene defects using a multiplex
PCR and CSGE strategy – a first report. *J Thromb
Haemost* 2003; **1**: 2051–2054.

14 Habart D, Kalabova D, Novotny M, Vorlova Z. Thirty-
four novel mutations detected in factor VIII gene by
multiplex CSGE: modeling of 13 novel amino acid substitutions. *J Thromb Haemost* 2003; **1**: 773–781.

15 Schouten JP, McElgunn CJ, Waaijer R, Zwijnenburg D,
Diepvens F, Pals G. Relative quantification of 40 nucleic
acid sequences by multiplex ligation-dependent probe
amplification. *Nucleic Acids Res* 2002; **30**: e57.

16 Bowen DJ, Keeney S. Unleashing the long-distance PCR
for detection of the intron 22 inversion of the factor VIII
gene in severe haemophilia A. *Thromb Haemost* 2003;
89: 201–202.

17 Liu Q, Nozari G, Sommer SS. Single-tube polymerase
chain reaction for rapid diagnosis of the inversion
hotspot of mutation in hemophilia A. *Blood* 1998; **92**:
1458–1459.

18 Frusconi S, Passerini I, Girolami F, *et al.* Identification of seven novel mutations of F8C by DHPLC. *Hum Mutat* 2002; **20**: 231–232.

19 Jayandharan G, Shaji RV, Baidya S, Nair SC, Chandy M, Srivastava A. Identification of factor VIII gene mutations in 101 patients with haemophilia A: mutation analysis by inversion screening and multiplex PCR and CSGE and molecular modelling of 10 novel missense substitutions. *Haemophilia* 2005; **11**: 481–491.

20 Peyvandi F. Carrier detection and prenatal diagnosis of hemophilia in developing countries. *Semin Thromb Hemost* 2005; **31**: 544–554.

21 Peake IR, Lillicrap DP, Boulyjenkov V, *et al.* Haemophilia: strategies for carrier detection and prenatal diagnosis. *Bull World Health Organ* 1993; **71**: 429–458.

22 Gigarel N, Frydman N, Burlet P, *et al.* Single cell co-amplification of polymorphic markers for the indirect preimplantation genetic diagnosis of hemophilia A, X-linked adrenoleukodystrophy, X-linked hydrocephalus and incontinentia pigmenti loci on Xq28. *Hum Genet* 2004; **114**: 298–305.

23 Michaelides K, Tuddenham EG, Turner C, Lavender B, Lavery SA. Live birth following the first mutation specific pre-implantation genetic diagnosis for haemophilia A. *Thromb Haemost* 2006; **95**: 373–379.

24 Peyvandi F, Jayandharan G, Chandy M, *et al.* Genetic diagnosis of haemophilia and other inherited bleeding disorders. *Haemophilia* 2006; **12** (Suppl 3): 82–89.

25 Mannucci PM, Duga S, Peyvandi F. Recessively inherited coagulation disorders. *Blood* 2004; **104**: 1243–1252.

26 Acharya SS, Coughlin A, Dimichele DM. Rare Bleeding Disorder Registry: deficiencies of factors II, V, VII, X, XIII, fibrinogen and dysfibrinogenemias. *J Thromb Haemost* 2004; **2**: 248–256.

27 Peyvandi F, Duga S, Akhavan S, Mannucci PM. Rare coagulation deficiencies. *Haemophilia* 2002; **8**: 308–321.

28 Asselta R, Duga S, Tenchini ML. The molecular basis of quantitative fibrinogen disorders. *J Thromb Haemost* 2006; **4**: 2115–2129.

29 Girolami A, Ruzzon E, Tezza F, Allemand E, Vettore S. Congenital combined defects of factor VII: a critical review. *Acta Haematol* 2007; **117**: 51–56.

30 Franchini M, Veneri D, Lippi G. Inherited factor XI deficiency: a concise review. *Hematology* 2006; **11**: 307–309.

11 Standardization of D-dimer testing

G. Reber & P. de Moerloose

The rationale of D-dimer measurement as an indicator of coagulation activation and fibrin digestion was provided by the studies of Gaffney[1] more than 30 years ago. Until monoclonal antibodies were available, fibrin and fibrinogen degradation products were measured in serum, mainly with either polyclonal antifibrinogen antibodies or with the staphylococcal clumping test. The results of these tests were obscured by many artefacts.[2] In the early 1980s, monoclonal antibodies obtained by immunization with D-dimer were raised, and this was the milestone of a novel area in hemostasis.[3] Indeed, monoclonal antibodies allow the measurement of soluble fibrin fragments (even in the presence of fibrinogen and its degradation products), opening new insights in the coagulation and fibrinolysis fields. In particular, D-dimer measurement provided an important contribution to the diagnostic work-up of venous thromboembolic (VTE) disease[4] and disseminated intravascular coagulation (DIC).[5,6] The test is now widely used in clinical laboratories and there are more than 30 assays available designed in various assay formats, using more than 20 monoclonal antibodies. The numerical assay results can vary widely among assays because in patients' plasma the analyte is highly heterogeneous and the specificity of the monoclonal antibodies differs depending on if the mixture of fragments in the sample or the calibrators are different.[7] Because

the efforts for standardization of the assays were unsuccessful,[8] harmonization procedures have been proposed.[9–12] This is an important issue particularly because each commercial assay has its own cut-off value for VTE exclusion that may confuse clinicians. In the DIC field, clinical scores have been proposed by the International Society of Thrombosis and Haemostasis (ISTH)[5] and the Japanese Ministry of Health and Welfare for overt DIC[6] in which a D-dimer value is included. However, as shown by a recent study,[11] the numerical value of a patient's sample may differ by about 20 times depending on the assay used. As a consequence, the amount of points related to D-dimer value computed in the patient's DIC score may range from 0 to 3.[5,6]

Heterogeneity of D-dimer containing fragments

After thrombin removal of the fibrinopeptide A, the N-terminal sequence of the α-chain becomes the site of polymerization in fibrinogen domain E. This polymerization site interacts with a corresponding site located in the D domain of another fibrin or fibrinogen molecule.[13] The double-stranded fibrin polymer grows and results in a protofibril. The lateral association of the protofibrils forms fibrin fibrils. Each γ chain contains two binding sites in the appendage linked to the D domain. Thrombin activation of factor XIII is catalyzed by polymerized fibrin. Upon factor XIII action, two covalent bonds form between adjacent D domains which result in cross-linked fibrin. The velocity of the

Quality in Laboratory Hemostasis and Thrombosis, 1st edition. By Steve Kitchen, John D. Olson and F. Eric Preston. Published 2009 by Blackwell Publishing. ISBN: 978-1-4051-6803-8

polymerization process, which is a function of fibrinogen and thrombin concentrations, governs the structure of the polymers. Because the presence of two cross-linking sites per γ chain, in addition to D-dimers, D-trimers and D-tetramers, are formed which ensure the branching between adjacent fibrin fibrils.[14]

Fibrin catalyzes plasminogen conversion to plasmin by tissue plasminogen activator (tPA), which results in localized fibrinolytic activity. Therefore, fibrin formation and breakdown occurs concomitantly and part of the fibrin measured consists of soluble plasmin-degraded fibrin. Patients' plasma samples contain a mixture of intravascular and extravascular clot derived fibrin as well as circulating soluble fibrin including D-dimer, D-trimers and D-tetramer motifs.[15] The terminal product of plasmin digestion is the fragment D-dimer whose molecular weight is about 195 kDa. In the circulation it is found as a complex with fragment E (DD/E).[16,17] Because of the variable degree of plasmin proteolysis, patients' plasma samples contain a mixture of fibrin fragment complexes containing one or several D-dimer motifs whose molecular weights range from 228 kDa (DD/E) to several thousands KDa (X-olimers).[8] In addition, fibrinogen (as shown by the presence of fibrinopeptide A) is also found in high molecular weight fibrin fragments.[18] As shown in Fig. 11.1, the current "D-dimer measurement" means a mixture of D-dimer containing fibrin fragments measurement.

Specificity of monoclonal antibodies directed to D-dimer motif

The first monoclonal antibody (3B6/22) was reported by Rylatt et al. in 1983.[3] Since then more than 20 monoclonal antibodies have been developed. In theory, they should react minimally with fibrinogen or fibrinogen degradation products. In addition, they should not react with fibrin and fibrinogen fragments from elastase proteolysis.[19] The assay format is important because proper combination of two monoclonal antibodies (catcher and tag) displaying some cross-reactivity with fibrinogen degradation products may paradoxically result in an enzyme-linked immunosorbent assay (ELISA) specific for cross-linked fibrin degradation products.[20]

The characterization of differences between the commercial tests concerning analyte reactivity has been studied in depth in the FACT study.[10] In this study, 23 quantitative D-dimer assays were evaluated in order to develop common calibrators. The 39 patients' samples were measured with six ELISA, 15 latex-enhanced photometric immunoassays and two membrane-based immunoassays. Depending on the assay, the mean values for the 39 samples varied from 0.63 µg/mL (range 0.01–3.42 µg/mL) to 13.35 µg/mL (range 0.07–258 µg/mL). Increasing amounts of tPA digested cross-linked fibrin diluted into normal plasma were measured with all assays. The slope of the response differed widely between assays (from 1 to 48). When replacing cross-linked fibrin by fibrinogen degradation products, two assays gave a high response indicating marked cross-reactivity with fragment D. Slopes of dilutions of plasma pools from DIC and deep venous thrombosis (DVT) patients into normal plasma differed between assays and for some assays between the two pools. To evaluate the response of assays to the type of fibrin species, high molecular weight fibrin (HMWF) was extracted from DIC pool and diluted into normal plasma. The slopes obtained varied from 1 to 5. This HMWF material was digested with plasmin in order to obtain low molecular weight cross-linked fibrin (LMWF) and was tested in the same way. The ratio of the slopes (native HMWF:plasmin-treated HMWF) showed that some assays react better to HMWF whereas others perform better with LMWF. This suggests that plasmin treatment may reveal additional epitopes that are the preferred target of some assays, especially ELISA type. Conversely, longer fibrin fragments could favor particle agglutination in latex-enhanced immunoassays because of the distance between latex particles.[10]

Calibrators for D-dimer assays

Manufacturers of D-dimer assays choose the type of calibrator that fits best with their assay. The majority of assays are calibrated with material obtained by controlled lysis of fibrin clots. Accordingly, calibrators' concentrations are often expressed as the amount of fibrinogen present in the mixture used to prepare the calibrator material. Thus, results may be expressed as fibrinogen equivalent units (FEU; µg/L).

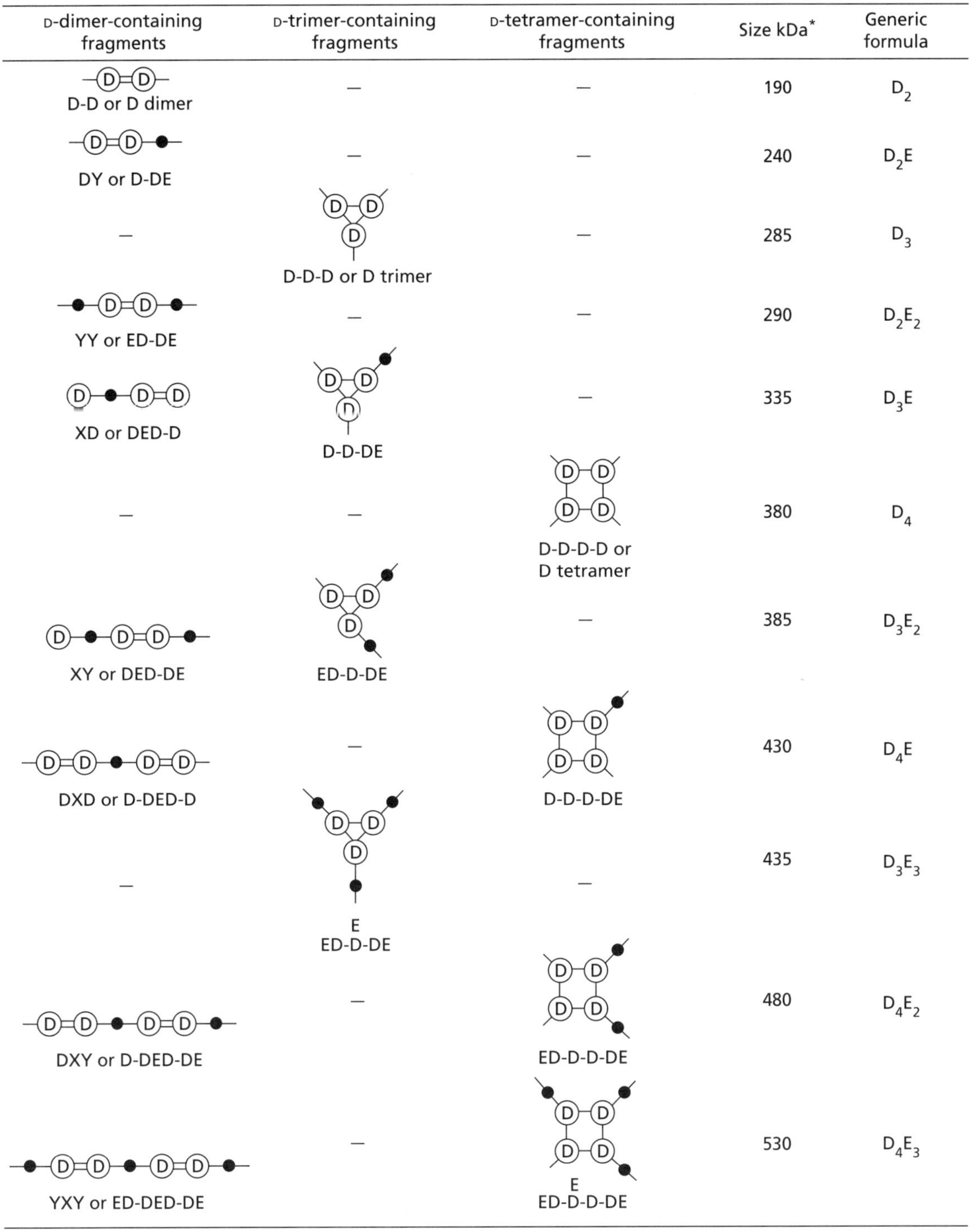

D-dimer-containing fragments	D-trimer-containing fragments	D-tetramer-containing fragments	Size kDa*	Generic formula
D-D or D dimer	—	—	190	D_2
DY or D-DE	—	—	240	D_2E
—	D-D-D or D trimer	—	285	D_3
YY or ED-DE	—	—	290	D_2E_2
XD or DED-D	D-D-DE	—	335	D_3E
—	—	D-D-D-D or D tetramer	380	D_4
XY or DED-DE	ED-D-DE	—	385	D_3E_2
DXD or D-DED-D	—	D-D-D-DE	430	D_4E
—	E ED-D-DE	—	435	D_3E_3
DXY or D-DED-DE	—	ED-D-D-DE	480	D_4E_2
YXY or ED-DED-DE	—	E ED-D-D-DE	530	D_4E_3

* Assumed sizes for monomolecular core constituents: E [—●—], 50 kDa; D [—Ⓓ], 95 kDa; Y [—●—Ⓓ], 145 kDa; X [Ⓓ—●—Ⓓ], 240 kDa

Fig. 11.1 Macromolecular fragments from plasmic digests of cross-linked fibrin. From Mosesson.[15]

Experimental conditions have to be carefully controlled in order to ensure the reproducibility of the mixture (HMWF and LMWF) in the final product. Some assays are calibrated with purified fibrin fragment D-dimer equivalents. Again, the experimental conditions of the purification have to be carefully controlled to avoid variability in antibody response.[21] According to their respective molecular weight (340 and 195 kDa), D-dimer values expressed in FEU should theoretically be about twice as high as those expressed in D-dimer units. However, it has to be taken into account that fibrin digests do not only contain D-dimer fragments but also HMWF depending on the lysis procedure. One assay is calibrated with plasma pools with different D-dimer levels prepared from DIC patients' samples.[22]

In the FACT study,[10] all assays were calibrated with:
1 Terminal fibrin fragments;
2 HMWF fragments; or
3 Dilutions of DIC patients' plasma pools in normal plasma.
Individual patients' plasma ($n = 39$) were measured with the three calibration curves. With terminal fibrin fragments, one assay could not be calibrated and two others overestimated patients' samples. Calibration with HMWF fragments resulted in either underestimation (three assays) or overestimation (three assays) of samples values. Calibration with DIC patients' plasma resulted in a better uniformity. When DIC plasma cannot be used, calibration with HMWF fragments is preferred because they mirror better the mixture contained in patients' samples as compared with terminal fibrin fragments.

Standardization of D-dimer assays

The first attempt towards D-dimer assay standardization was conducted by the National Institute for Biological Standard and Control (NIBSC).[8] Purified D-dimer preparations from three laboratories as well as a preparation of HMWF fragments were tested with three monoclonal antibodies. If the same epitopes were present on the different fragments then binding would be similar and standardization of measurements might be easier. Two antibodies bound similarly to all preparations immobilized on polyvinyl chloride wells, whereas the binding of the third one varied widely depending on the preparation. When tested as catcher antibodies in an ELISA format, two showed marked differences in the response to the four preparations whereas the responses of the third were more comparable. These data rule out the possibility that the same epitopes would be present irrespective of the type of fibrin fragments.

From a formal perspective, a standardization process has to meet some requirements. The analyte to be measured has to be fully characterized. Obviously, this cannot be the case for D-dimer assays because the analyte in plasma samples is a mixture of fibrin degradation products containing different structures and a wide range of molecular weights. Therefore, this heterogeneity precludes the preparation of a primary standard. This heterogeneity and the various responses of monoclonal antibodies (and their combinations) impede the establishment of a reference method. That is why a less stringent approach was tested, known as the harmonization procedure. This approach was, for example, applied successfully to the prothrombin time for monitoring oral anticoagulation and resulted, despite some limitations, in the worldwide accepted International Normalized Ratio (INR).

Harmonization of D-dimer assays

Harmonization relies on the use of a mathematical model in order to render the results obtained with different assays more comparable.

The first attempt was conducted in the framework of the Scientific and Standardization Committee of the ISTH.[9] The goal was to investigate whether it was possible to establish an international reference material (not a standard) for the harmonization of D-dimer assays. Two plasma pools from 20 patients with various diseases were prepared (i.e. not only patients with VTE or DIC). A third pool was prepared by mixing equal volumes of the two pools. These pools were tested with five D-dimer assays (four microplate ELISA and one microlatex) from four manufacturers. For each pool, the average of the numerical values obtained by each assay was computed and assigned as "pool consensus" value (Table 11.1). For each assay, the numerical result

Table 11.1 Reported values (mean ± SD) per assay (in µg/mL) and consensus values of the pools. After Nieuwenhuizen.[9]

Assay	1	2	3	4	5	Consensus
Pool						
A	6.22 ± 0.21	1.24 ± 0.30	7.80 ± 0.01	1.46 ± 0.04	1.21 ± 0.04	3.60
B	2.15 ± 0.06	0.31 ± 0.02	2.31 ± 0.02	0.63 ± 0.01	0.48 ± 0.01	1.24
C	3.94 ± 0.04	0.65 ± 0.14	5.24 ± 0.05	1.20 ± 0.06	0.88 ± 0.01	2.46

Table 11.2 Ratio of the consensus over the reported values. After Nieuwenhuizen.[9]

Assay	Pool	Ratio	Mean ± SD
1	A	0.58	0.59 ± 0.02
	B	0.58	
	C	0.62	
2	A	2.90	3.56 ± 0.48
	B	4.00	
	C	3.78	
3	A	0.46	0.49 ± 0.04
	B	0.54	
	C	0.47	
4	A	2.47	2.16 ± 0.22
	B	1.97	
	C	2.05	
5	A	2.98	2.79 ± 0.16
	B	2.18	
	C	2.80	

obtained with each pool was divided by the corresponding "pool consensus" value, and the three values (corresponding to the three pools) were averaged (Table 11.2). To ascertain whether this model, based on pool measurements, was applicable at individual level, the 40 samples used to prepare the pools were measured. Results were processed with the same model, i.e. 40 "sample consensus" values were computed and each sample result was divided by the corresponding "sample consensus" value. For each assay, these 40 "individually harmonized values" were plotted against the values obtained by dividing the 40 original results by the mean value of the three pools ("pool harmonized values"). The squared regression coefficient values ranged from 0.7 to 0.92. From this study it was concluded that a conversion factor, computed from patients' plasma pools, rendered comparable individual D-dimer numerical results obtained with different assays and that this conversion factor was independent of a pool.[9]

A second attempt at harmonization has been reported in the framework of the FACT study.[10] The approach differed somewhat from that of Nieuwenhuizen because individual samples were used instead of plasma pools. In addition, median instead of mean values were used for the computation of conversion factors. As already mentioned, 39 samples were tested with 23 assays, including ELISA, microlatex-enhanced and membrane-based D-dimer assays. A conversion factor was computed using the median of the median values obtained for each sample with all assays, and for each assay the median value obtained with all samples. Multiplication of the individual sample assay result with the assay-specific conversion factor led to an adjustment of the scales of the assays. The median values of these converted values for each individual sample were used as a single sample consensus value (SSCV). As shown in Table 11.3, the correlation of the between-individual assay results and the corresponding SSCV were analyzed by regression analysis and by Spearman rank correlation. Good correlations were observed with most assays, especially when Spearman rho coefficient was considered because it attenuated the influence of outliers and ceiling effects in some assays.

Table 11.3 Mean, median, minimum and maximum values of 39 clinical samples. Conversion factor, linear correlation with median of converted values of samples, including y-intercept, slope and numerical coefficient of correlation and Spearman rank correlation rho of individual assay results with the single sample consensus value (SSCV). After Dempfle et al.[10]

Assay	Mean (µg/mL)	Median (µg/mL)	Min (µg/mL)	Max (µg/mL)	Conversion factor	Linear correlation with SSCV			Spearman rank correlation coefficient rho
						y-intercept	Slope	Regression coefficient R^2	
AGEN Dimertest Gold	0.63	0.41	0.01	3.42	4.95	0.260	0.106	0.842	0.963
BioMérieux Vidas D-dimer	3.52	3.54	0.09	30.00	0.57	3.256	0.660	0.353	0.843
Biopool TintElize D-dimer	3.49	0.91	0.04	50.56	2.10	−0.890	1.278	0.970	0.969
Dade Behring Enzygnost D-dimer	1.31	0.49	0.01	19.73	3.99	−0.339	0.489	0.947	0.892
Organon Teknika Fibrinostika FbDP	8.42	2.29	<0.22	98.02	0.90	−1.908	3.017	0.962	0.883
Stago Asserachrom D-dimer	9.76	4.17	0.13	86.95	0.49	1.160	2.513	0.864	0.802
AGEN Autolatex D-dimer	1.22	0.81	<0.065	>2.00	2.48	0.635	0.170	0.579	0.955
Biopool AutoDimer LPIA	3.43	1.09	0.02	50.00	1.89	−0.834	1.247	0.964	0.984
Biopool Miniquanr D-dimer	3.53	1.54	0.01	57.98	1.32	−0.264	1.108	0.687	0.968
Dade Behring D-dimer PLUS	1.06	0.46	0.06	12.04	4.29	−0.005	0.312	0.982	0.916
Dade Behring Advanced D-dimer	9.20	4.18	0.53	103.00	0.48	0.104	2.657	0.981	0.921
Dade Behring Turbiquant D-dimer	1.13	0.65	<0.20	6.28	3.03	0.537	0.173	0.695	0.963
Diamed D-dimer LPIA	3.61	1.59	<0.10	43.50	1.30	−0.217	1.117	0.980	0.963
Helena D-dimer LPIA	1.47	1.1	0.01	5.58	1.82	1.091	0.107	0.233	0.972
Iatron D-dimer LPIA	11.35	5.15	0.10	123.80	0.33	1.983	2.677	0.816	0.938
Instrumentation Laboratories IL-Test D-dimer ACL	3.77	1.62	0.16	40.24	1.25	−0.211	1.164	0.991	0.993
Instrumentation Laboratories IL-Test D-dimer TurbILab	4.87	1.32	0.01	63.87	1.46	−1.081	1.737	0.988	0.978
AGEN Autolatex D-dimer LPIA, Organon Teknika Thrombolyzer	0.99	0.89	0.05	2.97	2.35	0.690	0.088	0.557	0.975
Organon Teknika MDA D-dimer	13.35	1.52	0.07	258.00	1.34	−8.927	6.508	0.941	0.928
Roche Diagnostics TINAquant D-dimer	5.95	3.01	0.10	35.69	0.57	2.107	1.122	0.877	0.948
Stago STA LIATest D-dimer	9.06	3.37	<0.22	89.50	0.60	−0.003	2.648	0.915	0.794
Nycomed Nycocard D-dimer	3.08	1.40	<0.10	30.00	1.49	0.309	0.809	0.963	0.975
Roche Diagnostics Cardiac Reader D-dimer	4.12	3.20	<0.10	10.00	0.55	3.629	0.188	0.064	0.815

Table 11.4 Method-specific consensus values (ng/mL ± SEM) of eight different D-dimer methods of five different samples (A–E). After Meijer *et al.*[11]

Method/sample	n	A	B	C	D	E
BioMérieux Vidas D-dimer	52	321 ± 8.2	655 ± 11.2	942 ± 14.7	2409 ± 32.3	4118 ± 44.8
BioMérieux Latex	25	64 ± 12.8	212 ± 38.8	251 ± 12.0	978 ± 112.8	1235 ± 24.9
Dade Behring D-dimer PLUS	75	28 ± 3.5	56 ± 3.0	88 ± 3.0	230 ± 2.9	421 ± 5.7
Dade Behring Turbiquant	16	11 ± 6.2	35 ± 7.9	89 ± 9.4	328 ± 26.4	638 ± 41.6
Diagnostica Stago	50	40.2 ± 11.2	945 ± 11.0	1336 ± 14.8	2863 ± 34.7	5551 ± 202
IL D-dimer	35	118 ± 9.3	269 ± 9.8	413 ± 52.9	1197 ± 52.9	2159 ± 97.4
Nycomed Nycocard D-dimer	60	212 ± 29.7	246 ± 33.9	454 ± 57.7	1089 ± 71.5	2004 ± 105
Roche Tinaquant	65	522 ± 11.7	1155 ± 13.9	1677 ± 18.0	4282 ± 42.0	7480 ± 76.5
Overall median value	252	425	736	1733	2816	

A third procedure for D-dimer results harmonization has been proposed.[11] This model takes into account the possible variation among test results and consensus values at different D-dimer levels. It relies on the transformation of an assay-specific regression line to a reference regression line, both obtained by measuring a set of five samples. These samples were prepared by dilutions of a patient's plasma pool (n = 50) into normal plasma. These samples were distributed to participants (n = 502) of the external quality control surveys of the European Concerted Action on Thrombosis Foundation and the German INSTAND Institute. After outlier exclusion, seven methods were analyzed. The mean value for each sample with each method was computed (Table 11.4). For each sample, the median values of the mean values obtained with the seven assays were plotted against the amount of pool added in order to obtain the reference line. For each assay, the mean values of each sample were also plotted against the amount of pool added in order to obtain the assay-specific line (Fig. 11.2). Using the slope (b) and the intercept (a) of the assay-specific line (A) and the reference line (H), the harmonized results (Y_H) can be computed from the measured result (Y_A) with the following equation:

$$Y_H = a_H \left[\frac{Y_A - b_A}{a_A} \right] b_H$$

Using this model, the between-assays coefficient of variations of the five plasma measured showed a dramatic decrease (Table 11.5). This model applies

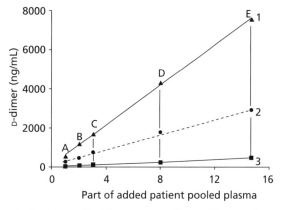

Fig. 11.2 Example of harmonization by transforming the regression line through the method-specific consensus values (1, Roche Tinaquant; 3, Dade Behring D-dimer PLUS to the regression line through the overall median values [2], using the residual slope and intercept of both regression equations). A–E, calibrator samples. After Meijer *et al.*[11]

to the whole measuring range of the assays provided that a linear relationship is obtained. Further validation of this model with more assay systems is necessary.

Another procedure for D-dimer results harmonization has been tested in the framework of the UK National External Quality Assessment Scheme (NEQAS) surveys.[12] Five samples were distributed to more than 500 participants. For statistical reasons, only assays ($n = 9$) used by more than 10 participants were taken into account, the results of three assays being expressed in FEU and the others in ng/mL. Three of the samples served as calibrators and two served as test samples. For these three samples, individual laboratory results were plotted against the median values obtained with all methods. All but three laboratories had correlation coefficients $r > 0.95$. The values obtained with the two tests samples by each laboratory were converted in harmonized values using the laboratory's own regression line. As shown in Table 11.6, this model resulted in an important decrease in coefficients of variation compared to those obtained with the original values. Unfortunately, the model was applied separately to assays calibrated in D-dimer ng/mL and to assays calibrated in FEU and therefore it cannot be ascertained whether this model can be generalized to all kinds of assays.

New studies on harmonization of D-dimer results are ongoing.

Problems in daily practice

The lack of standardization and/or harmonization of D-dimer results may be misleading in daily laboratory and clinical practice, particularly because of the different cut-off values and units among assays. In a European survey, nearly 90% of laboratories used D-dimer assay for the exclusion of VTE, 52% for diagnosis and monitoring of DIC, this test being available 24 h/day in 81% of laboratories.[23] A recent D-dimer proficiency testing by the College of American Pathologists showed that many laboratories were unclear about the units they reported (8% of

Table 11.5 Coefficients of variation for the method-specific consensus values of all methods included before and after harmonization for the five different plasma samples. After Meijer et al.[11]

Sample	Overall median value (ng/mL)	Before harmonization (%)	After harmonization (%)
A	252	91.0	18.2
B	425	92.3	7.4
C	736	86.8	6.1
D	1733	83.6	5.9
E	2816	82.3	1.5

Table 11.6 Improvement in between-center agreement after calibration. Overall results. After Jennings et al.[12]

	Sample D6			Sample D7		
	N	Median (ng/mL)	CV (%)	N	Median (ng/mL)	CV (%)
Fibrinogen equivalent units						
Original data	118	1252	25.9	116	950	22.4
Original data (outliers removed)	118	1252	25.9	115	960	22.0
All calibrated data	118	1162	11.6	116	918	8.9
Calibrated data, $r > 0.95$	118	1162	11.6	116	918	8.9
Calibrated data, $r > 0.95$, outliers removed	118	1161	11.6	115	920	7.7
Non-fibrinogen equivalent units						
Original data	302	411	45.3	302	348	40.8
Original data (outliers removed)	293	412	45.3	294	350	39.8
All calibrated data	302	427	34.3	302	356	111.5
Calibrated data, $r > 0.95$	299	426	22.7	299	356	13.0
Calibrated data, $r > 0.95$, outliers removed	293	427	21.6	284	358	11.6

CV, coefficient of variation.

laboratories did not know the type of units they were using).[24] The cut-off value for VTE exclusion is also a matter of concern; in this survey more than one-third of laboratories (488/1506) reported VTE cut-off values above those recommended by the manufacturer or by the literature (10–71% of the recommended value) which probably results in erroneous exclusion of VTE in patients. In the European survey, 55% of participants reported VTE cut-off values higher and 24% lower than the recommended cut-off. This can be explained in part by the fact that some manufacturers recommend the assessment of a local cut-off, although such a task is usually above the possibilities of small hospitals and private laboratories. In addition, for several assays, prospective validation studies are not available because in some countries such trials are not a precondition for launching tests into the market.[23] Depending on the prevalence of VTE in the population referred to the diagnostic center, several hundreds of patients suspected of VTE have to be tested in order to determine the VTE exclusion cut-off. The established cut-off has then to be validated in a prospective study, with a similar number of patients, based on the local diagnostic decision scheme; patients in whom anticoagulation is withheld on the basis of D-dimer (and possibly other criteria) have to be followed during several months to exclude an ulterior VTE. When testing D-dimer with closed assay systems (such as VIDAS, Stratus, AxSYM and others) or with the couple reagent/device from the same manufacturer, cut-off values indicated in the reagent insert should be used, provided that there is no significant batch-to-batch variability and that accurate validation studies have been conducted to assess it. When using reagents and devices from different manufacturers, the recommended cut-off should be carefully checked because of the possible effect of the device on assay results. With closed systems, within- and between-laboratories coefficients of variation, as found in reports of external quality control surveys, are useful tools to estimate the analytical performances of the assays.

For DIC categorization and monitoring, the absence of standardization and/or harmonization of D-dimer results obscures the adequate use of clinical scores. In both the ISTH and Japanese scores, D-dimer values contribute from zero to three points.[5,6] No point is added for D-dimer values ≤1.0 µg/mL

in the ISTH score and for <10 µg/mL in the Japanese one. In the Japanese score, one point is added for D-dimer values ≥10 and ≤25 µg/mL but two points in the 1.0–5.0 µg/mL range in the ISTH score. Three points correspond to values >5.0 µg/mL in the ISTH and 25 µg/mL in the Japanese scores, respectively. It has to be noted that for both scores no precision is given about the test to be used, which is critical when we know that numerical D-dimer values may vary as many as 20 times depending on the assay used.[11] Therefore, users of assay systems yielding relatively low D-dimer values are likely to underscore the Japanese score and users of assays yielding high values will overestimate the ISTH score. Harmonization of D-dimer results would provide some uniformity to D-dimer contribution in DIC scores even if the mathematical model used yields up to 20% variability in numerical values.

Conclusions

The availability of assays able to measure cross-linked fibrin fragments in the presence of fibrinogen and its degradation products has been an important step for clinical laboratories and a useful tool for diagnostic purposes. Unfortunately, the numerical results of D-dimer measurements obtained with various assays are different because of the nature of the analyte to be measured, the diversity of monoclonal antibodies and the calibration process. For these reasons, standardization of D-dimer assay is unlikely. In order to attain a better comparability of results, harmonization procedures appear as valuable surrogates. However, it is important to keep in mind that they carry some inherent imprecision and that the assessment of an unique cut-off value for VTE exclusion for all assays seems more particularly difficult because of the potential consequences of a false negative result which may be life-threatening. In contrast, the relative imprecision of harmonization procedures seems more acceptable for clinical scores such as those used for DIC patients. With the present assays the values measured in a high positive sample may vary from 2.97 µg/mL to 258 µg/mL (Table 11.3); even if harmonization induces a variation as high as 20%, this is far better than any result obtained without harmonization.

These harmonization procedures have to be validated with a large number of samples. This should be performed in collaboration with the manufacturers. If scientists and manufacturers agree on the suitability of one of the models, manufacturers should provide a chart with the correspondences between measured and harmonized values. Finally, this must be endorsed by scientific authorities such as the ISTH.

References

1 Gaffney PJ. Distinction between fibrinogen and fibrin degradation products in plasma. *Clin Chim Acta* 1975; 65: 109–115.

2 Gaffney PJ, Perry MJ. Unreliability of current serum fibrin degradation product (FDP) assays. *Thromb Haemost* 1985; 53: 301–302.

3 Rylatt DB, Blake AS, Cottis LE, Massingham DA, Fletcher WA, Masci PP, *et al.* An immunoassay for human D-dimer using monoclonal antibodies. *Thromb Res* 1983; 31: 767–778.

4 Bounameaux H, de Moerloose P, Perrier A, Miron MJ. D-dimer testing in suspected venous thromboembolism: an update. *Q J Med* 1997; 90: 437–442.

5 Taylor FB Jr, Toh CH, Hoots WK, Wada H, Levi M; Scientific Subcommittee on Disseminated Intravascular Coagulation (DIC) of the International Society on Thrombosis and Haemostasis (ISTH). Towards definition, clinical and laboratory criteria, and a scoring system for disseminated intravascular coagulation. *Thromb Haemost* 2001; 86: 1327–1330.

6 Wada H, Gabazza EC, Asakura H, Koike K, Okamoto K, Maruyama I, *et al.* Comparison of diagnostic criteria for disseminated intravascular coagulation (DIC): diagnostic criteria of the International Society of Thrombosis and Hemostasis and of the Japanese Ministry of Health and Welfare for overt DIC. *Am J Hematol* 2003; 74: 17–22.

7 Reber G, de Moerloose P. D-dimer assays for the exclusion of venous thromboembolism. *Semin Thromb Hemost* 2000; 26: 619–624.

8 Gaffney PJ, Edgell T, Creighton-Kempsford LJ, Wheeler S, Tarelli E. Fibrin degradation product (FnDP) assays: analysis of standardization issues and target antigens in plasma. *Br J Haematol* 1995; 90: 187–194.

9 Nieuwenhuizen W. A reference material for harmonisation of D-dimer assays. Fibrinogen Subcommittee of the Scientific and Standardization Committee of the International Society of Thrombosis and Haemostasis. *Thromb Haemost* 1997; 77: 1031–1033.

10 Dempfle CE, Zips S, Ergül H, Heene DL; Fibrin Assay Comparative Trial study group. The Fibrin Assay Comparison Trial (FACT): evaluation of 23 quantitative D-dimer assays as basis for the development of D-dimer calibrators. FACT study group. *Thromb Haemost* 2001; 85: 671–678.

11 Meijer P, Haverkate F, Kluft C, de Moerloose P, Verbruggen B, Spannagl M. A model for the harmonisation of test results of different quantitative D-dimer methods. *Thromb Haemost* 2006; 95: 567–572.

12 Jennings I, Woods TA, Kitchen DP, Kitchen S, Walker ID. Laboratory D-dimer measurement: improved agreement between methods through calibration. *Thromb Haemost* 2007; 98: 1127–1135.

13 Olexa SA, Budzynski AZ. Effects of fibrinopeptide cleavage on the plasmic degradation pathways of human cross-linked fibrin. *Biochemistry* 1980; 19: 647–651.

14 Mosesson MW, Siebenlist KR, Meh DA. The structure and biological features of fibrinogen and fibrin. *Ann N Y Acad Sci* 2001; 936: 11–30.

15 Mosesson MW. On behalf of the Subcommittee on Fibrinogen of the Scientific and Standardization Committee of the ISTH. Terminology for macromolecular derivatives of crosslinked fibrin. *Thromb Haemost* 1995; 73: 725–726.

16 Gaffney PJ, Lane DA, Kakkar VV, Brasher M. Characterisation of a soluble D-dimer–E complex in crosslinked fibrin digests. *Thromb Res* 1975; 7: 89–99.

17 Marder VJ, Budzynski AZ, Barlow GH. Comparison of the physicochemical properties of fragment D derivatives of fibrinogen and fragment D-D of cross-linked fibrin. *Biochim Biophys Acta* 1976; 427: 1–14.

18 Pfitzner SA, Dempfle CE, Matsuda M, Heene DL. Fibrin detected in plasma of patients with disseminated intravascular coagulation by fibrin-specific antibodies consists primarily of high molecular weight factor XIIIa-crosslinked and plasmin-modified complexes partially containing fibrinopeptide A. *Thromb Haemost* 1997; 78: 1069–1078.

19 Francis CW, Marder VJ. Degradation of cross-linked fibrin by human leukocyte proteases. *J Lab Clin Med* 1986; 107: 342–352.

20 Pittet JL, de Moerloose P, Reber G, Durand C, Villard C, Piga N, *et al.* VIDAS D-dimer: fast quantitative ELISA for measuring D-dimer in plasma. *Clin Chem* 1996; 42: 410–415.

21 Wylie FG, Walsh TP. Variable immunoreactivity of D-dimer preparations for monoclonal antibody DD-3B6/22. *Blood Coagul Fibrinolysis* 1995; 6: 738–742.

22 Adema E, Gebert U. Pooled patient samples as reference material for D-dimer. *Thromb Res* 1995; **80**: 85–88.

23 Spannagl M, Haverkate F, Reinauer H, Meijer P. The performance of quantitative D-dimer assays in laboratory routine. *Blood Coagul Fibrinolysis* 2005; **16**: 439–443.

24 Olson J, Cunningham M, Brandt J, Chandler W, Eby C, Hayes T, *et al*. Use of the D-dimer for exclusion of VTE: Difficulties uncovered through the Proficiency Testing Program of the College of American Pathologists (CAP). *J Thromb Haemost* 2005; **3** (suppl 1): OR303 (abstract).

12 Diagnostic assessment of platelet function

P. Nurden & A. Nurden

Platelets are small anucleate blood cells produced in large numbers in the bone marrow by mature megakaryocytes (MKs).[1] In the event of blood vessel injury, platelets are rapidly recruited to the area of damage where they accumulate to prevent blood loss. In this way they are essential elements in the arrest of bleeding and hemostasis. Included in this process are platelet adhesion, aggregation, thrombin generation with the formation of a clot and wound healing.

Adhesion is the process whereby platelets attach through membrane receptors to cellular and extracellular matrix constituents of the subendothelial tissue. For example, the GPIb-IX-V complex binds to multimers of von Willebrand factor (VWF) exposed within the injured vessel wall.[2] This step occurs at high shear and is responsible for transient platelet tethering. It is followed by the activation-dependent stable attachment of platelets to collagen and other extracellular matrix constituents. The $\alpha2\beta1$ integrin and GPVI are the principal receptors involved in the platelet–collagen interaction promoting platelet spreading and activation including secretion.[3] Platelet aggregation occurs through the interaction of soluble proteins such as VWF and fibrinogen (Fg) with the $\alpha IIb\beta3$ integrin and the cross-linking of adjacent platelets.[4] Aggregation is promoted by soluble cofactors or metabolites released from platelets such as adenosine diphosphate (ADP) and thromboxane A_2

(TXA_2), and by thrombin formed on the newly procoagulant platelet surface.[4,5] Thrombin initiates fibrin polymerization leading to clot formation and retraction, while released substances and α-granule stored proteins accelerate tissue repair.[6]

All platelet functional responses must be tightly regulated to ensure that the newly formed blood clot is of sufficient size to seal off the damaged area while not disrupting blood flow to vital organs by causing vessel occlusion. The consequences of abnormal platelet regulation can be either bleeding or the development of arterial thrombosis. Bleeding develops when there are qualitative or quantitative defects in platelets. Thrombotic complications involving platelets are mostly seen in the context of cardiovascular-related diseases such as myocardial infarction and stroke which are often associated with atherosclerosis.[7]

Bleeding syndromes arising through an inherited defect of platelet production constitute a heterogeneous group of rare diseases.[8,9] Some, including the Bernard–Soulier syndrome (BSS) and Wiskott–Aldrich syndrome (WAS), associate a thrombocytopenia with a deficiency in a functional protein. In many familial thrombocytopenias (FT), platelet dysfunction is secondary and the cause of bleeding is the inability of MKs to produce platelets in sufficient numbers. Recent evidence on the way that platelet lifespan is regulated suggests the existence of FT with accelerated platelet destruction.[10] Other syndromes associate defects of platelet function with a normal platelet count. In Glanzmann thrombasthenia (GT) an absence of aggregation is caused by a deficiency or a functional abnormality of the $\alpha IIb\beta3$ integrin.[11] Other

Quality in Laboratory Hemostasis and Thrombosis, 1st edition. By Steve Kitchen, John D. Olson and F. Eric Preston. Published 2009 by Blackwell Publishing. ISBN: 978-1-4051-6803-8

pathologies concern agonist receptors such as P2Y$_{12}$ (ADP), TPα (TXA$_2$) or GPVI (collagen). Intracellular defects include the storage pool deficiencies where defects in the biogenesis of dense granules or α-granules give rise to the Hermansky–Pudlak and Chédiak–Higashi syndromes or the Gray platelet syndrome.[12,13] An emerging field concerns intracellular signaling pathways and/or enzymes essential for energy or active metabolite production.[8]

Platelet adhesive properties are central to a variety of pathophysiologic processes which extend from inflammation to host defense and cancer. Platelets are also causally implicated in many acquired conditions including autoimmune diseases such as idiopathic thrombocytopenic purpura (ITP) and drug-dependent thrombocytopenias,[14,15] major diseases (e.g. kidney and liver disease, diabetes, microbial and viral infections, Alzheimer's disease) and the response to treatment with drugs or chemotherapy.[16] Tests are performed to explain the origin of a bleeding syndrome, to evaluate the risk of bleeding prior to surgery or during pregnancy, or to monitor the efficiency of antiplatelet treatment in thrombotic or inflammatory syndromes. The use of aspirin to prevent thrombosis has become generalized, while new, more potent, antiplatelet drugs have been developed such as the powerful αIIbβ3 inhibitors (abciximab, eptifibatide or tirofiban) and prodrugs such as clopidogrel or

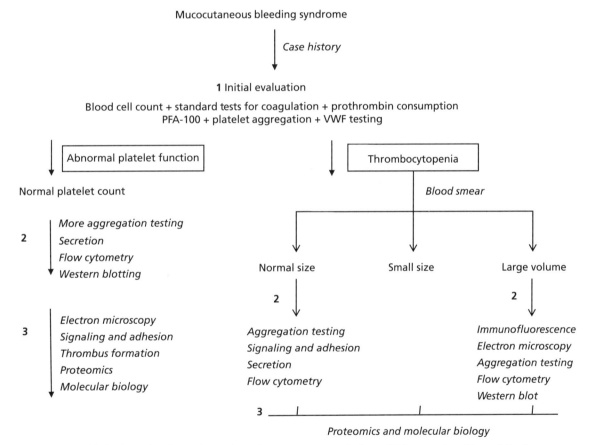

Fig. 12.1 Simplified schema for the work-up of a patient with an inherited bleeding disorder. This is a personalized view in which the patient is examined three times and which requires that non-specialized laboratories progressively establish networks with specialized centers perhaps through national societies or, as in France, by the national health ministry.

prasugrel whose metabolites specifically block ADP-induced platelet aggregation and which can be used as long-term maintenance anticoagulation.[17,18] Assessment of the clinical efficacy of such drugs is a new discipline.

Bleeding time

The skin bleeding time (BT) was introduced some 50 years ago as an *in vivo* test used for assessing primary hemostasis.[19] Historically, the Duke procedure was first used, the earlobe being pierced with a lancet. This was later replaced with the Ivy BT, where a small incision was made in the forearm. This was later modified into the template BT, in which the size and depth of the cut was standardized by placing a template on the skin. A spring-loaded blade within the device makes a standardized cut through a slit in the template. Cessation of bleeding is dependent on an adequate number of platelets and of the ability of platelets to form the hemostatic plug. Many variables influence the BT, including hematocrit, skin thickness, temperature, blood vessel anatomy, location of the incision and the skill of the operator. No study has clearly established the ability of BT measurement to predict the risk of hemorrhage in individual patients; it is not sensitive for the diagnosis of type I von Willebrand disease (type I VWD) while neonates may react differently from adults. The establishment of a reference range and/or control values is essential. For practical reasons, the BT is being replaced by such tests as the Platelet Function Analyzer-100 (PFA-100; see p. 114). Because of difficulty with variability, the BT test is now used less frequently and is not included in the algorithm shown in Fig. 12.1.

Prothrombin consumption

This simple procedure assesses residual prothrombin (PT) levels after coagulation is complete when whole blood is coagulated in a non-siliconized glass tube at 37°C.[20] The test depends on platelets and, in particular, on the availability of membrane phospholipid (formerly called platelet factor 3). Expressed as a percentage, PT is abnormal in BSS and in the very rare Scott syndrome.[7] The test suffers from a lack of reproducibility but can highlight defects in the platelet contribution to coagulation that are not detected by other procedures.

Platelet counting and morphology

Platelet counting is mostly performed automatically with hematology analyzers.[21] A normal platelet count ranges $150–400 \times 10^9$/L in whole blood. Counting is usually performed in ethylenediaminetetraacetic acid (EDTA) anticoagulated blood. The analyzers use impedance, optical or immunologic methods. A problem with impedance is to distinguish between small red cells and platelets (with an underestimation of large platelets). The use of analyzers identifying platelets with fluorochrome-labeled monoclonal antibodies (MoAbs) directed against markers of the MK lineage has been limited because of the high cost. It is recommended that an unexpectedly low platelet count is verified manually to look for agglutinates or platelet satellitism and that the count is repeated using a citrate-based anticoagulant to exclude pseudothrombocytopenia caused by natural antibodies acting after Ca^{2+}-chelation.

Platelet volume measurements can help diagnose the origin of a thrombocytopenia. Nevertheless, interpretation of results remains difficult because the analyzers are infrequently standardized. A blood smear should also be examined. Coloration with Wright's or May–Grünwald–Giemsa (MGG) stain and examination using a light microscope will confirm the presence of large platelets; the absence of α-granules causes a pale gray color and identifies gray platelet syndrome, while the presence of platelet agglutinates can suggest type 2B VWD or the Montreal platelet syndrome.[22,23] Of diagnostic importance for *MYH9*-related macrothrombocytopenias is the detection of abnormal inclusions, namely Döhle bodies, in neutrophils. A low platelet count and a small platelet volume is suggestive of X-linked thrombocytopenia and defects in the *WAS* gene if the thrombocytopenia is isolated. *WAS* is to be considered if the major clinical signs include repeated infections and eczema.

Electron microscopy (EM), a sophisticated technique requiring special training, allows a precise ultrastructural analysis of platelet morphology and of the activation mechanisms including exocytosis.[23,24]

EM is very useful for characterizing certain inherited platelet disorders. A distinguishing feature of giant platelet syndromes (e.g. *MYH9*-related disease and BSS) is the presence of enlarged round platelets. Often they have a heterogeneous distribution of α-granules with zones enriched in membranes and/or the dense tubular system. In the gray platelet syndrome, EM shows how the α-granules in the somewhat enlarged platelets are replaced by vacuoles.[25] Fused α-granules are a characteristic of the Paris–Trousseau syndrome. Figure 12.2 shows a gallery of photographs obtained with patients with different types of thrombocytopenia. When required, EM can be combined with immunogold labeling (I-EM) to localize specific membrane or granular components.[25] Immunofluorescence or confocal microscopy can be used to specifically identify α-granules in platelets,[26] while evaluating the distribution of non-muscle myosin heavy chain IIA in

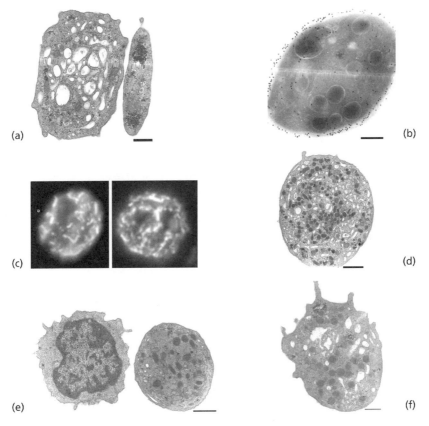

Fig. 12.2 Inherited disorders of platelets. A gallery of photographs to illustrate different aspects of platelet morphology as seen by electron microscopy (EM) (a,b,d–f) or by immunofluorescence microscopy (c). (a) Two platelets from a patient with the gray platelet syndrome.[13] One platelet is enlarged, round and full of vacuoles, the second is discoid and of normal size. Neither platelet has α-granules. (b) A platelet from a variant form of Paris–Trousseau syndrome. Note the large vesicular structure composed of fused α-granules. Electron microscopy with immunogold labeling (I-EM) has been performed, and the gold beads show the normal presence of the αIIbβ3 integrin. (c) The immunofluorescence staining of leukocytes for the myosin-IIA isoform. The patch-like distribution is typical of the May–Hegglin anomaly.[22] (d) A typical enlarged platelet from a patient with the May–Hegglin anomaly. Note the non-uniform distribution of the α-granules and the presence of membrane complexes. (e,f) Enlarged round platelets from two patients with type 2B von Willibrand disease (VWD). A leukocyte is shown in (e) for comparison. Bars = 1 μm.

leukocytes has become a standard test for *MYH9*-related disorders.[22]

Platelet Function Analyzer-100

The Platelet Function Analyzer-100 (PFA-100) closure time (CT) provides a simple and rapid assessment of high shear-dependent platelet function.[27,28] The apparatus is commercially available from Dade-Behring (Newark, DE, USA). Two types of cartridges are used: one containing an artificial membrane coated with collagen and epinephrine (C-EPI), the second is impregnated with collagen and ADP (C-ADP). Each membrane has a 150 μm central aperture. Platelet aggregates will block the central aperture when citrate-anticoagulated normal blood is aspirated across the membrane. Platelet dysfunction will prolong the CT or even prevent closure (defined as >300 seconds). Each laboratory should establish its own reference range. Like the BT, the PFA-100 CT is sensitive to changes in the platelet count or hematocrit. This test is particularly dependent on VWF and therefore is often used in initial evaluation for VWD. In congenital platelet disorders, the test lacks sensitivity and the CT varies with the severity and nature of the platelet defect.[28] Plug formation does not occur for patients with GT and BSS. For patients with $P2Y_{12}$ deficiency as well as for patients with granule deficiencies the results are variable;[28] for aspirin-like defects and SPD the collagen + epinephrine cartridge is the most sensitive. Care must be taken with neonates who have shorter CT because of higher hematocrit and VWF levels.

The PFA-100 is often used to predict bleeding risk in patients about to undergo surgery (e.g. cardiopulmonary bypass, management of coronary syndromes) and to evaluate the efficacy of antiplatelet drugs in patients with cardiovascular disease.[29,30] It is excellent for monitoring the action of the powerful anti-αIIbβ3 drugs that prolong or prevent closure of either cartridge. However, it is less effective in monitoring milder acting drugs such as aspirin where only the C-EPI cartridge is recommended. Controversy has arisen as to whether it will allow the so-called aspirin resistance seen in a significant proportion of patients.[30,31] The PFA-100 is relatively insensitive for monitoring treatment with drugs blocking the action of ADP on platelets, a situation illustrated by the fact

that the CT was normal for a patient with a total lack of $P2Y_{12}$ (P.N., personal communication). It may be considered when monitoring therapy in patients undergoing bleeding (e.g. 1-desamino-8-D-arginine vasopressin [DDAVP], recombinant factor VIIa, platelet or VWF transfusions) although there is as yet no hard evidence linking changes in the PFA-100 CT with clinical outcome. In conclusion, this test offers the relative comfort of a rapid testing; nevertheless, not all platelet abnormalities are detected. In rare patients with a bleeding diathesis, a prolonged CT is seen in the absence of other indications (normal coagulation, normal platelet aggregation) suggesting that as yet unknown causes can contribute to alterations in CT and possibly bleeding.

Point-of-care tests

Much effort has gone into producing machines that offer a rapid evaluation of bleeding risk. We have already dealt with the PFA-100, but other approaches are available. Excellent reviews of these technologies exist and the reader is referred to these for more detailed information.[29,30] The VerifyNow (formerly called the Ultegra rapid platelet function analyzer; Accumetrics, San Diego, CA) is a cartridge-based whole blood assay designed to measure directly the effects of anti-aggregants. It falls into the category of point-of-care tests designed for use at the patient's bedside. Different cartridges allow the evaluation of the efficacy of aspirin, thienopyridines or anti-αIIbβ3 drugs in a cardiovascular context. The device measures the agglutination of Fg-covered latex beads by platelets activated *in situ*. The percentage of drug inhibition for ADP or arachidonic acid is calculated relative to that obtained with a strong agonist, thrombin receptor activating peptide (TRAP).[32,33] Plateletworks (Helena Laboratories, Beaumont, TX) compares platelet counts in whole blood anticoagulated with EDTA and citrate using ADP and collagen as agonists. It is mostly used to monitor antiplatelet therapy.[34,35] The thromboelastograph PlateletMapping System (Haemoscope Corporation, Niles, IL) studies blood clotting in an oscillating cup, the clot's strength being measured through force transmitted to a central piston. Addition of platelet agonists enhances clot strength. It has been used to evaluate antiplatelet therapy as well as the efficacity of transfused platelets to restore hemostatic function in patients.[32,35,36] Through its ability to provide information on clotting and fibrinolysis, it has been used in studies on the Quebec platelet syndrome where there is increased platelet expression of urokinase-type plasminogen activator.[37] Finally, there is the Impact Cone and platelet analyzer (Diamed Cressier, Switzerland) where blood is exposed to uniform shear by the spinning of a cone in a standardized cup. Platelet adhesion and thrombus formation are subsequently analyzed by computer software. Again, the monitoring of anti-aggregant therapy has been the principal use.[38]

Platelet aggregometry

Analysis of platelet aggregation in citrated platelet-rich plasma (PRP) has become the gold standard for platelet function testing and is a key part of any initial diagnosis of a platelet defect (Fig. 12.3).[9] Whole blood aggregometers working on the principles of electrical impedance or particle counting are available and while they have the advantage of:

1 Testing the platelet response in the presence of other blood cells.

2 Eliminating artefacts resulting from the preparation of PRP.

3 Allowing testing with smaller sample size.

Their use has never become widespread.[39]

For optical platelet aggregometry, venous blood is usually taken into vacutainers with trisodium citrate (3.2% or 3.8%) as anticoagulant; PRP is obtained by centrifuging the tubes at a low speed (150–180 g for 10 or 15 minutes at room temperature). The PRP is aspirated from the tubes and platelet-poor plasma (PPP) prepared by subjecting the remaining blood to a new centrifugation at

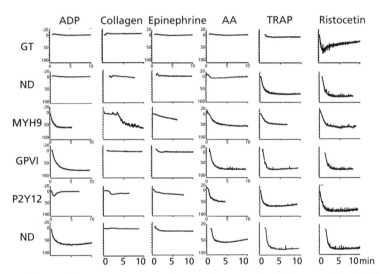

Fig. 12.3 Illustrations of the use of aggregometry to study rare disorders of platelets. Citrated platelet-rich plasma (PRP) has been challenged with the following agonists: adenosine diphosphate (ADP) (10 µmol/L), high dose collagen (2 µg/mL), epinephrine (4 µmol/L), arachidonic acid (AA; 0.5 mg/mL), thrombin receptor activating peptide (TRAP; 50 µmol/L) and ristocetin (1.5 mg/mL). Tracings are shown for a Glanzmann thrombasthenia (GT) patient with no aggregation to all agonists except for ristocetin where aggregation was reversible. The response of the large platelets of a patient with *MYH9*-related disease was basically normal despite thrombocytopenia. A newly characterized patient with a GPVI deficiency specifically failed to respond to collagen while a patient lacking the P2Y$_{12}$ ADP receptor showed a characteristic reduced and rapidly reversible aggregation to ADP and a reduced response to collagen (under conditions where secreted ADP plays a major part). Also shown are the tracings for two non-diagnosed patients (ND) where purported defects in a signaling pathway affect the response to specific agonists but not TRAP.

1500 g for 10 minutes. Commercially available aggregometers often permit the analysis of multiple samples simultaneously. Light transmittance is measured in stirred suspensions at 37°C; the aggregation tracing is calibrated between 0% and 100%, 0% corresponding to the PRP and 100% to the PPP (Fig. 12.2). As aggregation proceeds, the amount of light that passes across the stirred suspension is recorded. There is no consensus about the need for standardizing the platelet count prior to testing; indeed, platelet refractoriness may be induced by adding PPP to dilute the PRP.[40] The initial screening of platelet function disorders requires a panel of agonists which include: ADP (1–10 μmol/L), fibrillar collagen (1–5 μg; equine type 1 Horm, Nycomed, Munich), epinephrine (5–10 μmol/L), arachidonic acid (0.5–1 mg/mL), TRAP-6 mer or TRAP-14 mer (2–50 μmol/L). Both high and low doses of collagen should be tested while care should be taken in establishing control values when using different commercial collagen preparations; they may show different reactivities depending on the type of collagen that is present. Ristocetin is also used at low and high concentrations (0.5 and 1.5 mg/mL); low doses are used to verify the absence of spontaneous GPIb/VWF interactions as in platelet-type VWD or type 2B VWD while an absent response at 1.5 mg/mL points to BSS.[41] Reference values need to be established for each agonist.[42] A biphasic response, as seen with low doses of ADP, consists of an initial aggregation that is supplemented by the release of storage pool ADP and newly synthesized TXA_2.[42] An initial platelet shape change after the addition of agonist is recognized by the presence of a prompt and brief increase of light transmittance. Shape change is not given by epinephrine. Figure 12.2 shows profiles that are characteristic for patients belonging to a series of well-characterized inherited disorders such as GT or $P2Y_{12}$ or GPVI deficiencies.

Initial results should be confirmed for a second blood sample taken at a later date. Other agonists can also be tested (Fig. 12.2). For example, if the collagen response is abnormal and particularly when used at low doses, the snake venom protein, convulxin or collagen-related peptides that directly activate platelets through the GPVI receptor should be included.[25,42] An "aspirin-like" response suggests use of:

1 The TXA_2 analog U46619 which acts through the TPα receptor;
2 Phorbol 12-myristate 13-acetate (PMA) which interacts directly with protein kinase-C leading to diacylglycerol and inositol triphosphate formation; and
3 The ionophore A23187 which directly mobilizes intracellular pools of Ca^{2+}.
Information gained from such agonists is particularly important if the defect concerns intracellular signaling or secretory pathways.

Platelet aggregation can also be performed using washed platelets separated from plasma by differential centrifugation and resuspended in buffers that maintain the platelet functional response.[43,44] Gel filtration on Sepharose 2B and centrifugation on inert density gradients (albumin, stractan) are alternative procedures but are infrequently used. The use of washed platelets allows the concentration of platelets from thrombocytopenic patients and permits an evaluation of the platelet functional response at physiologic extracellular Ca^{2+} levels. The absence of plasma fibrinogen facilitates an analysis of the aggregation response to thrombin. Typical doses are 0.05 IU/mL for a low concentration of thrombin and 0.5–1 IU/mL for maximal activation and secretion. For testing other agonists with washed platelets, the addition of fibrinogen (300 μg/mL) is necessary. Use of washed platelets is a good way of controlling for the presence of plasma inhibitors of platelet aggregation. For example, antibodies in idiopathic thrombocytopenic purpura (ITP) patients reactive with surface receptors can block the functional response as well as induce thrombocytopenia. Incubating patient's plasma with washed control platelets prior to stimulation can confirm inhibitor activity. A rapid microtiter assay for screening potential drugs on platelet aggregation has recently been proposed.[45]

Platelet secretion

Dense granules can be visualized using the fluorescent dye mepacrine and counted by fluorescence microscopy or by examining whole mounts by EM.[46] If a dense granule abnormality is suspected then the releasable and total platelet pools of ADP and adenosine triphosphate (ATP) should be quantified and their ratio calculated. An alternative approach is to assess platelet capacity to take up and then release serotonin. As well as a qualitative storage pool deficiency, defects may concern a block in the secretory mechanism.[8] Dense granule secretion can be determined by measuring the release of ATP during platelet aggregation in a lumiaggregometer (Chronolog, Havertown, PA) by adding luciferin-luciferase reagent to the platelet samples.[42] Secretion is measured at 37°C with stirring, and step changes in the luminescence recording can be used to calculate the amount of ATP released by comparison to a calibration curve. Only the intra-granular pool of ATP is secreted and measured, the metabolic pool remains in the cytoplasm. Incubation of platelets with agonists (e.g. ADP, collagen, thrombin) with or without stirring for different times will allow an evaluation of the kinetics of secretion. The release of selected α-granule proteins such as platelet factor 4 (PF4) and platelet-derived growth factor (PDGF) can be quantified using commercial enzyme-linked immunosorbent assay (ELISA) procedures or radioimmunosassay.[25,47] The evaluation of platelet secretion by flow cytometry is discussed in the next section.

Flow cytometry

Flow cytometry (FC) is a powerful and often used tool that can provide much information on the functional status of platelets.[48] FC assesses cell size and granularity within a large population of cells, while simultaneously quantifying the fluorescence emitted from cell-bound fluorochrome-labeled antibodies and ligands. It allows a precise assessment of the physical and antigenic properties of platelets (e.g. surface expression of receptors, bound ligands, secretion, platelet aggregates, leukocyte–platelet aggregates). It facilitates the diagnosis of inherited (e.g. BSS, GT, storage pool disease) or acquired platelet disorders (e.g. ITP). Studies on platelets of a GT variant are shown in Fig. 12.4. FC also allows an assessment of:

1 The pathologic activation state of platelets (e.g. in the setting of acute coronary syndromes, cerebrovascular ischemia, peripheral vascular disease, cardiopulmonary bypass, diabetes).
2 The efficacy of antiplatelet drugs to combat thrombosis.

3 The efficacy of platelet transfusion in the event of bleeding as well as controlling the functional state of stored platelets.[49–51]

Using a panel of antibodies, the structure of membrane glycoprotein receptors can be studied in detail; for example, for αIIbβ3 there are not only MoAbs recognizing epitopes on each subunit, but also epitopes specific for the complex. The immunoglobulin M (IgM) MoAb, PAC-1 is able to recognize the activated form of the complex; while to detect the binding of ligands, there are two categories of MoAbs: the anti-RIBS (receptor-induced binding site) and anti-LIBS (ligand-induced binding site).[49] To quantify binding, antibodies can be conjugated directly with fluorochromes such as fluorescein isothiocyanate (FITC) or phycoerythrin (PE). Assessment can also be indirect with bound primary antibodies recognized by a species-specific second antibody coupled to one of a large panel of fluorochromes.[48] Results are printed in the form of histograms, with mean fluorescent intensity (MFI) (x axis) plotted against cell number (y axis). Prior fixation of platelets with paraformaldehyde (PFA) stabilizes surface antigens and allows transport of samples. Analyses can be performed on PRP or in whole blood, in the latter the use of a double-labeling procedure can permit an evaluation of an antigen on MoAb-identified cells and on mixed cell aggregates.[52] Commercially available quantification kits (Biocytex, Marseille, France) allow precise assessment of the number of bound MoAbs. Access to cytoplasmic proteins and to storage organelles is achieved by fixing the platelets with PFA, and permeabilizing them with agents such Triton X-100 or saponin. Use of the membrane-permeable dye, mepacrine, allows an indirect assessment of the platelet-dense granule content in suspected storage pool disease. Use of thiazole orange allows the analysis of reticulated platelets (newly released platelets), a technique that is proposed for evaluating platelet production and/or turnover.[53]

A new application for drug surveillance involves the use of permeabilized PFA-fixed platelets to measure the phosphorylation state of VASP protein by way of a MoAb that specifically recognizes the phosphorylated form of this protein (kit commercialized by Biocytex). VASP is dephosphorylated after ADP activates $P2Y_{12}$. The assay uses prostaglandin E_1 to increase intraplatelet cAMP and fully phosphorylate VASP, making the assay more sensi-

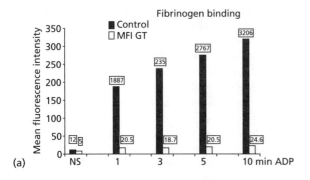

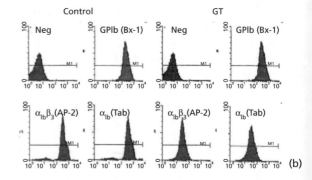

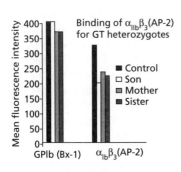

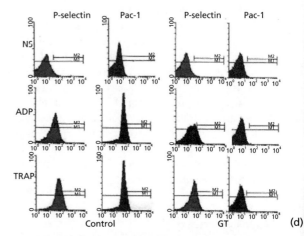

Fig. 12.4 A series of analyses to show the usefulness of flow cytometry (FC) in diagnosing the platelet defect in a patient with a variant form of Glanzmann thrombasthenia (GT) with a β3 L196P mutation. Part (a) shows the inability of the platelets to bind fluorescein isothiocyanate (FITC)-labeled fibrinogen (Fg) after stimulation with ADP. Part (b) shows the binding of a monoclonal antibody (MoAb) to GPIbα (Bx-1), to a complex-dependent determinant on the αIIbβ3 integrin (AP-2) and to the αIIb subunit (Tab). Note the normal presence of GPIb and the presence of small amounts of residual non-functional αIIbβ3. Part (d) shows the ability of flow cytometry (FC) to detect reduced amounts of αIIbβ3 in family members known to carry the mutation. Part (d) illustrates the ability of the patient's platelets to express P-selectin when stimulated (ADP and TRAP) and the inability of the patient's residual αIIbβ3 to bind the conformation-dependent MoAb PAC-1 – a result that agrees with the absence of Fg binding.

tive and specific for the effects of ADP. Assuming that the degree of dephosphorylation reflects the interaction between ADP and its receptor, this test is used to evaluate the clinical efficacy of antiplatelet drugs such as clopidogrel and prasugrel.[54] In a patient with a total P2Y$_{12}$ deficiency, ADP was without effect on VASP phosphorylation (P.N., personal communication).

Another application of FC is the study of platelet procoagulant activity. Phosphatidylserine (PS) is an essential platelet membrane phospholipid that is exposed at the platelet surface after activation and forming a procoagulant surface and promoting thrombin generation. The placental protein, annexin-V, binds specifically to PS and is used in FC to identify PS at the platelet surface. The mechanisms that induce the flip-flop phenomenon of PS during platelet activation also result in the liberation of microparticles (MPs) by a mechanism that involves the Ca^{2+}-dependent protease, calpain.[55] Annexin can bind PS only in the presence of Ca^{2+}, meaning that activation is realized *in vitro* using washed platelets. To obtain maximal amounts of annexin-V binding, platelets need to be stimulated by a thrombin and collagen mixture or by the ionophore A23187. A total lack of surface PS expression and MP formation is seen in the Scott syndrome.[8] Others have called the procoagulant platelets, "coated-platelets" based on the presence of surface-bound and secreted proteins covalently bound by a mechanism that involves serotonin.[56] Platelet-derived MPs can be measured in plasma by ELISA as well as by FC.[57] By using cell-specific MoAbs during the analysis, the cells from which the MPs are derived can be identified.[58] The MPs are said to be prothrombotic, but they can also have major roles in the development of atherosclerotic plaques, in wound healing and in inflammation.

Flow cytometry is especially useful in the diagnosis of inherited disorders of platelet function if combined with Western blotting (WB). Suspensions of washed platelets are solubilized by the ionic detergent sodium dodecyl sulfate (SDS) and the soluble proteins separated by polyacrylamide gel electrophoresis in the presence of the detergent (SDS-PAGE). Transfer of proteins to nitrocellulose membrane followed by their renaturation with non-ionic detergent permits their identification through antibody binding. Proteins suspected to be absent in platelets of diseases such as GT and BSS can be evaluated in this way, while alterations in protein structure (e.g. truncated proteins, degraded proteins) can also be identified provided that antibody-binding epitopes are retained.[59] With the use of chemiluminescent antibody detecting procedures, this is a very sensitive assay that can be applied to minor platelet proteins.

Clot retraction

Blood coagulation is followed by clot retraction resulting from the association of fibrin fibers with activated platelets. The retraction is brought about by the platelet contractile system with surface receptors forming a bridge with the fibrin.[60] Clot retraction is essential for thrombus stability and proceeds through a β3 and myosin IIA-dependent signaling pathway probably regulated by myosin light chain phosphorylation itself under the control of RhoA. In the absence or non-functioning of αIIbβ3, clot retraction does not occur; in some patients with GT with residual αIIbβ3 receptors it occurs partially.[11] It may also be abnormal in *MYH9*-related diseases. Clot retraction can be measured by simply incubating non-anticoagulated blood in a non-siliconized glass tube at 37°C. Retraction is a slow process which can take several hours. It is more rapid when using calcification of citrated PRP as a mode of thrombin generation.

Signaling pathways

As we have seen, agonist binding to platelet receptors mediates functional responses such as adhesion, activation, secretion and aggregation. The signaling network in platelets that brings about these processes is complex, involving multiple pathways that often converge. As well as being a receptor for VWF, GPIbα participates in thrombin-induced signaling.[2] GPVI and the α2β1 integrin harmonize to assure a stable platelet adhesion to collagen. GPVI associates with the FcRγ-chain which signals through its immunoreceptor-tyrosine-based activation motif (ITAM) via the adaptor LAT leading to the activation of phospholipase (PL) Cγ2.[3,61] Many of the primary agonists of platelets have more than one receptor belonging to the seven transmembrane domain receptor family: ADP, P2Y$_1$ and P2Y$_{12}$; thrombin, PAR-1 and PAR-4. Each receptor is linked to a specific G-protein whose subunits (α, β/γ) can lead to bidirectional signaling.[62] Diverse signaling routes have been characterized, in particular those involving specific tyrosine kinases (Syk, Src and Fyn), phospholipase A$_2$ (with TXA$_2$ generation), PLCγ2 (involving Cbl, LAT), PLC-β (adenylyl cyclase), protein kinase C (diacyl glycerol, IP$_3$) and the PI 3-kinases often involving Akt.[61,63] Studying these pathways requires collaborations with specialist laboratories. Phosphorylation on serine or threonine residues, or on tyrosine residues, can be studied using immunologic tools often involving immunoprecipitation and/or WB with the use of specific MoAbs reactive with the phosphorylated amino acids. As well as involving newly bound secreted proteins such as thrombospondin-1, aggregate stability also appears to involve a whole new generation of membrane receptors such as the ephrins and eph kinases, semaphorin 4D.[61] Many patients with bleeding disorders where the platelet receptors are present and appear to act normally are suspected to have defects within a signaling pathway.[8]

In vitro studies on thrombus formation

Requiring specialist procedures, platelet reactivity can be studied under static or flow conditions.

Platelet adhesion to collagen and other adhesive proteins under static conditions

A suggested approach is to compare the interaction of platelets with collagen, Fg and VWF coated on glass coverslips.[64–66] After blocking protein-free sites with BSA, a drop containing a suspension of washed platelets is added and the platelets left in contact with the surface for 30 minutes prior to their observation by differential interference contrast (DIC) microscopy with a wide-field objective. Real-time imaging can also be performed. The procedure can be adapted to the use of fluorochrome-labeled probes whose localization is determined by confocal microscopy following PFA fixation. Surface receptors can be visualized directly, while actin polymerization can be followed using fluorochrome-labeled phalloidin after cell permeabilization. The attachment of platelets to collagen first promotes the formation of long filopodia, while spreading is accompanied by secretion and the formation of distinct wave-like lamellipodia. Changes in intracellular Ca^{2+} can be followed using the calcium reporter dye Oregon Green-BAPTA 1-AM. Platelet adhesion and spreading on VWF involves both GPIb and $\alpha IIb\beta 3$; spreading is blocked by integrin inhibitors but can be restored by ristocetin or botrocetin where GPIb-mediated signaling now predominates.[66] This adhesion test is potentially very useful for detecting signaling defects in platelets and is recommended for thrombocytopenias where the platelet count is too low for aggregometry.

Thrombus formation on immobilized collagen under flow conditions

Various procedures have been developed in which anticoagulated blood from patients is perfused *ex vivo* through flow chambers or glass capillaries containing surfaces that have been coated with an adhesive protein, often type I collagen from equine tendon but also VWF and Fg.[67–69] Platelets can be labeled with a fluorescent dye such as mepacrine, allowing direct evaluation by epifluorescent videomicroscopy. Alternatively, evaluation is by light microscopy and computer analysis after fixation of the thrombi. Flow chambers have been designed to allow direct visualization of the platelet adhesion and aggregation process by, for example, reflexion interference contrast microscopy which is recorded with a video camera.[68] Image sequencing of the time-lapse recording and analysis of surface coverage can be compared from controls and patients at controlled shear rates. After fixation, the use of fluorochrome-labeled antibodies and confocal microscopy can provide information on the localization and role of specific proteins.[68] The use of such dyes as Oregon Green 488 BAPTA-1 and FURA Red AM, allows the study of calcium signaling during aggregation and thrombus build-up.[69]

New technologies

Proteomics and genomics

These are powerful tools for studying platelets. Proteomics allows large-scale study of the platelet proteome. It involves the separation of detergent-soluble platelet extracts by high-resolution two-dimensional gel electrophoresis or by sophisticated chromatographic procedures. Proteins are often identified by mass spectroscopy, usually by the analysis of peptides obtained by proteolyic digestion. Upwards of 641 proteins compose the platelet proteome.[70] While some groups have attempted to resolve the whole platelet proteome, others have confined themselves to specifically studying membrane glycoproteins, the secretome (i.e. proteins released from the storage pool) or the phosphoproteome (proteins involved in signaling pathways).[70–72] Although anucleate, platelets retain sufficient mRNA to allow transcription profiling using microarray.[73,74] In total, transcripts of 1526 genes were identified in one study.[74] In identifying pathologic changes in a cell, profiling of mRNA levels has the potential to identify not only defective genes, but also those abnormally regulated by a mutated protein. An example is the decreased platelet expression of myosin regulatory light chain polypeptide (*MYL9*) and other genes associated with platelet dysfunction in a patient with FT and a *CBFA2/RUNX1* mutation.[75] A major use of genomics and microarrays will be to study single nucleotide polymorphisms (SNPs) which affect virtually all genes.[76] Arguments can be put forward that a global assessment of the SNPs of platelet genes will provide much information to explain the biologic functional activity of platelets and its variation from individual to individual.

Gene sequencing

Any diagnosis of an inherited platelet disorder is incomplete without knowledge of the molecular defect that is responsible for the disease. In more frequently encountered diseases such as GT, gene sequencing has become commonplace and population studies are being performed.[77] While in past years prescreening for gene defects using PCR-SSCP or DGGE was commonplace, the preference now is for direct sequencing of gene promoters, exons and splice sites. BSS results from mutations affecting the *GPIBA*, *GPIBB* and *GP9* genes; as these are single exon genes (except for *GPIBB* which has two exons) direct sequencing is the rule. Genotyping of human platelet alloantigens associated with *ITGB3*, *ITGA2B* and *GPIBA* as major immunologic targets is important in the diagnosis and treatment of neonatal alloimmune thrombocytopenic purpura, post-transfusion purpura and refractoriness to platelet transfusion therapy.[78] Mutations in transcription factor genes are often responsible for FTs.[23] One example is the *GATA-1* gene where morphologically enlarged platelets may have a decreased GPIbα and α-granule content, while some patients also show red cell defects typical of β-thalassemia.[79] Notwithstanding this progress, many of the molecular defects giving rise to FTs remain without a classification. There is a need for gene sequencing on a large scale.

References

1 Patel SR, Hartwig JH, Italiano JE Jr. The biogenesis of platelets from megakaryocyte proplatelets. *J Clin Invest* 2005; **115**: 3348–3354.

2 Andrews, RK, Berndt, MC, Lopez JA. The glycoprotein Ib-IX-V complex. In *Platelets*, 2nd edn. Michelson A, (ed.). San Diego, CA: Academic Press, 2007: 145–163.

3 Sarratt KL, Chen H, Zutter MM, Santoro SA, Hammer DA, Kahn ML. GPVI and α2β1 play independent critical roles during platelet adhesion and aggregate formation to collagen under flow. *Blood* 2005; **106**: 1268–1277.

4 Jackson SP. The growing complexity of platelet aggregation. *Blood* 2007; **109**: 5087–5095.

5 Balasubramanian Y, Grabowski E, Bini A, Nemerson Y. Platelets, circulating tissue factor, and fibrin colocalize in *ex vivo* thrombi: real-time fluorescence images of thrombus formation and propagation under defined flow conditions. *Blood* 2002; **100**: 2787–2792.

6 Nurden AT, Nurden P, Sanchez M, Andia I, Anitua E. Platelets and wound healing. *Front Biosci* 2008; **13**: 3532–3548.

7 Choudhury RP, Fuster V, Fayad ZA. Molecular, cellular and functional imaging of atherothrombosis. *Nat Rev Drug Discov* 2004; **3**: 913–925.

8 Nurden P, Nurden AT. Congenital disorders associated with platelet dysfunctions. *Thromb Haemost* 2008; **99**: 253–263.

9 Bolton-Maggs PHB, Chalmers EA, Collins PW, Harrison P, Liesner RJ, Minford A, *et al.* A review of inherited platelet disorders with guidelines for their management on behalf of the UK HCDO. *Br J Haematol* 2006; **13**: 603–633.

10 Mason KD, Carpinelli MR, Fletcher JI, Collinge JE, Hilton AA, Ellis S, *et al.* Programmed anuclear cell death delimits platelet lifespan. *Cell* 2007; **128**: 31,173–31,186.

11 Nurden AT, George JN. Inherited abnormalities of the platelet membrane: Glanzmann thrombasthenia, Bernard–Soulier syndrome, and other disorders. In *Hemostasis and Thrombosis*, 5th edn. Colman RW, Marder VJ, Clowes AW, George JN, Goldhaber S, (eds). Philadelphia, PA: Lippincott, Williams & Wilkins, 2006: 987–1010.

12 Gunay-Aygun M, Huizing M, Gahl WA. Molecular defects that affect platelet dense granules. *Semin Thromb Hemost* 2004; **30**: 537–547.

13 Nurden AT, Nurden P. The Gray platelet syndrome: clinical spectrum of the disease. *Blood Rev* 2007; **21**: 21–36.

14 Bussel JB. Immune thrombocytopenic purpura. In *Platelets*, 2nd edn. Michelson A, (ed.). San Diego, CA: Academic Press, 2007: 831–846.

15 Aster RH, Bougie DW. Drug-induced thrombocytopenia. *New Engl J Med* 2007; **357**: 580–587.

16 Rao AK. Acquired disorders of platelet function. In *Platelets*, 2nd edn. Michelson A, (ed.). San Diego, CA: Academic Press, 2007: 1051–1076.

17 Agah R, Plow EF, Topol EJ. αIIbβ3 (GPIIb-IIIa) antagonists. In *Platelets*, 2nd edn. Michelson A, (ed.). San Diego, CA: Academic Press, 2007: 1145–1163.

18 Jakubowski JA, Winters KJ, Naganuma H, Wallentin L. Prasugrel: a novel thienopyridine antiplatelet agent. A review of preclinical and clinical studies and the mechanistic basis for its distinct antiplatelet profile. *Cardiovasc Drug Rev* 2007; **25**: 357–374.

19 Rodgers RP, Levin J. A critical appraisal of the bleeding time. *Semin Thromb Haemost* 1990; **16**: 1–20.

20 Quick AJ, Favre-Gilly JE. The prothrombin consumption test: Its clinical and theoretic implications. *Blood* 1949; **4**: 1281–1289.

21 Briggs C, Harrison P, Machin SJ. Platelet counting. In *Platelets*, 2nd edn. Michelson A, (ed.). San Diego, CA: Academic Press, 2007: 465–483.

22 Balduini CL, Cattaneo M, Fabris F, Gresele P, Iolascon A, Pulcinelli FM, et al. Italian Gruppo di Studio delle Piastrine. Inherited thrombocytopenias: a proposed diagnostic algorithm from the Italian Gruppo di Studio delle Piastrine. *Haematologica* 2003; **88**: 582–592.

23 Nurden P, George JN, Nurden AT. Inherited thrombocytopenias. In *Hemostasis and Thrombosis*, 5th edn. Colman RW, Marder VJ, Clowes AW, George JN, Goldhaber S, (eds). Philadelphia, PA: Lippincott, Williams & Wilkins, 2006: 975–986.

24 White JG. Platelet structure. In *Platelets*, 2nd edn. Michelson A, (ed.). San Diego, CA: Academic Press, 2007: 45–73.

25 Nurden P, Jandrot-Perrus M, Combrié R, Winckler J, Arocas V, Lecut C, et al. Severe deficiency of glycoprotein VI in a patient with gray platelet syndrome. *Blood* 2004; **104**: 107–114.

26 Italiano JE Jr, Richardson JL, Patel-Hett S, Battinelli E, Zaslavsky A, Short S, et al. Angiogenesis is regulated by a novel mechanism: Pro- and anti-angiogenic proteins are organized into separate platelet α-granules and differentially released. *Blood* 2008: **111**: 1227–1233.

27 Harrison P. The role of PFA-100® testing in the investigation and management of haemostatic defects in children and adults. *Br J Haematol* 2005; **130**: 3–10.

28 Hayward CP, Harrison P, Cattaneo M, Ortel TL, Rao AK on behalf of the Platelet Physiology Committee of the Scientific and Standardization Committee of the International Society on Thrombosis and Haemostasis. Platelet function analyzer (PFA)-100 closure time in the evaluation of platelet disorders and platelet function. *J Thromb Haemost* 2006; **4**: 312–319.

29 Michelson AD, Frelinger AL 3rd, Furman MI. Current options in platelet function testing. *Am J Cardiol* 2006; **98**: 4N–10N.

30 Gurbel PA, Becker RC, Mann KG, Steinhubl SR, Michelson AD. Platelet function monitoring in patients with coronary artery disease. *J Am Coll Cardiol* 2007; **50**: 1822–1834.

31 Podda GM, Bucciarelli P, Lussana F, Lecchi A, Cattaneo M. Usefulness of PFA-100 testing in the diagnostic screening of patients with suspected abnormalities of hemostasis: comparison with the bleeding time. *J Thromb Haemost* 2007; **5**: 2393–2398.

32 Steinbuhl SR, Talley JD, Braden GA, Tcheng JE, Castella PJ, Moliterno DJ, et al. Point-of-care measured platelet inhibition correlates with a reduced risk of an adverse cardiac event after percutaneous coronary intervention: results of the GOLD (AU-Assessing Ultegra) multicenter study. *Circulation* 2001; **103**: 2572–2578.

33 Jakubowski JA, Payne CD, Li YG, Brandt JT, Small DS, Farid NA, et al. The use of the VerifyNow P2Y12 point-of-care device to monitor platelet function across a range of P2Y12 inhibition levels following prasugrel and clopidogrel administration. *Thromb Hemost* 2008; **99**: 409–415.

34 Van Werkum JW, Gerritsen WB, Kelder JC, Hackeng CM, Ernst SM, Deneer VH, et al. Inhibition of platelet function by abciximab or high-dose tirofiban in patients with STEMI undergoing primary PCI: a randomized trial. *Neth Heart J* 2007; **15**: 375–381.

35 Craft RM, Chavez JJ, Snider CC, Muenchen RA, Carroll RC. Comparison of modified thromboelastograph and PlateletWorks whole blood assays to optical platelet aggregation for monitoring reversal of clopidogrel inhibition in elective surgery patients. *J Lab Clin Med* 2005; **145**: 309–315.

36 Male C, Koren D, Eichelberger B, Kaufmann K, Panzer S. Monitoring survival and function of transfused platelets in Glanzmann thrombasthenia by flow cytometry and thromboelastography. *Vox Sang* 2006; **91**: 174–177.

37 Diamandis M, Adam F, Kahr WH, Wang P, Chorneyko KA, Arsenault AL, et al. Insights into abnormal hemostasis in the Quebec platelet disorder from analysis of clot lysis. *J Thromb Haemost* 2006; **4**: 1086–1094.

38 Osende JL, Fuster V, Lev EI, Shimbo D, Rauch U, Marmur JD, et al. Testing platelet activation with a shear-dependent platelet function test versus aggregation-based tests: relevance for monitoring long-term glycoprotein IIb/IIIa inhibition. *Circulation* 2001; **103**: 1488–1491.

39 Jarvis GE. Platelet aggregation in whole blood: impedence and particle counting methods. *Methods Mol Biol* 2004; **272**: 77–87.

40 Cattaneo M, Lecchi A, Zighetti ML, Lussana F. Platelet aggregation studies: autologous platelet-poor plasma inhibits platelet aggregation when added to platelet-rich plasma to normalize platelet count. *Haematologica* 2007; **92**: 694–697.

41 Federici AB, Mannucci PM. Management of inherited von Willebrand disease in 2007. *Ann Med* 2007; **39**: 346–358.

42 Ban B, Dawood A, Wilde JB, Watson SP. Reference curves for aggregation and ATP secretion to aid diagnosis of platelet-based bleeding disorders: effect of inhibition of ADP and thromboxane A2 pathways. *Platelets* 2007; **18**: 329–345.

43 Cazenave J-P, Ohlmann P, Cassel D, Eckly A, Hechler B, Gachet C. Preparation of washed platelet suspensions from human and rodent blood. *Methods Mol Biol* 2004; **272**: 13–28.

44 Kim S, Jin J, Kunapuli SP. Akt activation in platelets depends on Gi signaling pathways. *J Biol Chem* 2004; **279**: 4186–4195.

45 Moran N, Kiernan A, Dunne E, Edwards RJ, Shields DC, Kenny D. Monitoring modulators of platelet aggregation in a microtiter plate assay. *Anal Biochem* 2006; **357**: 77–84.

46 Enders A, Zieger B, Schwartz K, Yoshimi A, Speckmann C, Knoepfle C-M, et al. Careful clinical and molecular diagnosis is essential to discriminate between Griscelli syndrome and Hermansky–Pudlak syndrome type II. *Blood* 2006; **108**: 81–87.

47 Weiss HJ, Witte LD, Kaplan KL, Lages BA, Chernoff A, Nossel HL, et al. Heterogeneity in storage pool deficiency: studies on granule-bound substances in 18 patients including variants deficient in α-granules, platelet factor 4, β-thromboglobulin, and platelet-derived growth factor. *Blood* 1979; **54**: 1296–1319.

48 Michelson AD, Linden MD, Barnard MR, Furman MI, Frelinger AL III. Flow cytometry. In *Platelets*, 2nd edn. Michelson A, (ed.). San Diego, CA: Academic Press, 2007: 545–563.

49 Bihour C, Durrieu-Jais C, Macchi L, Poujol C, Coste P, Besse P, et al. Expression of markers of platelet activation and the interpatient variation in response to abciximab. *Arterioscler Thromb Vasc Biol* 1999; **19**: 212–219.

50 Frehlinger AL 3rd, Jakubowski JA, Li Y, Barnard MR, Fox ML, Linden MMD, et al. The active metabolite of prasugrel inhibits ADP-stimulated thrombo-inflammatory markers of platelet activation: influence of other blood cells, calcium and aspirin. *Thromb Haemost* 2007; **98**: 192–200.

51 Linden MD, Furman MI, Frelinger AL 3rd, Fox ML, Barnard MR, Li Y, et al. Indices of platelet activation and the stability of coronary artery disease. *J Thromb Haemost* 2007; **4**: 761–765.

52 Barnard MR, Linden MD, Frelinger AL 3rd, Li Y, Fox ML, Furman MI, et al. Effects of platelet binding on whole blood flow cytometry assays of monocyte and neutrophil procoagulant activity. *J Thromb Haemost* 2005; **3**: 2563–2570.

53 McCabe DJ, Harrison P, Sidhu PS, Brown MM, Machin SJ. Circulating reticulated platelets in the early and late phases after ischaemic stroke and transient ischaemic attack. *Br J Haematol* 2004; **126**: 861–869.

54 Aleil B, Ravanat C, Cazenave JP, Rochoux G, Heitz A, Gachet C. Flow cytometric analysis of intraplatelet VASP phosphorylation for the detection of clopidogrel resistance in patients with ischemic cardiovascular disease. *J Thromb Haemost* 2005; **3**: 85–92.

55 Dachary-Prigent J, Pasquet J-M, Freyssinet J-M, Nurden AT. Calcium involvement in aminophospholipid exposure and microparticle formation during platelet activation: a study using Ca^{2+}-ATPase inhibitors. *Biochemistry* 1995; **34**: 11,625–11,634.

56 Dale GL. Coated-platelets: an emerging component of the procoagulant response. *J Thromb Haemost* 2005; **3**: 2185–2192.

57 Lynch SF, Ludlam CA. Plasma microparticles and vascular disorders. *Br J Haematol* 2007; **137**: 36–48.

58 Morel O, Toti F, Hugel B, Bakouboula B, Camoin-Jau L, Dignat-George F, et al. Procoagulant microparticles: disrupting the vascular homeostasis equation. *Arterioscler Thromb Vasc Biol* 2006; **26**: 2594–2604.

59 Milet-Marsal S, Breillat C, Peyruchaud O, Nurden P, Combrie R, Nurden AT, et al. Glanzmann thrombasthenia secondary to a Glu[324] to Lys substitution in the αIIb subunit of the fibrinogen receptor: analysis of the amino acid requirement for a normal αIIbβ3 maturation. *Thromb Haemost* 2002; **88**: 655–662.

60 Schoenwaelder SM, Yuan Y, Cooray P, Salem HH, Jackson SP. Calpain cleavage of focal adhesion proteins regulates the cytoskeletal attachment of integrin αIIbβ3 (platelet glycoprotein IIb/IIIa) and the cellular retraction of fibrin clots. *J Biol Chem* 1997; **272**: 1694–1702.

61 Brass LF, Stalker TJ, Zhu L, Woulfe DS. Signal transduction during platelet plug formation. In *Platelets*, 2nd edn. Michelson A, (ed.). San Diego, CA: Academic Press, 2007: 319–346.

62 Offermanns S. Activation of platelet function through G protein-coupled receptors. *Circ Res* 2006; **99**: 1293–1304.

63 Kahner BN, Shankar H, Murugappan S, Prasad GL, Kunapuli SP. Nucleotide receptor signaling in platelets. *J Thromb Haemost* 2006; **4**: 2317–2326.

64 Pula G, Schuh, K, Nakayama K, Nakayama KI, Walter U, Poole A. PKCδ regulates collagen-induced platelet aggregation through inhibition of VASP-mediated filopodia formation. *Blood* 2006; **108**: 4035–4044.

65 Thornber K, McCarty, Watson SP, Pears CJ. Distinct but critical roles for integrin αIIbβ3 in platelet lamellipodia formation on fibrinogen, collagen-related peptide and thrombin. *FEBS Letts* 2006; **273**: 5032–5043.

66 McCarty OJT, Calaminus SDJ, Berndt MC, Machesky LM, Watson SP. Von Willebrand factor mediates platelet spreading through glycoprotein Ib and αIIbβ3 in the presence of botrocetin and ristocetin, respectively. *J Thromb Haemost* 2006; **4**: 1367–1378.

67 Goto S, Tamura N, Arai M, Kodama R, Takayama H. Involvement of glycoprotein VI in platelet thrombus formation on both collagen and von Willebrand factor surfaces under flow conditions. *Circulation* 2002; **106**: 266–272.

68 Reininger AJ, Heijnen HF, Schumann H, Specht HM, Schramm W, Ruggeri ZM. Mechanism of platelet adhesion to von Willebrand factor and microparticle formation under high shear stress. *Blood* 2006; **107**: 3537–3545.

69 Nesbitt WS, Giuliano S, Kulkarni S, Dopheide SM, Harper IS, Jackson, SP. Intracellular calcium communication regulates platelet aggregation and thrombus growth. *J Cell Biol* 2003; **160**: 1151–1161.

70 Garcia A, Prabhakar S, Brock CJ, Pearce AC, Dwek RA, Watson SP, *et al.* Extensive analysis of the human platelet proteome by two-dimensional gel electrophoresis and mass spectrometry. *Proteomics* 2004; **4**: 656–668.

71 Coppinger JA, O'Connor R, Wynne K, Flanagan M, Sullivan M, Maguire PB. Moderation of the platelet release response by aspirin. *Blood* 2007; **109**: 4786–4792.

72 Maguire PB, Wynne KJ, Harney DF, O'Donoghue NM, Stephens G, Fitzgerald DJ. Identification of the phosphotyrosine proteome from thrombin activated platelets. *Proteomics* 2002; **2**: 642–648.

73 Gnatenko DV, Dunn JJ, McCorkle SR, Weissmann D, Perrotta PL, Bahou WF. Transcript profiling of human platelets using microarray and serial analysis of gene expression. *Blood* 2003; **101**: 2285–2293.

74 Bugert P, Dugrillon A, Günaydin A, Eichler H, Klüter H. Messenger RNA profiling of human platelets by microarray hybridization. *Thromb Haemost* 2003; **90**: 738–748.

75 Sun L, Gorospe JR, Hoffman EP, Rao AK. Decreased platelet expression of myosin regulatory light chain polypeptide (MYL9) and other genes with platelet dysfunction and CBFA2/RUNX1 mutation: insights from platelet expression profiling. *J Thromb Haemost* 2007; **5**: 146–154.

76 Jones CI, Garner SF, Angenent W, Bernard A, Berzuini C, Burns P, *et al.* Mapping the platelet profile for functional genomic studies and demonstration of the effect size of the GP6 locus. *J Thromb Haemost* 2007; **5**: 1756–1765.

77 Nelson EJ, Nair SC, Peretz H, Coller BS, Seligsohn U, Chandy M, *et al.* Diversity of Glanzmann thrombasthenia in Southern India: 10 novel mutations identified among 15 unrelated patients. *J Thromb Haemost* 2006; **4**: 1730–1737.

78 Castro V, Kroll H, Origa AF, Falconi MA, Marques SBD, Marba ST, *et al.* A prospective study on the prevalence and risk factors for neonatal thrombocytopenia among 9332 unselected Brazilian newborns. *Transfusion* 2007; **47**: 59–66.

79 Freson K, Devriendt K, Matthijs G, Van Hoof A, De Vos R, Thys C, *et al.* Platelet characteristics in patients with X-linked macrothrombocytopenia because of a novel GATA1 mutation. *Blood* 2001; **98**: 85–92.

13

Laboratory evaluation of von Willebrand disease: phenotypic analysis

E.J. Favaloro

Background

Von Willebrand disease and von Willebrand factor

Von Willebrand disease (VWD) is now recognized to be the most common inherited bleeding ailment. Individuals with VWD have defects in, or reduced levels of, von Willebrand factor (VWF), an adhesive plasma protein essential for primary hemostasis.[1-5] In plasma, VWF exists in a multimeric dimer configuration, ranging in size from small ("low molecular weight"; LMW) to "intermediate molecular weight" (IMW) to very large "high molecular weight" [HMW] forms. The larger the VWF molecule, the greater the overall number of individual adhesion sites, and thus the greater the overall adhesive capacity. VWD is very heterogeneous and may be characterized by quantitative or qualitative defects in VWF. Comprehensive laboratory testing is therefore required to define specific defects. The current VWD classification scheme is detailed elsewhere,[1] and summarized below. Although genetic testing is available in some geographic localities and useful for some selective clinical investigations, it is not indicated for most. Genetic testing for VWD is the subject of another chapter (Chapter 14). For practical purposes, a diagnosis of VWD, consistent with clinical findings and confirmed by phenotypic hemostasis testing, is accepted as sufficient evidence for VWD.

Quality in Laboratory Hemostasis and Thrombosis, 1st edition. By Steve Kitchen, John D. Olson and F. Eric Preston. Published 2009 by Blackwell Publishing. ISBN: 978-1-4051-6803-8

Type 1 VWD is caused by partial deficiency in VWF, whereas type 3 VWD occurs when VWF is essentially absent (i.e. both are "quantitative" defects).[1-5] In contrast, individuals with qualitative defects are classified as type 2, of which there are four subtypes: 2A, 2B, 2M and 2N.[1-5] Type 2A individuals have decreased VWF-dependent adhesion that is associated with a loss of HMW VWF multimers. Type 2B variants show an increased affinity for platelet glycoprotein Ib α (GPIBA), and sometimes also a loss of HMW VWF and mild thrombocytopenia. Type 2M variants have decreased platelet-dependent adhesion associated with evidence of a dysfunctional VWF molecule (activity decreased relative to antigen) that is not caused by a loss of HMW VWF. Type 2N variants have normal VWF platelet function; however, they demonstrate a markedly decreased affinity of VWF for factor VIII, usually causing a reduced circulating factor VIII. The correct classification of an individual's VWD is important not only because the presenting biologic activity of VWF determines the hemorrhagic risk, but also because subsequent clinical management may differ accordingly.

A number of other disorders can mimic VWD, because of similarities in clinical presentation and/or laboratory results. These disorders include "platelet-type" (PT-, or "pseudo-") VWD (a hereditary platelet GPIBA disorder caused by mutations in the *GPIBA* gene) and acquired VWD-like disorders associated with myeloproliferative disease or presenting as auto-anti-VWF antibody syndromes.[1-5]

Fundamental problems with the phenotypic evaluation of VWD

VWD heterogeneity and assay limitations
Because of individual assay limitations and evident VWD heterogeneity, no single laboratory procedure is able to detect all forms of VWD. For example, a normal level of plasma VWF protein ("antigen"; measured by the VWF:Ag assay) does not discount VWD, as many type 2 VWD individuals will have levels that fall within the normal reference range; these cases will therefore only be identified by performance of additional *functional* VWF assays.[1-7] Secondly, a low plasma level of VWF:Ag will suggest VWD, but cannot, in isolation, identify the underlying subtype. Accordingly, overall laboratory investigation for VWD requires a panel of tests. The classically used "VWD-screening" panel normally comprises factor VIII coagulant (FVIII:C), VWF:Ag *and* VWF function, typically using the ristocetin cofactor (VWF:RCo) assay, and, in some laboratories, the collagen binding (VWF:CB) assay and/or other VWF "activity" assays.[1-7]

The test panel of FVIII:C, VWF:Ag, VWF:RCo and VWF:CB will *identify* the majority of VWD cases, and supplementary tests can then be used to further *classify* the identified VWD. These include ristocetin-induced platelet aggregation (RIPA), VWF:Multimer analysis and VWF:FVIII binding assays. Other more recent diagnostic developments are also influencing VWD diagnostics.

Preanalytical variables
It is important to be aware of preanalytical variables,[8] as these cause substantial problems for the identification of VWD. In brief, collection of blood into inappropriate tubes, delayed transport of blood or of separated plasma, inappropriate transport of refrigerated whole blood or of non-frozen plasma, and inappropriate processing of whole blood or separated plasma (e.g. by filtration) can potentially lead to false identification of VWD in non-VWD individuals, or to false identification of type 2 VWD in type 1 VWD individuals. Poor collection techniques or difficult collections may also lead to partial sample clotting, and loss of HMW VWF because of entrapment or platelet activation.

VWF is an acute phase reactant causing levels to vary considerably in the same patient when studied on different occasions. Plasma levels of VWF may be related to inflammation, stress, diurnal variation (higher levels later in the day) and hormonal influences (e.g. fluctuations within menstrual cycles and higher levels in pregnancy). ABO blood groups also influence VWF levels, with lower levels in O blood group individuals compared to non-O blood group. VWF levels also increase with age. A diagnosis of VWD must take all these potential factors into account. At the very least, all tests should be repeated for confirmation using a freshly collected sample, taken some weeks apart, before making or excluding a definitive diagnosis of VWD. The investigations should also be repeated when normal results are obtained in individuals with a convincing clinical history of bleeding (e.g. the stress of a hospital visit may temporarily correct the abnormality).

Clinical evaluation, personal and family histories
A diagnosis of VWD should also not be made without a full and comprehensive clinical and family history and physical evaluation. Although important in the work-up of VWD, this aspect of diagnosis is not covered by this report, and the reader is referred elsewhere for details.[2]

Phenotypic assays used in the diagnosis of VWD

Routine coagulation tests

The prothrombin time (PT) and activated partial thromboplastin time (aPTT) are the two most widely used clot-based assays. The PT is not sensitive to deficiencies or defects in either FVIII:C or VWF. The aPTT is sensitive to deficiencies or defects in FVIII:C and because FVIII:C levels might be low in individuals with VWD, the aPTT has some limited value as a screening test for VWD. However, a normal aPTT will not exclude VWD. If VWD is suspected, appropriate specific and sensitive assays should always be performed.

Skin bleeding times and PFA-100®

Skin bleeding times (SBT) procedures are neither specific for, nor highly sensitive to the presence of VWD,[9,10] and are thus not recommended for this purpose. If the laboratory has a PFA-100®, this might be a better option for use as a VWD-screening tool in selected test cases as highlighted elsewhere.[9–11]

Platelet counts and platelet morphology

This is often worthwhile, especially when the individual initially presents and the clinical history is unclear. Both platelet count and platelet size should be evaluated. Individuals with type 2B VWD and PT-VWD will sometimes present with mild thrombocytopenia. Alternatively, platelet counts and platelet morphology may differentially define an alternate platelet-related disorder or deficiency to explain a bleeding propensity.[12–14]

Platelet function analysis

Ristocetin-induced platelet agglutination is a useful diagnostic test for VWD (see p. 128), otherwise standard platelet function testing *per se* is of no value in the diagnosis of VWD. Nevertheless, comprehensive platelet function would be indicated to define potential platelet abnormalities in the event that VWD investigations prove to be negative in individuals with strong clinical histories.[12–14]

Sensitive and specific laboratory assays for VWD

FVIII:C
Testing for FVIII:C should always be included in a phenotypic work-up for possible VWD. Although a number of methodologies are available, the "one-stage" clot-based assay is that most generally employed by laboratories for technical simplicity. Generally, the lower the FVIII:C, the more severe the VWD and the hemorrhagic risk. However, FVIII:C testing alone is insufficient to identify, diagnose or exclude VWD (i.e. a normal level of FVIII:C will not always exclude VWD, and an abnormal level will not necessarily define VWD, nor give information on the VWD subtype). Details regarding assays for coagulation factors are found elsewhere in this book (Chapter 9).

VWF:Ag
Many methods are available, although most laboratories now perform an enzyme-linked immunosorbent assay (ELISA) procedure or newer automated technologies such as immunoturbimetric or latex immunoassays (LIA).[3–7] Although LIA-based methodologies will continue to gain popularity because of automation, one drawback is the potential interference of rheumatoid factor. Interestingly, LIA assays also tend to provide higher values for VWF:Ag than do ELISA assays.[15] Importantly, assays will also differ in relative sensitivity at low VWF levels.[3–7] Used alone, determination of VWF:Ag will help *detect* all type 3 VWD, and *identify* most type 1 VWD, but will miss many type 2 VWD individuals. Also, while a low level may suggest VWD, it will provide no information on disease subtype.

Functional VWF assays I: VWF:RCo and VWF:Act assays
VWF:RCo is the original functional VWF assay,[16] and is classically performed using a platelet agglutination procedure, but has also now been automated. VWF:RCo assesses the ability of plasma VWF to bind to normal platelets in the presence of ristocetin, and has some capacity to preferentially recognize HMW forms. Thus, plasma from individuals with types 2A, 2B and usually 2M VWD will tend to give lower VWF:RCo results than VWF:Ag (i.e. show functional VWF discordance), because of the absence of HMW VWF (type 2B VWD), IMW and HMW VWF (type 2A VWD), or functionally defective VWF (type 2M VWD). However, there are notable assay problems that diminish the overall effectiveness of VWF:RCo, including assay reproducibility (i.e. high variability; intra-assay, inter-assay and inter-laboratory) and low level VWF sensitivity issues.[3–7] What this means in practice is that the test needs to be repeated several times for confirmation, and levels under 20% cannot be accurately determined by some methods. This is a serious assay limitation, given that most severe cases of VWD present with levels of VWF:RCo below 20%.

Because of the above, and because of the labor intensiveness of the classic VWF:RCo assay, several functional VWF alternatives continue to evolve.[3–7] Some methodologies include the incorporation of monoclonal antibodies (MAB) to functional epitopes in VWF, binding of VWF to collagen, and use of recombinant platelet receptor binding (e.g. using glycocalicin, which is a plasma analog of GPIBA) or MAB to these receptors. Only some of these assays use ristiocetin. One method, now commercially marketed as a VWF "activity" (VWF:Act) assay, utilizes a MAB against VWF in an ELISA. Several versions have been developed, none of which incorporate ristocetin, and these are not considered suitable as alternatives to classic VWF:RCo.[3–7,17,18]

More recently, two different versions of a "genuine" VWF:RCo ELISA have been described.[19–21] The first utilizes recombinant glycocalicin in an ELISA procedure that incorporates ristocetin to facilitate binding of added plasma VWF.[19] The assay correlates well with classic VWF:RCo, and has since been independently validated.[20] The alternative (newer) version utilizes a MAB to GPIBA to capture plasma glycocalicin and then a similar procedure (incorporating ristocetin) to facilitate VWF adhesion.[21] This assay also correlates well with classic VWF:RCo, and unpublished data from our own laboratory would support its potential utility in VWD, but otherwise the assay remains to be independently validated. Cross-laboratory studies for both these assays are also lacking at this time. Finally, the most recent entry into the VWF "Activity" assay group is an automated LIA-based assay. At this time, there are limited data on the assay's utility in VWD diagnostics, although such studies are encouraging.[15,22–24] Also encouraging are attempts to develop better ristocetin-based assays using flow cytometry.[25,26]

Functional VWF assays II: VWF:CB assays
The VWF:CB is typically performed by ELISA, although a flow cytometry based method has been described.[3,7] A number of different commercial ELISA-based kits are available. VWF:CB gives some estimate of the level of VWF present, but its greatest strength, when appropriately optimized, is its ability to selectively detect primarily HMW VWF (i.e. most functional, adhesive and hemostatically potent forms of VWF).[3,7,27] The VWF:CB is generally more sensitive to HMW forms of VWF than VWF:RCo, although efficacy depends on various factors, and not all VWF:CB assays behave identically. This standardization issue has delayed their more general incorporation into laboratory practice, and has been extensively discussed in previous reviews.[3,7] In brief, the following can be emphasized:
1 Type I/III collagen-mixture preparations (from equine or bovine tendon) are generally better able to preferentially detect HMW VWF than either purified

human derived type III collagen or purified animal derived type I collagen
2 The purified human derived type III collagen systems appear to bind VWF too well, and thus may not show selective discrimination of HMW VWF, and the purified type I collagen systems appear to bind VWF too poorly, leading to poor reproducibility issues, particularly at low levels of VWF
3 HMW VWF discrimination findings from factor concentrate studies seem to mimic those in plasma systems

Technically, VWF:CB ELISA assays use similar procedural steps to VWF:Ag ELISA assays, but rely on the ability of VWF to adhere to collagen. Although the potential significance of this as an *in vivo* correlate has yet to be fully evaluated. However, VWF binding to tissue matrix proteins including collagen is a primary hemostatic mechanism following injury, and it needs to be recognized that this adhesive activity is distinct to that identified by VWF:RCo assays. The potential importance of this is explored in more detail elsewhere.[6,7]

Ristocetin-induced platelet agglutination procedure
The RIPA assay assesses an individual's platelet-rich plasma (PRP) for sensitivity to ristocetin at various concentrations (typically, using at least two to three distinct concentrations over the range 0.5–1.5 mg/mL).[2–5] Ristocetin sensitivity in RIPA is dependent on both the level and functional activity of VWF. Normal individuals show platelet agglutination at (and above) 1.0–1.5 mg/mL ristocetin, but typically not at or below 0.5 mg/mL. Patients with type 3 VWD will typically not show any platelet agglutination even using high concentrations because they essentially lack VWF. The level of platelet agglutination using PRP from individuals with type 1 VWD will depend on the presenting plasma level of VWF. However, RIPA is somewhat insensitive to mild quantitative deficiencies, and individuals with moderate loss of VWF (e.g. presenting with levels above 30% VWF) may show normal RIPA. Alternatively, individuals with severe type 1 VWD (i.e. <15% VWF) or severe type 2A VWD will tend to show no agglutination (or only mild agglutination) with ≤1.5 mg/mL ristocetin. In contrast, individuals with type 2B VWD (and those with PT-VWD) show an enhanced agglutination response, and PRP will typically agglutinate with ≤0.5 mg/mL ristocetin.[2–5] RIPA is recom-

mended for use to confirm or subtype VWD in all patients showing a consistent discordance in VWF: Ag versus functional VWF (i.e. VWF:RCo and/or VWF:CB) and to differentially diagnose type 2B and PT-VWD.[2-5]

VWF:multimer assay

This gel eletrophoresis procedure identifies VWF of differing molecular weight, as well as identifying certain VWF structural abnormalities.[28,29] Because of test complexity, time and cost, it is now only performed by a limited number of expert laboratories (e.g. <5% of Australian laboratories). Although this procedure still has a place in VWD testing and diagnosis, its use is diminishing as alternative (easier to perform and faster) tests are improving. Nevertheless, VWF:multimers still form a part of the classification process,[1] and if it is locally available can be used to help confirm the diagnosis (i.e. to confirm or subtype VWD, particularly for qualitative VWD variants).

My personal view is that it is not generally appropriate to assess VWF:multimers during the initial VWD investigation process unless there is compelling clinical compulsion. VWF:multimers are not generally indicated when previous VWF testing using FVIII:C, VWF:Ag and functional VWF assays are consistently normal, and platelet function testing has excluded a platelet dysfunction, unless there is compelling evidence of mucocutaneous bleeding (in this case, a VWF structural abnormality is still feasible, although unlikely). VWF:multimers are also not generally indicated when previous VWF testing is suggestive of a quantitative VWF defect (i.e. type 1 or 3 VWD), because this will merely act to confirm the loss of VWF already identified by previous testing.

However, VWF:multimer testing may be useful when evident functional discordance has been identified (i.e. low VWF:RCo/VWF:Ag and/or low VWF: CB/VWF:Ag). The first approach here is to perform RIPA analysis (see p. 128). VWF:multimers may then be useful to help identify, distinguish or confirm type 2A VWD (loss of HMW and IMW VWF), type 2B VWD (loss of HMW and occasionally IMW VWF) and type 2M VWD (no significant loss of HMW or IMW VWF). Other qualitative defects (abnormal triplet patterns or smearing) may also be visible in the

gel pattern and potentially useful to identify unusual subtypes of VWD.

VWF:FVIII binding assay

This assay assesses the ability of an individual's VWF to bind FVIII and is used to differentially diagnose type 2N VWD. In the normal individual, factor VIII circulates bound to VWF and has a half-life of 8–12 hours. When VWC is structurally abnormal (e.g. type 2N VWD) or absent (i.e. type 3 VWD), the half-life of factor VIII is reduced to minutes, lowering the plasma concentration. Clinical manifestations of type 2N VWD are those of hemophilia. The VWF:FVIII binding assay is most frequently used for the differential diagnosis of hemophilia and type 2N VWD, rather than for the usual clinical presentations of VWD. This assay is typically performed as an ELISA procedure, and may also involve a chromogenic assay step.[30-32] A disproportion of bound VWF and bound FVIII identified in this assay (i.e. FVIII:VWF ratio <0.6) is suggestive of a type 2N VWD defect. This diagnosis can also be addressed with molecular methods, discussed in Chapter 14.

The VWF:FVIII binding assay should always be performed for newly identified individuals that give a clinical presentation of hemophilia, particularly where the genetic inheritance does not fit the classic pattern of hemophilia (which is sex-linked, whereas type 2N VWD is not). The penetrance of type 2N VWD may also be geographically based; for example, the disorder appears to be very common in north Europe (particularly in France, where it was originally identified),[33] but is less common in more distant localities (e.g. relatively rare in Australia).[32]

A diagnostic laboratory process for VWD

If VWD is suggested by clinical review the performance of routine coagulation tests such as PT and aPTT is optional, as is the performance of the PFA-100®.[2-7] However, performance of a platelet count is indicated together with FVIII:C plus VWF:Ag plus at least one (but preferably multiple) VWF functional assay(s). If only a single functional VWF assay is able to be supported by laboratories, then the VWF:CB appears to have some advantage over the VWF:RCo, for the following reasons:

1 The VWF:CB more consistently and correctly identifies types 2A and 2B VWD.

2 Is generally less variable in terms of intra-assay, inter-laboratory and inter-assay results.

3 Is usually more sensitive to low levels of VWF (important for proper identification of severe types 1, 2 and 3 VWD).

4 Uses similar methodology to VWF:Ag and thus is 'easier' to perform.[3,6,7]

Nevertheless, a diagnostic test panel that excludes the VWF:RCo may miss some patients with platelet function discordant type 2M VWD. However, it is no longer appropriate for laboratories to deploy the VWF:RCo as the sole VWF functional assay, because this approach will lead to the misdiagnosis of up to one-quarter of VWD cases being investigated, as well as potentially missing some (matrix-binding function-discordant) type 2M VWD cases.[7]

Based on the initial test findings, plus the degree of clinical evidence, further evaluation may or may not be required. Although the recommended steps outlined in this chapter will cover most situations appropriately, VWD does not always present in "textbook" fashion. Clinicians should at all times be guided by their patient's clinical history, and their local expert hemostasis laboratory's advice.

Possible outcomes

Exclusion of VWD

If all initial phenotypic test results are normal, and if the clinical suspicion is low, then further investigation may not be warranted, as VWD is highly unlikely. Alternatively, if results are normal, but the clinical suspicion is high, then test processes should be repeated for confirmation to discount a potential laboratory testing or collection artefact. Repeat testing is also required if the initial sampling occurred at an inappropriate time (e.g. during pregnancy or during acute stress when VWF levels might be falsely elevated). The supplementary tests of VWF:multimers and RIPA might be indicated if there is a strong clinical history of mucocutaneous bleeding even if the standard phenotypic tests (FVIII:C, VWF:Ag, VWF:RCo, VWF:CB) are all consistently normal, because an unusual or rare presentation of VWD is still fea-

sible, as recently illustrated.[34] VWF is a complex molecule, with multiple functional domains. We simply do not have all the required tools to identify all possible types of VWD. Although current testing should identify all currently known forms of VWD, there is no doubt that some forms of VWD are yet to be discovered, and potentially represented by abnormalities in VWF structure that current tests cannot identify.[7]

Similarly, the supplementary test of VWF:FVIII binding might also be indicated where there is a strong clinical history of hemophilia-like bleeding, even if the standard phenotypic tests (FVIII:C, VWF:Ag, VWF:Rco, VWF:CB) are all consistently normal, because the standard testing will occasionally miss some forms of type 2N VWD.[32] Finally, should all currently available VWF tests be normal, platelet function testing would then be indicated to identify potential platelet dysfunctions.[12-14]

Making a diagnosis of VWD

If test results are abnormal, then follow-up testing is indicated and is dependent on the initial pattern of phenotypic test results. Repeat testing for confirmation is usually indicated to exclude potential testing and/or collection artefacts, and because of assay variability and sampling issues. Repeat confirmation is particularly important when VWF:RCo is being employed as the sole functional VWF assay. It is important to repeat *all* the assays (i.e. VWF:Ag, VWF:RCo, VWF:CB, FVIII:C) on the second sample.

Identification of type 1 VWD

If all initial phenotypic tests (VWF:Ag, VWF:RCo, VWF:CB, FVIII:C) show low levels, but are proportionally similar (i.e. concordant test patterns obtained on initial *and* repeat testing), then type 1 VWD is most likely (Table 13.1). VWF:multimers are generally unnecessary (as the VWF distribution pattern will typically be normal and the overall relative intensity of multimer bands will simply correlate with the level of VWF). Further confirmation of severity using RIPA or a desmopressin challenge (or deamino D-arginine vasopressin [DDAVP] trial) may be useful in some cases.[35] The PFA-100® may also have a role in the setting of DDAVP trials.[36]

Table 13.1 Typical laboratory patterns in von Willebrand disease. Values within the table are approximate guide values only; different laboratories may derive different reference ranges. After Favaloro.[3-5]

Laboratory assay	VWD subtype					
	1	2A	2B[a]	2N	2M	3
Screening tests						
PT	Normal	Normal	Normal	Normal	Normal	Normal
aPTT	Raised (/normal)	Raised (/normal)	Normal (/raised)	Raised (/normal)	Normal (/raised)	Raised
Platelet count	Normal	Normal	Low (/normal)	Normal	Normal	Normal
PFA-100® (closure time; CT)	Prolonged/ (normal)	Prolonged/no closure	Prolonged/no closure	Normal	Prolonged/no closure	Prolonged/no closure
Diagnostic assays[b,c,d]						
FVIII:C	Low/ (normal)	Low/ (normal)	Low/normal	Proportional low	Normal/low	Low ("<20%")
VWF:Ag	Low ("<50%")	Low/(normal)	Low/normal	Normal (/low)	Normal/low	Very low ("<5%")
VWF:RCo	Low/(occasionally normal)	Low ("<30%")	Low/(occasionally normal)	Normal (/low)	Low (/normal)	Very low ("<5%")
VWF:CB	Low/(occasionally normal)	Very low ("<15%")	Low ("<40%")	Normal (/low)	Low (/normal)	Very low ("<5%")
VWF:RCo to VWF:Ag ratio[e,f,g,h]	Normal ("<0.7")	Low ("<0.7")	Low ("<0.7")	Normal ("<0.7")	Low/normal	Variable – do not use
VWF:CB to VWF:Ag ratio[e,f,g,h]	Normal ("<0.7")	Low ("<0.7")	Low ("<0.7")	Normal ("<0.7")	Low/normal	Variable – do not use

(Continued)

Table 13.1 *Continued*

Laboratory assay	VWD subtype					
	1	2A	2B[a]	2N	2M	3
Confirmative/VWD subtyping assays						
VWF:FVIII binding assay bound FVIII/bound VWF ratio	Normal (">0.6")	Normal (">0.6")	Normal (">0.6")	Low ("<0.6")	Normal (">0.6")	Variable – do not use
1.0 mg/mL	Reduced/(normal)	Reduced	Normal	Normal	Reduced/(normal)	Absent
1.5 mg/mL	Reduced/(normal)	Reduced/(normal)	Normal	Normal	Reduced/(normal)	Absent
VWF:multimer pattern	Normal pattern, VWF reduced	Large to intermediate multimers missing	Large multimers missing	Normal	Normal VWF multimer distribution (but with possible abnormal bands)	Multimers "absent"

[a]Pseudo- or "platelet-type" VWD patterns are similar to those for Type 2B VWD.

[b]For VWF and FVIII: values >50% usually considered normal; however, single or individual "normal" assay results cannot ciscount VWD.

[c]For VWF and FVIII: values <50% usually considered abnormal; however, single or individual "abnormal" assay results do not diagnose VWD.

[d]Normal reference ranges vary between laboratories, tests and methods; lower VWF values expected in blood group O individuals.

[e]Some workers use the reciprocal ratios (i.e. VWF: Ag/functional VWF [e.g. Ag/RCo, Ag/CB]).

[f]For 2A VWD, CB/Ag ratio generally lower than RCo/Ag because VWF:CB generally more sensitive to loss of HMW VWF than VWF:RCo.

[g]For 2M VWD, discordance in RCo/Ag or CB/Ag depends on the specific defect defined by the 2M VWD (i.e. platelet adhesion or matrix adhesion).

However, most type 2M VWD so far defined show inherent VWF-platelet-adhesion defect (not inherent VWF-collagen adhesion defect); so, in these cases of type 2M, RCo/Ag ratio is lower than CB/Ag ratio.

Modified from references [3–5], viz: Favaloro EJ. Laboratory assessment as a critical component of the appropriate diagnosis and sub-classification of von Willebrand's disease. *Blood Reviews* 1999;13:185–204. Favaloro EJ. Appropriate laboratory assessment as a critical facet in the proper diagnosis and sub-classification of von Willebrand's disorder. *Ballieres Best Pract Res Clin Haematol* 2001;14:299–319. Favaloro EJ. Laboratory identification of von Willebrand disease: Technical and scientific perspectives. *Semin Thromb Hemost* 2006;32:456–71. Reproduced with respective permission of Elsevier and Thieme.

[h]The cut-off value of 0.7 for assay ratios given in the above table is based on internal local studies: these cut-off values may differ from laboratory to laboratory. The risk of false positives and false negatives can be reduced by repeating the tests for confirmation, and by performing multiple test (VWF:RCo and VWF:CB) instead of single tests (VWF:RCo or VWF:CB) alone.

Identification of type 2 VWD

A discordant pattern is obtained if functional test results (i.e. FVIII:C, VWF:CB and/or VWF:RCo) are substantially lower than VWF:Ag (Table 13.1). In this case, type 2A, 2B, 2N or 2M VWD is likely. It should be noted that discordance using a VWF:Ag and VWF:RCo test combination is not always apparent upon single testing; again, it is important to repeat the assays to confirm or discount previous findings. If discordance between VWF:Ag and "VWF:function" (i.e. VWF:RCo and/or VWF:CB) is confirmed upon repeat testing, there is an indication to perform RIPA analysis. If RIPA is reduced, then type 2A or 2M VWD is suggested. If RIPA is enhanced, then type 2B VWD or PT-VWD is suggested.

In types 2A and 2B VWD, VWF:CB/VWF:Ag ratios generally tend to be lower than VWF:RCo/VWF:Ag, because the VWF:CB is generally more sensitive to the loss of HMW VWF than VWF:RCo. In type 2M VWD, VWF:RCo/VWF:Ag ratios generally tend to be lower than VWF:CB/VWF:Ag because most type 2M VWD so far described show an inherent VWF-platelet-adhesion defect rather than a VWF-collagen-adhesion defect. If required, types 2A and 2M VWD can be differentiated using VWF:multimer analysis. Again, it might be more useful to perform RIPA testing, or a DDAVP trial.[3–7,35]

If RIPA analysis shows enhanced responsiveness (i.e. at ≤ 0.5 mg/mL), then type 2B or a PT-VWD is indicated.[1–5] Mixtures of platelets and plasma from patients and normal subjects can help to identify if the defect is plasma or platelet related. Thus, type 2B VWD will show enhanced ristocetin responsiveness in mixed samples comprising normal platelets and patient plasma, but generally not with patient platelets and normal plasma. PT-VWD will show the opposite pattern, and give enhanced ristocetin responsiveness in mixed samples comprising patient platelets and normal plasma, but not with normal platelets and patient plasma. Differentiation between type 2B and PT-VWD is generally considered important because these are differentially managed.

Phenotypic discordance between VWF:Ag and FVIII:C (i.e. FVIII/VWF ratio <0.7), confirmed by repeat testing, usually indicates hemophilia A, but type 2N VWD is possible. Some guidance will be offered by family history studies (i.e. sex-linked or not). If type 2N VWD is suspected then specific VWF:

FVIII binding studies should be performed. If the FVIII bound to VWF is reduced in this assay (ratio of FVIII/VWF <0.6) then type 2N VWD is likely.[30–33] Alternatively, if the FVIII bound to VWF in the VWF:FVIII binding assay is not reduced (ratio of bound FVIII/VWF >0.6) then type 2N VWD is unlikely, and hemophilia A is probable. Discrimination of type 2N VWD from hemophilia A is clinically important, both from the viewpoint of treatment modalities and also genetic counseling.[31] However, it is important to note that a lack of discordance between VWF and FVIII:C screening assays will not always exclude type 2N VWD,[32] so direct analysis using the specific VWF:FVIII binding assay should always be performed if there is a clinical suspicion of type 2N VWD, even if initial VWF and FVIII:C discordance is not observed.

Identification of type 3 VWD

If the initial test results reveal that VWF was not detectable using any VWF assay (i.e. VWF:Ag, VWF:CB and VWF:RCo), then type 3 VWD is suggested. Repeat testing should be performed to confirm the severity of the disease. Remember that low level sensitivity issues may be a problem, particularly with VWF:RCo.[7] Molecular manifestations of type 3 VWD are addressed in Chapter 14.

DDAVP challenge or factor concentrate pharmacokinetic studies

Although therapeutic management of VWD is not a focus of this review, it is also important to consider the potential value of a DDAVP challenge or factor concentrate pharmacokinetics (PK) to the diagnosis of VWD. Such studies may permit more clinically relevant diagnosis and better discriminate type 1 from types 2A, 2M or 3 VWD, as well as identify VWF "secretory" VWD defects versus "clearance" defects.[1,3,35–38]

Recommendations and conclusions

1 Assessment of VWD requires both a thorough clinical evaluation and appropriate laboratory testing.

2 All relevant clinical criteria should be considered, especially bleeding and family history, but also age, gender, recent drug history, ABO blood group, pregnancy and estrogen replacement therapy.

3 As a screening process, and to exclude the presence of other hypocoagulopathic disorders, it would be reasonable to perform PT, aPTT, fibrinogen, thrombin time, platelet count, FVIII:C and VWF:Ag plus at least one (but preferably two) functional VWF assays (i.e. VWF:CB and VWF:RCo). If time is critical, a more pragmatic approach (e.g. inclusion of PFA-100® and specific coagulation factors) might be indicated.

4 Alternatively, if VWD is strongly suggested by clinical history or previous testing, a more direct comprehensive laboratory assessment is indicated. This may include retesting of the initial test panel for confirmation, plus RIPA and/or VWF:multimers and/or VWF:FVIII binding studies as specifically indicated.

5 All abnormal laboratory results should be repeated at least once, for both confirmation of previous findings and to exclude potential specimen collection, or laboratory testing artefacts. Similarly, when there is a moderate or strong clinical index of suspicion, all borderline or normal laboratory findings should also be repeated for confirmation (because of assay variation and individual fluctuations). Tests should also be repeated if the original sampling period might have resulted in spurious findings (e.g. tested during pregnancy).

6 The possibility of a platelet defect, or some specific factor deficiency, should also be considered if clinically indicated.

Acknowledgments

The author would like to thank all personnel from his laboratory for ongoing technical support over the past years.

References

1 Sadler JE, Budde U, Eikenboom JCJ, Favaloro EJ, Hill FG, Holmberg L, et al. Working Party on von Willebrand Disease Classification. Update on the pathophysiology and classification of von Willebrand disease: a report of the Subcommittee on von Willebrand Factor. *J Thromb Haemost* 2006; **4**: 2103–2114.

2 Laffan M, Brown SA, Collins PW, Cumming AM, Hill FGH, Keeling D, et al. The diagnosis of von Willebrand disease: a guideline from the UK Haemophilia Centre Doctors' Organization. *Haemophilia* 2004; **10**: 199–217.

3 Favaloro EJ. Laboratory identification of von Willebrand disease: Technical and scientific perspectives. *Semin Thromb Hemost* 2006; **32**: 456–471.

4 Favaloro EJ. Laboratory assessment as a critical component of the appropriate diagnosis and sub-classification of von Willebrand's disease. *Blood Reviews* 1999; **13**: 185–204.

5 Favaloro EJ. Appropriate laboratory assessment as a critical facet in the proper diagnosis and sub-classification of von Willebrand's disorder. *Baillieres Best Pract Res Clin Haematol* 2001; **14**: 299–319.

6 Favaloro EJ. von Willebrand factor (VWF) collagen binding (activity) assay (VWF:CBA) in the diagnosis of von Willebrand's disorder (VWD): A 15-year journey. *Semin Thromb Hemost* 2002; **28**: 191–202.

7 Favaloro EJ. An update on the von Willebrand factor collagen binding assay: 21 years of age and beyond adolescence, but not yet a mature adult. *Semin Thromb Hemost* 2007; **33**: 727–744.

8 Favaloro EJ. Preanalytical variables in coagulation testing. *Blood Coagul Fibrinolysis* 2007; **18**: 86–89.

9 Fressinaud E, Veyradier A, Truchaud F, Martin I, Boyer-Neumann C, Trossaert M, et al. Screening for von Willebrand disease with a new analyser using high shear stress: A study of 60 cases. *Blood* 1998; **91**: 1325–1331.

10 Cattaneo M, Federici AB, Lecchi A, Agati B, Lombardi R, Stabile F, et al. Evaluation of the PFA-100® system in the diagnosis and therapeutic monitoring of patients with von Willebrand disease. *Thromb Haemost* 1999; **82**: 35–39.

11 Favaloro EJ. The utility of the PFA-100® in the identification of von Willebrand disease: A concise review. *Semin Thromb Hemost* 2006, **32**: 537–545.

12 Hayward CPM. Inherited platelet disorders. *Curr Opin Hematol* 2003; **10**: 362–368.

13 Quiroga T, Goycoolea M, Panes O, Aranda E, Martínez C, Belmont S, et al. High prevalence of bleeders of unknown cause among patients with inherited mucocutaneous bleeding: a prospective study of 280 patients and 299 controls. *Haematologica* 2007; **92**: 357–365.

14 Favaloro EJ. Investigating people with mucocutaneous bleeding suggestive of primary hemostatic defects: a low

likelihood of a definitive diagnosis? *Haematologica* 2007; **92**: 292–296.

15 Favaloro EJ, Bonar R, Meiring M, Street A, Marsden K. RCPA QAP in Haematology. 2B or not 2B? Disparate discrimination of functional VWF discordance using different assay panels or methodologies may lead to success or failure in the early identification of type 2B VWD. *Thromb Haemost* 2007; **98**: 346–458.

16 Howard MA, Firkin BG. Ristocetin. A new tool in the investigation of platelet aggregation. *Thromb Diath Haemorrh* 1971; **26**: 362–365.

17 Favaloro EJ, Henniker A, Facey D, Hertzberg M. Discrimination of von Willebrand's disease (VWD) subtypes: Direct comparison of von Willebrand factor: collagen binding activity/assay (VWF:CBA) with monoclonal Antibody (MAB) based ELISA VWF-detection systems. *Thromb Haemost* 2000; **84**: 541–547.

18 Favaloro EJ. Discrimination of von Willebrand's disease (VWD) subtypes: Direct comparison of commercial ELISA-based options used to detect qualitative von Willebrand factor (VWF) defects. *Am J Clin Pathol* 2000; **114**: 608–618.

19 Vanhoorelbeke K, Cauwenberghs N, Vauterin S, Schlammadinger A, Mazurier C, Deckmyn H. A reliable and reproducible ELISA method to measure ristocetin cofactor activity of von Willebrand factor. *Thromb Haemost* 2000; **83**: 107–113.

20 Federici AB, Anciani MTC, Forza I, Mannucci PM, Marchese P, Ware J, et al. A sensitive ristocetin co-factor activity assay with recombinant glycoprotein Ibα for the diagnosis of patients with low von Willebrand factor levels. *Haematologica* 2004; **89**: 77–85.

21 Vanhoorelbeke K, Pareyn I, Schlammadinger A, Vauterin S, Hoylaerts MF, Arnout J, et al. Plasma glycocalicin as a source of GPIb alpha in the von Willebrand factor in the ristocetin cofactor ELISA. *Thromb Haemost* 2005; **93**: 165–171.

22 De Vleeschauwer A, Devreese K. Comparison of a new automated von Willebrand factor activity assay with an aggregation von Willebrand ristocetin cofactor activity assay for the diagnosis of von Willebrand disease. *Blood Coagul Fibrinolysis* 2006; **17**: 353–358.

23 Sucker C, Senft B, Scharf RE, Zotz RB. Determination of von Willebrand factor activity: Evaluation of the HaemosIL™ assay in comparison with established procedures. *Clin Appl Thromb Hemost* 2006; **12**: 305–310.

24 Piñol M, Sales M, Costa M, Tosetto A, Canciani MT, Federici AB. Evaluation of a new turbidimetric assay for von Willebrand factor activity useful in the general screening of von Willebrand disease. *Haematologica* 2007; **92**: 712–713.

25 Chen D, Daigh CA, Hendricksen JI, Pruthi RK, Nichols WL, Heit JA, et al. A highly sensitive plasma von Willebrand factor ristocetin cofactor (VWF:RCo) activity assay by flow cytometry. *J Thromb Haemost* 2008; **6**: 323–330.

26 Giannini S, Mezzasoma AM, Leone M, Gresele P. Laboratory diagnosis and monitoring of desmopressin treatment of von Willebrand's disease by flow cytometry. *Haematologica* 2007; **92**: 1647–1654.

27 Favaloro EJ. Collagen binding assay for von Willebrand Factor (VWF:CBA): Detection of von Willebrand's disease (VWD), and discrimination of VWD subtypes, depends on collagen source. *Thromb Haemost* 2000; **83**: 127–135.

28 Budde U, Pieconka A, Will K, Schneppenheim R. Laboratory testing for von Willebrand disease: contribution of multimer analysis to diagnosis and classification. *Semin Thromb Hemost* 2006; **32**: 514–521.

29 Adcock DM, Bethel M, Valcour A. Diagnosing von Willebrand disease: A large reference laboratory's perspective. *Semin Thromb Hemost* 2006; **32**: 472–479.

30 Nishino M, Girma J-P, Rothschild C, Fressinaud E, Meyer D. New variant of von Willebrand disease with defective binding to factor VIII. *Blood* 1989; **74**: 1591–1599.

31 Casonato A, Pontara E, Zerbinati P, Zucchetto A, Girolami A. The evaluation of factor VIII binding activity of von Willebrand factor by means of an ELISA method: significance and practical implications. *Am J Clin Pathol* 1998; **109**: 347–352.

32 Rodgers SE, Lerda NV, Favaloro EJ, Duncan EM, Casey GJ, Quinn DM, et al. Identification of von Willebrand's disorder type 2N (Normandy) in Australia: A cross-laboratory investigation using different methodologies. *Am J Clin Pathol* 2002; **118**: 269–276.

33 Meyer D, Fressinaud E, Gaucher C, Lavergne JM, Hilbert L, Ribba AS, et al. Gene defects in 150 unrelated French cases with type 2 von Willebrand disease: From the patient to the gene. INSERM Network on Molecular Abnormalities in von Willebrand disease. *Thromb Haemost* 1997; **78**: 451–456.

34 Casonato A, Sartorello F, Pontara E, Gallinaro L, Bertomoro A, Grazia Cattini M, et al. A novel von Willebrand factor mutation (I1372S) associated with type 2B-like von Willebrand disease: An elusive phenotype and a difficult diagnosis. *Thromb Haemost* 2007; **98**: 1182–1187.

35 Michiels JJ, van de Velde A, van Vliet HHDM, van der Planken M, Schroyens W, Berneman Z. Response of von Willebrand factor parameters to desmopressin in patients with type 1 and type 2 congenital von Willebrand disease: Diagnostic and therapeutic implications. *Semin Thromb Hemost* 2002; **28**: 111–131.

36 Favaloro EJ. Laboratory monitoring of therapy in von Willebrand disease: efficacy of the PFA-100® and von Willebrand factor:collagen-binding activity as coupled strategies. *Semin Thromb Hemost* 2006; **32**: 566–576.

37 Brown SA, Eldridge A, Collins PW, Bowen DJ. Increased clearance of von Willebrand factor antigen post-DDAVP in type 1 von Willebrand disease. *J Thromb Haemost* 2003; **1**: 1714–1717.

38 van Schooten CJ, Tjernberg P, Westein E, Terraube V, Castaman G, van Mourik JA, *et al.* Cysteine-mutations in von Willebrand factor associated with increased clearance. *J Thromb Haemost* 2005; **3**: 2228–2237.

14 Laboratory analysis of von Willebrand disease: molecular analysis

A. Goodeve & I. Peake

The common inherited bleeding disorder, von Willebrand disease (VWD), results from deficient or defective plasma von Willebrand factor (VWF). There are two important hemostatic roles for VWF: binding to and thus protecting factor VIII (FVIII) from premature proteolytic degradation and binding platelets to subendothelium at sites of vascular damage. The disorder is divided into three types: types 1 and 3 are partial and complete quantitative deficiencies whereas type 2 represents qualitative defects and is further divided into four subtypes, 2A, 2B, 2M and 2N, dependent upon the function perturbed.[1] The VWF gene (*VWF*), located on chromosome 12, encodes the large 2813 amino acid VWF protein. Its repeated domain structure is illustrated in Fig. 14.1.

VWF comprises 52 exons that span 178 kb of genomic DNA. An incomplete pseudogene with 97% homology to the gene, *VWFP*, on chromosome 22[2] complicates molecular analysis and polymerase chain reaction (PCR) primer design must be biased towards amplification of the gene and not the pseudogene. *VWF* mutation analysis has been undertaken since the gene was first cloned in the 1980s.[3] The International Society on Thrombosis and Haemostasis Scientific and Standardization Committee (ISTH SSC) on VWF Database (http://www.vwf.group.shef.ac.uk/VWF Database) lists information on previously identified *VWF* mutations and currently has 508 entries, giving

an indication of the extent of analysis undertaken by many laboratories worldwide.

Mutation analysis has initially been undertaken to understand the molecular basis of VWD. Subsequently, some mutation analysis has moved into diagnostic laboratories and analysis is currently undertaken in both research and diagnostic locations. This article considers particularly quality control issues in molecular genetic analysis of VWD and so has relevance especially for diagnostic laboratories. However, many of the issues discussed also apply to research laboratories obtaining correct mutation results. Only a brief description of VWD types and mutations responsible is presented, as this information is abundantly available elsewhere.[1,4–8]

Type 3 VWD

This is the most severe form of VWD where plasma VWF levels are generally undetectable. It is autosomal recessively inherited and has a prevalence of 0.5–6 per million population.[9–11] Type 3 VWD is most common in populations where consanguineous relationships are common. Carriers are often asymptomatic but affected individuals have severe bleeding problems that may require the infusion of blood products containing VWF.

A number of population-based studies have sought mutations in patients with type 3 VWD.[12–16] The VWF Database lists reported mutations.[17] Sequence alterations associated with type 3 VWD are reported from codon 47 in exon 3 to codon 2804 in exon 52 (Fig. 14.1). Of the mutations 81% are predicted to

Quality in Laboratory Hemostasis and Thrombosis, 1st edition. By Steve Kitchen, John D. Olson and F. Eric Preston. Published 2009 by Blackwell Publishing. ISBN: 978-1-4051-6803-8

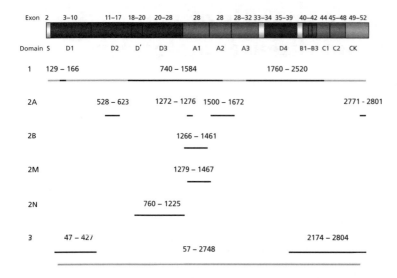

Fig. 14.1 Location of *VWF* point mutations in patients with von Willebrand disease (VWD). The top panel shows *VWF* domain structure with the exons encoding each domain indicated. The panels below show the main location of mutations identified in each VWD type. The black line in type 1 VWD denotes the most common mutation locations while the gray line denotes less commonly occurring mutations. In type 3 VWD, the black line denotes missense mutation locations while the gray line denotes null allele locations.

result in null (non-expressed) alleles and comprise nonsense (35%), small deletions (21%), splice mutations (13%), small insertions (8%) and large deletions (4%). The remaining 19% of mutations are missense and are largely located in the CK domain and propeptide where they are predicted to interfere with VWF dimerization and multimerization. Only a small number of large deletions have been reported, but this may partly result from difficulty in identifying heterozygous deletions. Point mutations are located throughout *VWF*.

A small number of diagnostic laboratories offer full analysis of *VWF* for mutations (exons 2–52 covering all of the protein coding region, plus intron–exon boundaries). Prenatal diagnosis in VWD is infrequently requested and is generally only carried out in cases of type 3 disease.[18]

Type 2 VWD

Type 2 VWD patients have plasma VWF that has abnormal function either in relation to the binding of VWF to platelets via the GP1b receptor or to circulating FVIII.

Type 2A VWD

Type 2A VWD is generally dominantly inherited and is usually a result of missense mutations within the A2 domain of *VWF* encoded by exon 28. These mutations can result in VWF that shows increased susceptibility to proteolysis by ADAMTS13, a plasma metaloprotease which moderates VWF function by cleavage, thus reducing the number of the largest, most active multimer forms of VWF in plasma.[19] Thus, VWF in the plasma of patients with type 2A has a reduced ability to bind to platelets and shows reduced proportions of high molecular weight (HMW) plasma VWF multimers. Phenotypic results in type 2A VWD reveal decreased platelet binding function (through the VWF:RCo assay).

Sequence analysis of exon 28 generally reveals a causative mutation that is highly penetrant and dominantly inherited. Type 2A VWD is a moderately severe bleeding condition and knowledge of the causative mutation within a family can be of value in genetic counselling and in confirming an individual's diagnosis when phenotypic tests are either unreliable or unavailable. If recessive inheritance is suspected or an exon 28 mutation is not identified, other regions of *VWF* may be analyzed (particularly exons 12–16 and 52; Fig. 14.1).

Type 2B VWD

Type 2B VWD is characterized by plasma VWD that shows increased ability to bind to platelets through the GP1b receptor. This can result in platelet microthrombi and a reduced platelet count (thrombocytopenia). As a result, and also because of enhanced ADAMTS13 cleavage resulting from the altered VWF conformation,[20] the plasma multimeric profile in type 2B VWD shows reduced levels of HMW VWF multimers. VWF mutations in type 2B VWD are found in the A1 domain at or close to the GP1b binding site. Analysis of *VWF* exon 28 will reveal mutations in most cases. However, the possibility of platelet type/pseudo VWD should also be contemplated if analysis of exon 28 does not identify any mutations. Mixing experiments can help phenotypically to clarify phenotype (Chapter 13).[21] Missense mutations affecting three *GPIBA* codons have been identified: p.Thr145Met, p.Gly233Val, p.Gly233Ser and p.Met239Val; these can readily be sought using a single PCR and sequence analysis. Mutations are listed on the Human Gene Mutation Database (HGMD; http://www.hgmd.cf.ac.uk/ac/index.php). The relative frequency of type 2B VWD and pseudo VWD is not yet established.[22] It is important to distinguish the disorders as treatment differs; VWF-containing concentrate should not be given to pseudo VWD patients.

Type 2B VWD is dominantly inherited with high penetrance, so knowledge of the causative mutation within a family can be of value in genetic counselling. It can also be important in diagnosis confirmation in relation to other type 2 conditions because any treatment that increases the level of the patient's plasma VWF (e.g. deamino D-arginine vasopressin [DDAVP]]) can result in increased platelet–platelet binding through VWF and an increased risk of thrombocytopenia.

Type 2M VWD

Type 2M is currently defined as occurring in individuals whose plasma VWF shows reduced ability to bind to platelets via GP1b but where HMW multimers are present (unlike type 2A). This type is generally poorly defined and on a functional level (reduced binding to platelet GP1b) could be considered as part of the type 2A subtype. Mutations are found within the carboxyl terminal of the A1 domain and very occasionally in the D4-CK domains.[17,23] and the condition is dominantly inherited with high penetrance. Typically, VWF levels in plasma do not respond to DDAVP and for this reason a precise diagnosis

based on causative mutation detection would seem appropriate.

Type 2N VWD

Type 2N VWD is characterized by reduced levels of plasma FVIII, considerably lower than the VWF levels, which can be completely normal. Mutations affect the ability of VWF to bind FVIII (VWF:FVIIIB). Recessive inheritance of the disorder results from one of three different scenarios:

1 Homozygous missense mutation affecting VWF:FVIIIB.
2 Compound heterozygous inheritance of two different missense mutations both affecting VWF:FVIIIB.
3 One missense mutation affecting VWF:FVIIIB plus a null allele.

The latter situation occurs most frequently. Missense mutations largely lie in the D′ domain encoded by exons 18–20, but case reports of mutations from exons 17–27 have been published. As in type 3 VWD, a second mutation resulting in a null allele can be anywhere in *VWF*. Heterozygotes for a single missense mutation can present with mildly reduced FVIII levels but are generally asymptomatic.

Phenotypically, the disorder appears very similar to mild hemophilia A and bleeding is largely brought about by the reduced FVIII level. A phenotypic VWF:FVIIIB assay can discriminate VWF that has a reduced ability to bind FVIII; however, the test is not widely available. Unless there is a reasonably extensive family history of bleeding, the two disorders cannot readily be discriminated by inheritance pattern and this can be further complicated as some hemophilia carrier females can have low FVIII levels and experience bleeding symptoms. *VWF* mutation analysis is most frequently requested in order to discriminate mild hemophilia A and 2N VWD.

Type 2 VWD summary

Overall, mutations in type 2 VWD have been well characterized and there is a close association between mutation location and VWF functional domain. Knowledge of the causative mutation within a family can add to the ability to predict bleeding risk within individuals and so will aid genetic counselling. Knowledge of the phenotype–genotype correlation of mutations also allows for targeted *VWF* analysis, so reducing cost and time.

Type 1 VWD

Type 1 VWD is the most common form of the disorder with about 70% of cases being so classified. Originally it was defined as those VWD patients with reduced plasma levels of normal VWF as assessed by a normal ratio of protein to function (VWF:RCo/ VWF:Ag as a specific activity) and a normal multimeric profile.[24] More recently[1] it has been accepted that subtle changes in the multimeric profile can be seen in the plasma VWF of some cases of type 1 VWD, notably those most severely affected with the lowest levels of plasma VWF. The VWF:RCo/VWF: Ag ratio can also be recorded as below 0.7[25] (the usually accepted limit between type 1 and type 2A or 2M patients) but the reliability of this assessment at low levels of VWF is poor.

Recently published multicenter studies on type 1 VWD from Europe and Canada[7,26,27] have revealed much information on the mutations that can be found in type 1 VWD. The EU study[26] used a non-selective recruitment strategy and consequently 38% of the recruited index cases showed some evidence of abnormal multimer structure but generally not typical of type 2A or 2B VWD. In over 90% of these cases a potentially causative mutation was identified and levels of plasma VWF:Ag were low (median 19 IU/ dL). Of the remaining index cases with normal multimers, 55% had a detected change in *VWF* (several had more than one). The Canadian study[27] was considerably more selective in its recruitment strategy and as a result the cohort resembled closely the group from the EU study having normal VWF multimers (see above) with 63% having detectable *VWF* alterations. In the UK study,[7] with the recruitment criteria intermediate between the above two studies, candidate mutations were identified in 53% of cases. Of identified mutations from the three studies 75% are missense, a small proportion result in in-frame deletions/insertions or exon skipping, the remainder are predicted to result in null alleles or are changes in the promoter region. Between 10 and 15% of patients had more than one mutation identified, which include both allelic (including gene conversions)[28] and compound heterozygous changes.[26]

The value of *VWF* analysis in type 1 VWD has been a matter of some debate particularly as it appears that mutations in this type of VWD, especially in the milder forms, are less frequent and when present demonstrate incomplete penetrance.[29,30] Based on the complete EU cohort and using levels of VWF:Ag as a descriptor, patients with <20 IU/dL VWF:Ag have a 96% chance of having a detectable *VWF* mutation with high penetrance. As such, knowledge of the mutation will have potential benefit in genetic counselling as for type 2 VWD. Patients with >40 IU/dL have 52% chance of having a *VWF* change, but these appear not to be highly penetrant and in many cases could be described as risk factors for bleeding. Their value in diagnosis and genetic counselling is probably limited. For those patients with 21–40 IU/dL VWF:Ag, 75% will have a detectable *VWF* change and it is likely that the penetrance and diagnostic significance of these "mutations" will be very variable. Further understanding of their significance through *in vitro* and *in vivo* expression studies is clearly indicated in this group.

Mutation analysis

Two different approaches have been applied to *VWF* mutation analysis: using a mutation screening technique to seek amplicons with sequence alterations followed by DNA sequencing of those that indicate a sequence change, for example confirmation sensitive gel electrophoresis (CSGE) or single-strand confirmation polymorphism analysis[16,26,31] and direct DNA sequencing of all exons and intron–exon boundaries.[7,13] The latter approach is becoming more common as DNA sequencing becomes cheaper and easier to undertake. In this instance, software that can help with identification of sequence alterations is vital.

Screening techniques, e.g. CSGE, are poor for many regions of *VWF* because of the high number of single nucleotide polymorphisms (SNPs). Some regions will frequently show a migration change indicating the presence of a sequence alteration caused by heterozygous SNPs and the amplicon will require sequencing, so such regions should be sequenced from the outset. Regions of *VWF* known to lack SNPs can be screened. The VWF Database and the single nucleotide polymorphism database (dbSNP; http://www.ncbi.nlm.nih.gov/projects/SNP/) can be used to identify SNP locations within the gene and highlight those where sequencing alone should be used.

Mutation analysis in VWD: When is it necessary?

For a condition such as VWD, where patients may have differing levels of severity and where the disease may show autosomal dominant or recessive inheritance, decisions on whether *VWF* gene analysis is necessary for the benefit of the patient and their family are complex. The additional well-reported feature of variable penetrance of clinical VWD within a family also adds to this complexity.

The following points should be considered when, in a diagnostic setting, *VWF* analysis is contemplated. The same considerations could also be addressed in the research environment when assessing the value of gene analysis in understanding the etiology of the condition:

1 The clinical severity of the condition in the index case and affected family members. It is clear that *VWF* mutations are highly prevalent in the most severe forms of VWD and that these mutations are highly penetrant. In milder cases of type 1 VWD, any candidate mutations identified are likely to display incomplete penetrance, where not all individuals inheriting the change have symptoms. Such sequence alterations should be treated as a risk factor for bleeding and decisions on whether to undertake genetic analysis based on likely findings in such cases.

2 The value of *VWF* analysis in relation to the desirability of early neonatal diagnosis or, in the most severe forms, prenatal diagnosis based on chorionic villus sample (CVS) analysis.

3 The possible association between a particular mutation and treatment.

4 The value of *VWF* analysis as a complement to phenotypic analysis where the latter results are unclear.

5 The cost–benefit of *VWF* analysis.

What to analyze?

Table 14.1 suggests regions of *VWF* that should be analyzed in each type of VWD.

Missing mutations and too many mutations

Mutations are not found in all VWD patients, even in phenotypically well-characterized VWD, and there are many possible explanations for this. In type 3 VWD about 90% of expected mutations are identified,[32] whereas in type 2 VWD more than 80% of expected mutations are identified (S. Enayat, personal communication, October 2007). In type 1 VWD a candidate mutation may be identified in about 60% of cases.[7,26,27] Mutations may be missed by the analysis, or lie outside the regions of the gene analyzed. *VWF* has an unusually large number of SNPs; PCR primers should be checked whenever there is a new build of the human genome to determine whether there are SNPs within the primer sequences used for PCR amplification. If only one allele and not both are amplified due to allele drop-out, an undetected candidate mutation on the non-amplified allele may be missed. Occasionally, the converse is seen; a "homozygous" mutation may apparently pass from one generation to the next due to allele drop-out of the normal allele.

A full or partial gene deletion should be suspected if a larger than expected number of contiguous homozygous SNPs are observed in an individual. Only a small number of full and/or partial *VWF* deletions have been described to date,[17,33–36] but this may reflect ascertainment bias; gene dosage analysis to seek deletions of one allele has not been described in VWD. In other genes, multiplex ligation-dependent probe amplification (MLPA)[37] and quantitative PCR from genomic DNA have been used to determine gene copy number.

Intronic sequence alterations leading to changes in splicing may occur. Although not yet reported in VWD, an example was described in hemophilia A of a point mutation deep in intron 1 creating a novel splice site and leading to an aberrant mRNA and lack of FVIII.[38] The mutation was detected using mRNA analysis and this may be helpful where *VWF* mutations cannot be identified in genomic DNA. Alterations in splicing may also result from changes to splice enhancers and repressors[39] whose role has not yet been explored in VWD.

The recent studies on type 1 VWD[7,26,27] analyzed the *VWF* promoter region and identified a number of sequence alterations. The majority were absent from normal individuals but their pathogenic significance

Table 14.1 Suggested extent of *VWF* analysis in patients with von Willebrand disease (VWD).

VWD type	Initial screen of exon no.	Additional screen of exon no./gene	Comments
1	18–28	Promoter-17 29–52	55% mutations located in central *VWF* region but significant proportion elsewhere
2A	28 (A2 domain)	12–16, 52	Screen additional exons if exon 28 mutation not identified or recessive inheritance suspected. In this case, second mutation may be a null allele, causative mutation can be anywhere in *VWF*
2B	28 (A1 domain)	*GP1BA*	Screen *GP1BA* for mutations resulting in pseudo VWD if exon 28 mutation not identified. Plasma mixing studies may also clarify phenotype
2M	28 (A2 domain)	35–52	Rarely, mutations more 3' than exon 28 have been identified[23]
2N	18–20	17, 21–27 *F8*	Screen additional exons if no missense mutation identified in exons 18–20. Phenotype analysis may indicate whether two VWF:FVIIIB missense mutations or missense plus null are expected. Mutation resulting in null allele can be anywhere in *VWF*. If no mutations identified, mild hemophilia A may be responsible for the phenotype
3	2–52		Mutations can be located anywhere in *VWF*, with no particular hotspot. Heterozygous large deletions difficult to identify. Linkage analysis possible for PND

has not yet been demonstrated. It is possible that some of these sequence alterations could result in reduced *VWF* expression from one allele. Promoter analysis may be justified in the future if such sequence alterations are shown to contribute significantly to reduced VWF levels.

In a small number of patients, more mutations than expected are detected; these may result from gene conversions[40] mediated by *VWFP*.[28] Up to five different single nucleotide substitutions have been reported to occur on a single allele as a result of gene conversion.[27] All of these possibilities should be borne in mind and mentioned where relevant when reporting mutations.

Prenatal diagnosis

Prenatal diagnosis is rarely requested in VWD, but type 3 VWD families who already have one affected child may wish to know the VWD status of further pregnancies. In these instances, where the familial mutation(s) has already been identified, the mutation(s) can be sought by targeted PCR and DNA sequencing. Where familial mutations have not been identified prior to pregnancy and time for mutation analysis is short, linkage analysis can be used. *VWF* has a number of short tandem repeat (STR) polymorphisms located in intron 40[18,41] and the promoter.[42] These can be analyzed singly using PCR amplification and gel electrophoresis or can be fluorescently labeled, amplified as a multiplex and analyzed using a DNA sequencer.[43]

Maternal and CVS DNA should be analyzed to confirm that maternal contamination of fetal material is absent. This can be achieved using for example the Powerplex 16 kit (Promega) where a number of STR loci from around the genome are analyzed. Two separate CVS fronds should be independently analyzed. This is particularly important where the fetal and maternal VWF genotypes are the same.

Internal quality control

A water blank should be included with every PCR amplification to ensure that there is no contamination of PCR reagents by exogenous DNA. No amplified product should be visible in this tube. Whenever any product is seen, all simultaneously amplified PCR products should be discarded.

Ensure that only *VWF* and not *VWFP* has been amplified. PCR primers should be designed with both gene and pseudogene sequences available and mismatches with *VWFP* incorporated at the 3′ end. Suspect that *VWFP* has also been amplified if a number of apparently heterozygous changes are seen within one amplicon. Gene–pseudogene mismatch positions may be responsible.

Always repeat the sequence of an amplicon in which a candidate mutation has been identified, preferably on a separately extracted DNA sample (from a blood sample taken on a different day if possible); if not, at least from a separate PCR amplification. A second scientist should independently check sequences, nucleotide number and base change and its predicted effect on the protein. When analyzing family members for a previously identified mutation, include a familial positive control plus a normal control lacking the familial mutation. If the mutation in the index case was not originally determined by the laboratory undertaking analysis of a subsequent family member and the DNA sample from the index case is not available, the report should highlight the name of the laboratory undertaking the original analysis and the report date. This is particularly important where the familial mutation is absent.

When a sequence alteration is identified, use the VWF Database and review the literature using both old and new VWF numbering (previous cDNA numbering was from the transcription start site, 250 bp 5′ to the currently used A of the ATG initiation codon. Protein numbering was from Ser764 of the mature VWF, rather than from the initiator methionine)[44] to seek previous reports of the mutation. If it has been previously reported, is the phenotype the same as in previous patients? If not, review the patient phenotype and be cautious.

For previously unreported missense mutations, a number of predictions of pathogenicity can be used,[45] these include SIFT,[46] PolyPhen[47] and Align GV GD.[48] Combined use of all three pieces of software is recommended to help predict the possible deleterious nature of any change.

Similarly, if a sequence alteration is suspected to have an effect on mRNA splicing, a number of prediction tools are available and the use of a number of these tools in combination is recommended before suggesting that an effect on splicing is likely; these include Fruit Fly (http://www.fruitfly.org/seq_tools/splice.html), NetGene2 (http://www.cbs.dtu.dk/services/NetGene2/) and Splice Site Finder (http://violin.genet.sickkids.on.ca/~ali/splicesitefinder.html). Where an effect on splicing is likely, follow-up by platelet mRNA analysis can confirm the prediction.[7]

External quality control

No materials are currently available for external quality control. Immortalized cell line DNA containing known *VWF* mutations may become available in the future through the UK National Institute for Biological Standards and Control (NIBSC).

External quality assessment

An external quality assessment (EQA) scheme is available through UK National External Quality Assessment Scheme (NEQAS) for Blood Coagulation on Hemophilia Genetics. This scheme runs twice yearly exercises that alternate between hemophilia A, hemophilia B and VWD;[49] other hemostasis genetic analysis EQA schemes may also be available. As with other molecular genetic EQA schemes, the three areas of clerical accuracy, genotyping and interpretation are examined. Marks are lost for errors in each of these three areas. Essential content for genetic analysis reports is given below.

Reporting

Develop standard templates for commonly used report types to avoid missing essential information. Reports should be written so that they can follow the patient and be interpreted by a number of healthcare professionals.

Nomenclature

Standard abbreviations for VWF and its activities should follow Mazurier and Rodeghiero.[50] Nucleotide and amino acid numbering, and nomenclature for sequence alterations should follow Human Genome Variation Society (HGVS) recommendations (http://www.hgvs.org/mutnomen/). GenBank reference sequences with version numbers should be stated for both cDNA and protein (currently NM_000552.3 and NP_000543.2).

Report inclusions

The following pieces of information are required by UK NEQAS to be present in genetic analysis reports, as they are necessary for complete understanding of patient mutation data and its interpretation:

1 The laboratory name and address and contact details for the individual(s) undertaking VWD genetic analysis.

2 Identity of the patient by first name, family name, date of birth plus at least one further unique identifier such as the hospital number.

3 Referring clinician's name and address.

4 Clinical question being investigated.

5 Patient's levels for VWF:Ag, VWF:RCo and FVIII:C. Where relevant also state result of other phenotypic assays such as VWF:FVIIIB, RIPA and multimer analysis.

6 Disease and gene being examined.

7 Extent of molecular analysis and if relevant, reference to the method. This can be added as a footnote.

8 Relationship between the patient and the index case where there is a family history of VWD.

9 Where a mutation(s) was identified, state whether the individual was homozygous heterozygous or compound heterozygous (if known).

10 The nucleotide change and predicted effect on the protein as a single block of text, following HGVS guidelines, e.g. c.2561G>A, predicted to result in p.Arg854Gln. This enables others transcribing the mutation data from the text the best chance of correctly copying the mutation.

11 Conclude whether a mutation(s) identified is commensurate with the phenotype. Be cautious with novel sequence alterations (check for SNPs, use relevant prediction software).

12 For previously reported mutations, reference the publication and include sufficient information for the reader to obtain the reference themselves.

13 If a mutation was identified, state that it has implications for family members.

14 If no mutation was identified, give possible reasons why (e.g. it could lie in unanalyzed regions of the gene) and suggest any further analysis that could be undertaken.

15 The interpretation must be succinct and accurate.

16 The report should be checked and signed by two suitably qualified healthcare professionals for accuracy of all information.

17 The reference cDNA and protein sequences used for comparison with the patient sequence should be stated. These can be added as footnotes.

18 The numbering scheme used should also be stated. VWF follows the HGVS conventions where nucleotide and amino acid numbering are from the 'A' of the methionine start codon.

19 Mention, where appropriate, the possibility of errors resulting from factors beyond the control of the laboratory (e.g. the need for family relationships as stated on the referral being correct).

Implementation of the above recommendations into both clinical reports and other descriptions of mutations where relevant should enhance the accuracy of the information transmitted.

References

1 Sadler JE, Budde U, Eikenboom JC, Favaloro EJ, Hill FG, Holmberg L, *et al.* Update on the pathophysiology and classification of von Willebrand disease: a report of the Subcommittee on von Willebrand Factor. *J Thromb Haemost* 2006; **42**: 103–114.

2 Mancuso DJ, Tuley EA, Westfield LA, Lester-Mancuso TL, Le Beau MM, Sorace JM, *et al.* Human von Willebrand factor gene and pseudogene: structural analysis and differentiation by polymerase chain reaction. *Biochemistry* 1991; **30**: 253–269.

3 Mancuso DJ, Tuley EA, Westfield LA, Worrall NK, Shelton-Inloes BB, Sorace JM, *et al.* Structure of the gene for human von Willebrand factor. *J Biol Chem* 1989; **264**: 19514–19527.

4 Goodeve A. Genetics of type 1 von Willebrand disease. *Curr Opin Hematol* 2007; **14**: 444–449.

5 James P, Lillicrap D. Genetic testing for von Willebrand disease: the Canadian experience. *Semin Thromb Hemost* 2006; **32**: 546–552.

6 James AH. Von Willebrand disease. *Obstet Gynecol Surv* 2006; **61**: 136–145.

7 Cumming A, Grundy P, Keeney S, Lester W, Enayat S, Guilliatt A, *et al*. An investigation of the von Willebrand factor genotype in UK patients diagnosed to have type 1 von Willebrand disease. *Thromb Haemost* 2006; **96**: 630–641.

8 Schneppenheim R, Budde U. Phenotypic and genotypic diagnosis of von Willebrand disease: a 2004 update. *Semin Hematol* 2005; **42**: 15–28.

9 Lak M, Peyvandi F, Mannucci PM. Clinical manifestations and complications of childbirth and replacement therapy in 385 Iranian patients with type 3 von Willebrand disease. *Br J Haematol* 2000; **111**: 1236–1239.

10 Berliner SA, Seligsohn U, Zivelin A, Zwang E, Sofferman G. A relatively high frequency of severe (type III) von Willebrand's disease in Israel. *Br J Haematol* 1986; **62**: 535–543.

11 Mannucci PM, Bloom AL, Larrieu MJ, Nilsson IM, West RR. Atherosclerosis and von Willebrand factor. I. Prevalence of severe von Willebrand's disease in western Europe and Israel. *Br J Haematol* 1984; **57**: 63–6

12 Schneppenheim R, Krey S, Bergmann F, Bock D, Budde U, Lange M, *et al*. Genetic heterogeneity of severe von Willebrand disease type III in the German population. *Hum Genet* 1994; **94**: 640–652.

13 Zhang ZP, Blomback M, Egberg N, Falk G, Anvret M. Characterization of the von Willebrand factor gene (VWF) in von Willebrand disease type III patients from 24 families of Swedish and Finnish origin. *Genomics* 1994; **21**: 188–193.

14 Eikenboom JC, Castaman G, Vos HL, Bertina RM, Rodeghiero F. Characterization of the genetic defects in recessive type 1 and type 3 von Willebrand disease patients of Italian origin. *Thromb Haemost* 1998; **79**: 709–717.

15 Baronciani L, Cozzi G, Canciani MT, Peyvandi F, Srivastava A, Federici AB, *et al*. Molecular characterization of a multiethnic group of 21 patients with type 3 von Willebrand disease. *Thromb Haemost* 2000; **84**: 536–540.

16 Baronciani L, Cozzi G, Canciani MT, Peyvandi F, Srivastava A, Federici AB, *et al*. Molecular defects in type 3 von Willebrand disease: updated results from 40 multiethnic patients. *Blood Cells Mol Dis* 2003; **30**: 264–270.

17 ISTH-VWF-SSC. International Society on Thrombosis and Haemostasis Scientific and Standardization Committee. http://www.vwf.group.shef.ac.uk/

18 Peake IR, Bowen D, Bignell P, Liddell MB, Sadler JE, Standen G, *et al*. Family studies and prenatal diagnosis in severe von Willebrand disease by polymerase chain reaction amplification of a variable number tandem repeat region of the von Willebrand factor gene. *Blood* 1990; **76**: 555–561.

19 Hassenpflug WA, Budde U, Obser T, Angerhaus D, Drewke E, Schneppenheim S, *et al*. Impact of mutations in the von Willebrand factor A2 domain on ADAMTS13-dependent proteolysis. *Blood* 2006; **107**: 2339–2345.

20 Rayes J, Hommais A, Legendre P, Tout H, Veyradier A, Obert B, *et al*. Effect of von Willebrand disease type 2B and type 2M mutations on the susceptibility of von Willebrand factor to ADAMTS-13. *J Thromb Haemost* 2007; **5**: 321–328.

21 Favaloro EJ. 2B or not 2B? Differential identification of type 2B, versus pseudo-von Willebrand disease: response to Whalley and Perry. *Br J Haematol* 2007; **136**: 345–346.

22 Enayat MS, Guilliatt AM, Lester W, Wilde JT, Williams MD, Hill FG. Distinguishing between type 2B and pseudo-von Willebrand disease and its clinical importance. *Br J Haematol* 2006; **133**: 664–666.

23 James PD, Notley C, Hegadorn C, Poon MC, Walker I, Rapson D, *et al*. Challenges in defining type 2M von Willebrand disease: results from a Canadian cohort study. *J Thromb Haemost* 2007; **5**: 1914–1922.

24 Sadler JE. A revised classification of von Willebrand disease. For the Subcommittee on von Willebrand Factor of the Scientific and Standardization Committee of the International Society on Thrombosis and Haemostasis. *Thromb Haemost* 1994; **71**: 520–52

25 Federici AB, Castaman G, Mannucci PM. Guidelines for the diagnosis and management of von Willebrand disease in Italy. *Haemophilia* 2002; **8**: 607–1.

26 Goodeve A, Eikenboom J, Castaman G, Rodeghiero F, Federici AB, Batlle J, *et al*. Phenotype and genotype of a cohort of families historically diagnosed with type 1 von Willebrand disease in the European study, Molecular and Clinical Markers for the Diagnosis and Management of Type 1 von Willebrand Disease (MCMDM-1VWD). *Blood* 2007; **109**: 112–121.

27 James PD, Notley C, Hegadorn C, Leggo J, Tuttle A, Tinlin S, *et al*. The mutational spectrum of type 1 von Willebrand disease: results from a Canadian cohort study. *Blood* 2007; **109**: 145–154.

28 Gupta PK, Adamtziki E, Budde U, Jaiprakash M, Kumar H, Harbeck-Seu A, *et al*. Gene conversions are a common cause of von Willebrand disease. *Br J Haematol* 2005; **130**: 752–758.

29 Keeney S, Cumming A, Hay C. Mutations in von Willebrand factor multimerization domains are not a common cause of classical type 1 von Willebrand disease. *Thromb Haemost* 1999; **82**: 1446–450.

30 Coughlan TC, Blagg JL, Abulola M, Daly ME, Hampton KK, Makris M, et al. Null alleles are not a common cause of type 1 von Willebrand disease in the British population. *Thromb Haemost* 1999; **82**: 1373–1375.

31 Soteh MH, Peake IR, Marsden L, Anson J, Batlle J, Meyer D, et al. Mutational analysis of the von Willebrand factor gene in type 1 von Willebrand disease using conformation sensitive gel electrophoresis: a comparison of fluorescent and manual techniques. *Haematologica* 2007; **92**: 550–553.

32 Eikenboom JC. Congenital von Willebrand disease type 3: clinical manifestations, pathophysiology and molecular biology. *Best Pract Res Clin Haematol* 2001; **14**: 365–379.

33 Ngo KY, Glotz VT, Koziol JA, Lynch DC, Gitschier J, Ranieri P, et al. Homozygous and heterozygous deletions of the von Willebrand factor gene in patients and carriers of severe von Willebrand disease. *Proc Natl Acad Sci U S A* 1988; **85**: 2753–2757.

34 Schneppenheim R, Castaman G, Federici AB, Kreuz W, Marschalek R, Oldenburg J, et al. A common 253-kb deletion involving VWF and TMEM16B in German and Italian patients with severe von Willebrand disease type 3. *J Thromb Haemost* 2007; **5**: 722–728.

35 Xie F, Wang X, Cooper DN, Chuzhanova N, Fang Y, Cai X, et al. A novel Alu-mediated 61-kb deletion of the von Willebrand factor (VWF) gene whose breakpoints co-locate with putative matrix attachment regions. *Blood Cells Mol Dis* 2006; **36**: 385–391.

36 Shelton-Inloes BB, Chehab FF, Mannucci PM, Federici AB, Sadler JE. Gene deletions correlate with the development of alloantibodies in von Willebrand disease. *J Clin Invest* 1987; **79**: 1459–1465.

37 Gille JJ, Hogervorst FB, Pals G, Wijnen JT, van Schooten RJ, Dommering CJ, et al. Genomic deletions of MSH2 and MLH1 in colorectal cancer families detected by a novel mutation detection approach. *Br J Cancer* 2002; **87**: 892–897.

38 Bagnall RD, Waseem NH, Green PM, Colvin B, Lee C, Giannelli F. Creation of a novel donor splice site in intron 1 of the factor VIII gene leads to activation of a 191 bp cryptic exon in two haemophilia A patients. *Br J Haematol* 1999; **107**: 766–771.

39 Wang GS, Cooper TA. Splicing in disease: disruption of the splicing code and the decoding machinery. *Nat Rev* 2007; **8**: 749–761.

40 Chen JM, Cooper DN, Chuzhanova N, Ferec C, Patrinos GP. Gene conversion: mechanisms, evolution and human disease. *Nat Rev Genet* 2007; **8**: 762–775.

41 van Amstel HK, Reitsma PH. Tetranucleotide repeat polymorphism in the vWF gene. *Nucleic Acids Res* 1990; **18**: 4957.

42 Zhang ZP, Deng LP, Blomback M, Anvret M. Dinucleotide repeat polymorphism in the promoter region of the human von Willebrand factor gene (vWF gene). *Hum Mol Genet* 1992; **1**: 780.

43 Vidal F, Julia A, Altisent C, Puig L, Gallardo D. Von Willebrand gene tracking by single-tube automated fluorescent analysis of four short tandem repeat polymorphisms. *Thromb Haemost* 2005; **93**: 976–981.

44 Goodeve AC, Eikenboom JC, Ginsburg D, Hilbert L, Mazurier C, Peake IR, et al. A standard nomenclature for von Willebrand factor gene mutations and polymorphisms. On behalf of the ISTH SSC Subcommittee on von Willebrand factor. *Thromb Haemost* 2001; **85**: 929–931.

45 Bhatti P, Church DM, Rutter JL, Struewing JP, Sigurdson AJ. Candidate single nucleotide polymorphism selection using publicly available tools: a guide for epidemiologists. *Am J Epidemiol* 2006; **164**: 794–804.

46 Ng PC, Henikoff S. Predicting deleterious amino acid substitutions. *Genome Res* 2001; **11**: 863–874.

47 Sunyaev S, Ramensky V, Koch I, Lathe W 3rd, Kondrashov AS, Bork P. Prediction of deleterious human alleles. *Hum Mol Genet* 2001; **10**: 591–597.

48 Tavtigian SV, Deffenbaugh AM, Yin L, Judkins T, Scholl T, Samollow PB, et al. Comprehensive statistical study of 452 BRCA1 missense substitutions with classification of eight recurrent substitutions as neutral. *J Med Genet* 2006; **43**: 295–305.

49 Perry DJ, Goodeve A, Hill M, Jennings I, Kitchen S, Walker I. The UK National External Quality Assessment Scheme (UK NEQAS) for molecular genetic testing in haemophilia. *Thromb Haemost* 2006; **96**: 597–601.

50 Mazurier C, Rodeghiero F. Recommended abbreviations for von Willebrand factor and its activities. *Thromb Haemost* 2001; **86**: 712.

15 Dilemmas in heritable thrombophilia testing

I.D. Walker & I. Jennings

Over the past decade, the number of requests for thrombophilia tests has risen dramatically, challenging resource allocation in already overstretched health budgets. This has led to serious discussions about who should be tested and why, what components and parameters should be measured, what methods should be used and how should results be interpreted? The purpose of this chapter is to debate some of these dilemmas in relation to testing for heritable thrombophilic defects.

What to include in the thrombophilia screen

The term thrombophilia "screen" is unfortunate because it implies testing or "screening" unselected subjects. Nonetheless, it is in widespread use and is useful shorthand for describing the list of tests a laboratory would usually perform in response to a request for thrombophilia testing. There is convincing evidence that antithrombin, protein C and S deficiencies are associated with an increased risk of venous thrombosis. Retrospective cohort analyses of family studies indicate a roughly 10-fold increase in risk compared to non-deficient subjects. There is also good evidence that factor V Leiden and the prothrombin G20210A mutation increase the risk of venous thrombosis

three- to sevenfold. The activated partial thromboplastin time (aPTT), prothrombin time and thrombin clotting time should be incorporated in the initial testing. The aPTT may identify some patients with antiphospholipid antibodies (depending on the sensitivity of the aPTT reagent used) but is not sufficient alone to exclude antiphospholipid antibodies. The thrombin clotting time will allow identification of dysfibrinogenemia (associated with increased thrombotic risk although the prevalence of fibrinogen abnormalities in patients with venous thrombosis is less than 1%) and heparin contamination. The prothrombin time is useful in the interpretation of low protein C or S results.

Some thrombophilias have a mixed etiology and are the result of environment interacting with underlying genetic factors. For activated protein C resistance (in the absence of factor V Leiden), elevated plasma factor VIII and hyperhomocysteinemia the best evidence is based on case–control studies which suggest a two- to threefold increased risk of venous thrombosis. Some authors recommend including an assay of clotting factor VIII in the thrombophilia screen and some also suggest including a test that will detect activated protein C resistance not resulting from factor V Leiden. Elevated homocysteine levels may be reduced by treatment with vitamins B_{12}, folic acid and B_6 but although elevated levels have been associated with an increased risk of venous thrombosis there is no evidence that reducing plasma homocysteine levels reduces recurrent venous thrombosis risk. Testing for the presence of the C677T methylene tetrahydrofolate reductase (MTHFR) mutation, which is associated with a mild elevation in plasma

Quality in Laboratory Hemostasis and Thrombosis, 1st edition. By Steve Kitchen, John D. Olson and F. Eric Preston. Published 2009 by Blackwell Publishing. ISBN: 978-1-4051-6803-8

homocysteine levels, is not clinically useful. Tests for fibrinolytic activity, widely used in early thrombophilia investigations, are considered too difficult to standardize and interpret to include in thrombophilia screening profiles. Their clinical utility in thrombophilia testing is now accepted as very limited. The tests that may be included in a thrombophilia screen are shown in Table 15.1. Possible additional tests are listed in Table 15.2. Diagnostic laboratories performing thrombophilia testing for heritable defects would usually include tests for the presence of acquired antiphospholipids – functional testing for lupus anticoagulant activity and immunologic testing for anticardiolipins and/or β_2-glycoprotein 1 – with their initial testing.

Which methods?

Given the general requirement to contain costs, routine diagnostic laboratories need to ensure that their testing profile includes methods that are as sensitive and specific as possible.

Antithrombin

Antithrombin (previously called antithrombin III) is the most important inhibitor of thrombin and also inhibits other coagulation serine proteases including activated factor X (factor Xa), factors IXa, XIa, XIIa and tissue factor bound factor VIIa. Antithrombin has two important functional regions: a thrombin-binding domain at Arg393-Ser394 (at the carboxyterminal end of the molecule) and a heparin binding site at its amino terminus. In the absence of heparin, antithrombin inactivates thrombin slowly – progressive antithrombin activity. Heparin binding to antithrombin produces a conformational change in antithrombin which accelerates by 4000-fold the rate of complex formation between antithrombin and serine proteases. This rapid inactivation of thrombin

Table 15.1 Suggested first line investigations. Discussion of the suggested methods is included in the text.

Test type		Method (see text for discussion)
Coagulation screen	Functional	Activated partial thromboplastin time, prothrombin time, thrombin clotting time
Antithrombin	Functional	Heparin cofactor activity with bovine thrombin or factor Xa substrate
Protein C	Functional	Chromogenic activity
Protein S	Immunologic	Free protein S antigen
Activated protein C resistance or	Functional	Predilution of test plasma in factor V depleted plasma
Factor V Leiden	DNA-based	
Prothrombin G20210A	DNA-based	

In addition, tests for acquired antiphospholipids are usually included

Lupus anticoagulant	Functional	Clotting-based tests
Anticardiolipins	Immunologic	

Table 15.2 Possible additional investigations.

Parameter	Method
Activated protein C resistance	Original (unmodified) test
Antithrombin antigen	Immunologic assay
Protein C antigen	Immunologic assay
Protein C activity	Clotting-based functional assay
Total protein S antigen	Immunologic assay
Protein S activity	Clotting-based functional assay
Fibrinogen	Clotting-based functional assay
Fibrinogen	Immunologic assay
FVIII, FIX, FXI	Clotting-based functional assays
Homocysteine	Functional or immunologic assay

and factor Xa in the presence of heparin is referred to as the heparin cofactor activity of antithrombin.

Two major types of heritable antithrombin deficiency are recognized. Type I deficiency is characterized by a quantitative reduction of qualitatively (functionally) normal antithrombin; antithrombin antigen and activity levels are concordantly reduced. Type II deficiency is brought about by the production of a qualitatively abnormal protein. Antithrombin activity is significantly reduced but antithrombin antigen levels are normal or near normal. Type II antithrombin deficiency is subclassified according to the site of the molecular defect. Reactive site variants have mutations near the thrombin-binding site and have decreased activity in both progressive antithrombin activity and heparin cofactor activity assays. Heparin binding site variants are caused by mutations at the amino terminus. Affected individuals generally have reduced heparin cofactor activity (approximately 50% of normal) but normal progressive antithrombin activity. Pleiotropic effect variants are the result of mutations at the carboxy terminal end of the antithrombin molecule. Affected individuals exhibit reductions in both heparin binding and progressive antithrombin activity.

Distinction between the types and subtypes of antithrombin deficiency is of clinical relevance because the incidence of thrombosis is higher in association with type I deficiency and type II reactive site defects than in type II heparin binding site defects. An initial classification into type I or II can be made by comparing the result of an immunologic assay with the result of the antithrombin heparin cofactor assay.

Antithrombin assays
Only functional assays of heparin cofactor activity will detect both type I and II antithrombin deficiencies. Type II defects, present in approximately 40% of subjects with antithrombin deficiency and a thrombotic history, may remain undetected if only an immunologic assay is used.

The incubation time of plasma with heparin and thrombin is critical. Maximal sensitivity of thrombin-based antithrombin assays to some heparin-binding defects occurs when the incubation time is reduced to 20 seconds, although incubation times up to 50 seconds will still detect other defects.[1] Because the majority of currently used antithrombin heparin cofactor activity assays utilize a long incubation,

heparin-binding defects are not detected by most routine diagnostic laboratories. This may be of no clinical significance, given the low prevalence of thrombotic events in subjects with these defects. Crossed immuno-electrophoresis with heparin is a simple tool which may be used to detect type II heparin-binding site variants.

Heparin cofactor II is a confounding factor in antithrombin heparin cofactor activity assays. Antithrombin heparin cofactor assays using human thrombin may overestimate antithrombin activity because 20–30% of the total activity measured may be brought about by heparin cofactor II activity. Bovine thrombin is minimally inhibited by heparin cofactor II. Heparin cofactor II does not inhibit factor Xa and requires concentrations of heparin of at least 1 unit/mL in the reaction mixture to function as an efficient inhibitor of thrombin.[2] Antithrombin heparin cofactor assay methods measuring plasma anti-factor Xa activity or those measuring anti-IIa activity in the presence of 0.22 mol NaCl exclude the influence of heparin cofactor II activity. An UK National External Quality Assessment Scheme (NEQAS) exercise demonstrated good sensitivity of bovine thrombin and Xa-based assays to a rare but clinically important antithrombin variant (antithrombin Wobble) but 40% of centers employing human thrombin-based assays failed to report reduced antithrombin activity in this plasma (unpublished data).

The missense substitution Ala384Ser (Cambridge II) is a relatively prevalent variant in the general population[3,4] but it is not detectable by assay of antithrombin antigen or by the anti-Xa heparin cofactor activity.[5] Although antithrombin Cambridge II has been associated with cases of venous thrombosis its clinical relevance is not clear.[6] In a recent study of 20 patients with antithrombin Cambridge II, antithrombin antigen and activity levels as measured by anti-Xa assay were within the normal ranges but, compared with controls, antithrombin activity measured in a chromogenic assay using bovine thrombin was mildly (but significantly) reduced.[3] This study also demonstrated an adjusted odds ratio of 9.75 of developing venous thrombosis associated with the Cambridge II variant – placing the thrombotic risk somewhere between that associated with a mild prothrombotic polymorphism (e.g. factor V Leiden) and that associated with severe thrombophilic mutations (e.g. type 1 antithrombin deficiency). In an exercise in which

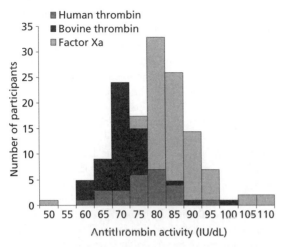

Fig. 15.1 Antithrombin activity assay results from an UK National External Quality Assessment Scheme (NEQAS) exercise in which participants were asked to test a sample from a donor heterozygous for antithrombin Cambridge II (Ala384Ser). The median antithrombin activity reported by 105 participants using factor Xa substrate was 83 IU/dL (range 50–110 IU/dL); by 25 participants using human thrombin substrate was 76 IU/dL (range 60–95 IU/dL); and by 59 participants using bovine thrombin substrate was 71 IU/dL (range 60–100 IU/dL).

the UK NEQAS for Blood Coagulation circulated a sample from a patient with antithrombin Cambridge II (Fig. 15.1), almost half of the centers using human thrombin-based assays and 80% of those using factor Xa-based assays reported antithrombin activity levels of 80 IU/dL or greater.

If it is considered necessary for a routine diagnostic laboratory to be able to detect antithrombin Cambridge II, an assay employing bovine thrombin would be preferable to an anti-Xa-based assay but antithrombin Cambridge II heterozygotes have only mildly impaired anti-IIa activity and even an assay using bovine thrombin may miss affected subjects.[7] Plasma methods for detection of antithrombin deficiency may have to be complemented with a genetic test for the point mutation to avoid underdiagnosing the Cambridge II variant.

Protein C

Activated protein C with its cofactor protein S inactivates the coagulation cascade cofactors factors Va

and VIIIa, reducing the thrombin generating capacity of blood. Protein C, the vitamin K dependent zymogen of activated protein C, is synthesized in the liver. Heritable protein C deficiency is usually an autosomal dominant trait. Homozygous protein C deficiency is an autosomal recessive disorder usually manifesting as neonatal purpura fulminans. Homozygotes with a milder phenotype have also been described.

As with antithrombin deficiency, familial protein C deficiency can be classified on the basis of phenotypic analysis employing functional and immunologic assays. Type I, accounting for 75% of heritable protein C deficiency, is characterized by concordant reductions of functional and immunoreactive protein C. In type II disease the functional protein C level is substantially lower than that of the antigen. Type II deficiencies may be subdivided into those with reduced function detectable in both coagulation and amidolytic assays (about 95% of type II protein C deficiencies) and those with reduced activity detectable only in coagulation-based assays. To detect both type I and II defects, a functional assay is required. The underlying genetic variant and associated phenotype are not predictive of thrombotic risk. Classification of protein C deficiency into types I and II therefore serves no useful clinical purpose.

The complexity of early protein C activity assays was avoided with the discovery of snake venoms capable of direct activation of protein C. The most widely used venom, available under the trade name Protac® (American Diagnostica), is isolated and purified from Agkistrodon contortrix contortrix (the southern copperhead snake). It activates protein C without affecting other components of hemostasis and without hydrolyzing to any significant extent chromogenic substrates for protein C. The activated protein C formed can be quantitated by clotting or chromogenic methods, the latter being more specific.

Protein C assays

There is a wide overlap in protein C activity between heterozygous carriers and their unaffected relatives in families with protein C deficiency.[8] For samples where clotting factor activation is suspected, e.g. pediatric samples and samples from patients with disseminated intravascular coagulation, a blank (water substituted for Protac®) tube should be included in chromogenic assays to avoid overestimation of protein C activity resulting from autohydrolysis of the chromogenic substrate.[9,10]

Some type II protein C defects, including some defects that impair the binding of protein C to protein S and calcium,[11] will not be detected by chromogenic assay but will be apparent only when a clot-based assay is performed. Early suggestions that 40% of type II protein C defects would be detectable only by clot-based assay[11] were an overestimate because they preceded knowledge of the effect of activated protein C (APC) resistance on some clot-based assays and it is likely that some individuals with factor V Leiden were erroneously diagnosed as having type II protein C deficiency. More recent estimates suggest that around 5% of type II protein C defects have normal amidolytic activity and are detectable only on clot-based assay.[12]

In an UK NEQAS for Blood Coagulation exercise in which a sample homozygous for factor V Leiden was distributed to participants, there was a significant difference in the median protein C activity reported by participants using chromogenic assays and those using a clotting-based assay (Fig. 15.2a) and more than half of the participants using a clotting-based assay erroneously diagnosed the sample as protein C deficient (Fig. 15.2b).[13] The effect of factor V Leiden may be avoided by predilution of plasma in protein C deficient plasma, or use of a chromogenic assay. In addition to the misleadingly low protein C activity levels that may be obtained with clotting-based assays in the presence of factor V Leiden, clotting-based assays are subject to interference by a number of other variables including elevated plasma factor VIII levels[14] or the presence of a lupus inhibitor[15] or heparin[16] or hyperlipidemia.

In patients on vitamin K antagonists, protein C antigen will be overestimated by Laurell rocket electrophoresis unless EDTA is present in the gel and buffer to ensure equal migration of carboxylated and non-carboxylated protein C.[17] More recently, other immunologic assays have been developed including the ELISA[18] and ELFA.

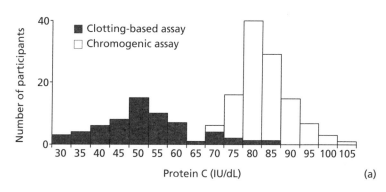

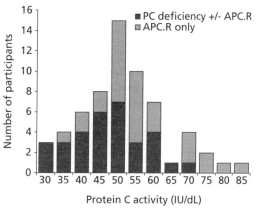

Fig. 15.2 (a) Protein C activity assay results from an UK National External Quality Assessment Scheme (NEQAS) exercise in which participants were asked to test a sample from a donor with no protein C defect but homozygous for factor V Leiden. The median protein C activity for 116 participants using chromogenic assays was 82.0 IU/dL and for 62 participants using clotting-based assays was 50 IU/dL. (b) Thirty-two of the 62 participants using clotting-based assays erroneously reported that the donor was protein C (PC) deficient with or without evidence of increased resistance to activated protein C (APC.R). The remaining 30 reported the donor had only increased resistance to activated protein C.

151

Protein S

Protein S is a vitamin K-dependent protein. Approximately 65% of the total plasma protein S is complexed with C4b-binding protein (C4bBP). Protein S that is bound to C4bBP has no cofactor activity. The remainder, designated free protein S, remains uncomplexed and is the active moiety – acting as a cofactor for APC in the degradation of factors Va and VIIIa.

Heritable protein S deficiency is classified into three subtypes. Type I protein S deficiency is a quantitative defect caused by genetic abnormalities that result in the reduced production of structurally normal protein, with reduced plasma levels of both total and free protein S antigen and a decrease in functional protein S. Type II protein S deficiency has been characterized as a qualitative defect with reduced protein S activity but normal (or near normal) levels of both total and free protein S antigen. In type III deficiency, although free protein S antigen and functional protein S are reduced, the total protein S antigen level is normal. Evaluation of the relationship between protein S and C4bBP in families with protein S deficiency has shown that types I and III may be phenotypic variants of the same disorder.[19]

Protein S assays

Accurate diagnosis of protein S deficiency is widely accepted as problematic. Overlap of total protein S antigen levels occurs between controls and subjects with heritable protein S variants. Types II and III protein S deficiency are not detected by total protein S antigen assay. It has even been suggested that some total protein S antigen assays will fail to detect type I deficiency. Free protein S antigen estimation is the preferred method for identifying protein S deficiency. Although free protein S antigen levels correlate well with protein S activity in subjects with types I and III protein S deficiency, they may not in patients with type II deficiency or an acquired deficiency.

Immunologic assays measure both fully carboxylated (active) and non-carboxylated (inactive) forms of free protein S and may overestimate the level of functional protein S. Free protein S antigen in a patient on warfarin will give higher values than those obtained using a functional assay. Total protein S antigen assays require conditions such that there is dissociation of the protein S–C4bBP complex, unless the antibodies used in the assay show equal affinity for bound and free protein S. Using ELISA methodology, high dilutions of plasma and long incubation times with primary antibody are required. If the dilution of the plasma or the incubation time is inadequate, total protein S levels may be underestimated. Measurement of free protein S antigen is required to distinguish type III protein S deficiency. Reduced free protein S antigen is the best indicator of a *PROS1* genetic defect.[20]

The original immunologic assays for protein S antigen used polyclonal antibodies that could not distinguish between the free and C4bBP bound protein S. Free protein S is measured in the supernatant fluid following precipitation of the C4bBP bound complexes by polyethylene glycol (PEG). This method is very cumbersome and poorly reproducible because standardization of the PEG precipitation step is difficult. The extra sample processing step was perceived to contribute to poor precision for this assay, and encouraged the development of methods for direct measurement of free protein S. With increasing understanding of the interaction between protein S and C4bBP it has become possible to prepare monoclonal antibodies against the protein S domain responsible for binding to C4bBP. These antibodies are relatively specific for free protein S and allow direct measurement of free protein S without the need for a precipitation stage. Latex immunoassays are now the most widely employed methods for measuring free protein S antigen but there may also be pitfalls related to the use of direct assays. It has been noted that when protein S levels are particularly reduced, monoclonal assays may overestimate free protein S concentration relative to the PEG method. Recently published data show that the incubation temperature for direct methods may be critical, and overestimation of free protein S in plasma from subjects with heritable protein S defects may occur.[21]

Type II (qualitative) protein S defects may be missed if an immunologic assay only is used and measuring protein S activity should, theoretically, be preferable to measurement of protein S antigen. Protein S activity may be measured by a number of prothrombin time or aPTT-based assays. These assays measure the effect that degradation of factors Va and VIIIa by APC with free protein S as a cofactor has on a clotting time test. Commercial kits employ different methodologies. In some, activation is mediated by bovine thromboplastin and in others by factors Va or Xa.

Ideally, these assays should reflect only free protein S activity but this is not always the case because separation of free protein S from C4bBP-complexed protein S is not performed in many of the available methods.

Although readily automated, protein S activity assays show considerable variation between methods, between laboratories and even within laboratories. Cut-off values vary between laboratories, instruments, reagent handling and other preanalytical variables and use of calibrant or reference plasmas from different sources may contribute to differences in results observed between methods. Some individuals with protein S deficiency will not be detected with some of the commercial kits for measuring protein S activity if the users employ the manufacturers' suggested reference ranges.[22]

Protein S activity assays may be sensitive to the inherited APC resistance associated with factor V Leiden (Fig. 15.3) and the acquired APC resistance observed in some patients with antiphospholipid antibodies. Protein S levels may be influenced by *in vitro* activation of factor VII, e.g. as a consequence of repeated freeze–thawing of samples. Without careful consideration of confounding factors, protein S activity assay use can lead to erroneous diagnosis of protein S deficiency. Where a functional protein S assay is used as an initial screening test for protein S deficiency, low results should always be further investigated with an immunoreactive assay of free protein S.[23]

Activated protein C resistance and factor V Leiden

APC resistance is defined as an impaired plasma anticoagulant response to APC added *in vitro*. APC with its cofactor protein S inactivates factors Va and VIIIa. APC cleaves factor Va at amino acid position Arg506 and subsequently at Arg306 and Arg 679. The majority of patients with familial APC resistance have factor V Leiden,[24] a point mutation in the gene for factor V which involves the 506 cleavage site.

Testing for APC resistance

Many factors including age, gender, pregnancy and estrogen use influence sensitivity to APC. The most commonly employed test system is aPTT-based. The aPTT is measured before and after the addition of exogenous APC and calcium to the test plasma. The resultant clotting times are expressed as a ratio the so-called APC sensitivity ratio (APC.R). The original aPTT test has a wide range of reported sensitivities and specificities. Methodologic variability can be reduced by "normalizing" the results by dividing the patient's APC.R by the APC.R of pooled normal plasma. If this system is adopted it is important to establish that the normal plasma pool does not include

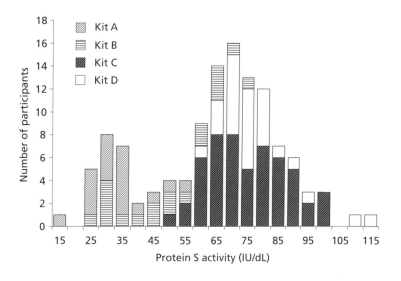

Fig. 15.3 Protein S activity assay results from an UK National External Quality Assessment Scheme (NEQAS) exercise in which participants were asked to test a sample from a donor with no protein S defect (median free protein S antigen 90.0 IU/dL; $n = 90$) but homozygous for factor V Leiden. The median protein S activity reported by 19 participants using kit A was 33.0 IU/dL; by 19 participants using kit B was 50.5 IU/dL; by 53 participants using kit C was 74.0 IU/dL; and by 28 participants using kit D was 75.4 IU/dL.

a contribution from an individual who carries the factor V Leiden mutation because even a single affected donation is sufficient to affect the APC.R of the pool. Although normalizing the result may reduce intra-laboratory and inter-laboratory variability, it does not significantly improve the diagnostic efficiency for APC resistance.

The originally described aPTT-based APC resistance test is not diagnostic of factor V Leiden because it is affected by plasma levels factor VIII and protein S and by the presence of antiphospholipids. It is also inaccurate if the patient has an elevated baseline aPTT because of deficiency of clotting factors or the presence of heparin. Predilution of the test plasma 1 in 5 in factor V deficient plasma reduces the number of confounding factors and increases the specificity of the aPTT-based APC.R as a screen for factor V Leiden.[25] This modification makes the test close to 100% specific and sensitive to factor V Leiden.[26] It may be expected that the factor V deficient plasma into which the test plasma is diluted would supply adequate levels of protein S to counteract the effect of protein S deficiency in the test plasma. However, it has been reported that protein S may become inactivated during the commercial preparation of factor V deficient plasma with the result that a test plasma may be erroneously classified as factor V Leiden positive.[27]

Because the modified test is also aPTT-based, it is subject to interference from lupus anticoagulant in the test plasma. Diluting the patient plasma 1 in 40 in factor V deficient plasma[28] or adding phospholipid to the test sample to neutralize the lupus anticoagulant activity[29] may overcome antiphospholipid interference. Prothrombin time or Russell Viper Venom-based tests have been described and are reported to be insensitive to lupus anticoagulants.[30] In practice, however, it is probably simpler to proceed directly to a genetic test for factor V Leiden in patients with antiphospholipids.

There is evidence that the APC.R determined with the original unmodified test correlates with venous thrombosis risk irrespective of whether or not factor V Leiden is present. The specificity of the modified APC.R test means that individuals who have increased APC resistance for reasons other than the possession of the factor V Leiden mutation will be overlooked if the original APC.R test is omitted from the screening procedure.

Detection of the factor V Leiden mutation

Factor V Leiden is a point mutation at nucleotide position 1691 that results in elimination of an *Mnl*I restriction site. Detection of the factor V Leiden mutation relies on amplification of the mutation site from either genomic DNA or from mRNA followed by digestion of the product with *Mnl*I.[31] The presence of the factor V Leiden mutation is indicated by the absence of an *Mnl*I site at position 1691. Testing by polymerase chain reaction (PCR) allows clear distinction of heterozygotes and homozgotes. Many other DNA-based assays for factor V Leiden have been described, including ELISA, melting curve analysis and fluorescence allele-specific discrimination methods.[32]

Prothrombin G20210A mutation

The G-A transition at nucleotide 20210 in the 3′ untranslated region of the prothrombin gene is associated with elevated plasma prothrombin levels and an increased risk of venous thrombosis.[33] In the absence of a specific phenotypic test for the presence of the variant 20210A allele, DNA-based procedures are required. The 20210A transition is not associated with the introduction or loss of a specific restriction enzyme recognition site and detection methods that do not require the use of restriction enzyme digestion of the amplified PCR product have been devised.

For both factor V Leiden and prothrombin G20210A investigations, studies have demonstrated errors are made by laboratories performing these complex tests, and it is important that robust assays with careful procedures and reporting systems are employed. Errors occur even in genetic testing and genetic tests are rarely repeated. Repeat testing should be considered at least for homozygous or doubly heterozygous patients where the thrombotic risk may be significantly increased.

Other tests

Homocysteine may be measured by a number of methods including fluorescence polarization immunoassay (FPIA) and high pressure liquid chromatography (HPLC). Between-center agreement in UK NEQAS for Blood Coagulation exercises is generally very good. Fibrinogen activity may be assessed by clotting-based methods and an immunologic assay may be used to confirm dysfibrinogenemia. Although some studies in which raised levels of factors VIII, IX or XI have been associated with thrombophilia were performed using immunologic methods, others have employed clotting methods to demonstrate an association.

What samples and when?

Sample quality is paramount. Although the thrombin time, antithrombin activity, aPTT and APC resistance test have been shown not to be influenced by sample collection into plastic tubes, statistically significant but clinically irrelevant differences were noted in the levels of protein S activity and chromogenic protein C activity between samples collected into glass and into plastic.[34] The choice of anticoagulant can also affect some tests, notably the APC. R test.[35]

Twenty-four hours' storage at either room temperature or 4°C has no significant effect on APC.R or assays of natural anticoagulants but artefactually increased APC resistance is seen in samples left for more than 24 hours post venepuncture.[36] Protein C and S levels may be reduced after 48 hours storage at either room temperature or 4°C so that subjects with borderline low normal levels may be misclassified as thrombophilic. In contrast, antithrombin levels may rise after storage at either room temperature or 4°C, so that subjects with a mutation associated with borderline antithrombin activity may be misclassified as normal.[36]

In general, antigen assays are unaffected by freeze–thawing of samples prior to analysis but functional assay results vary after freeze–thawing.[36] Platelet contamination or activation also results in artefactually increased resistance to APC.[37] Double centrifugation, and freezing of samples into multiple aliquots and storage at −40°C or below prior to testing is recommended.

There is seldom any point in striving to obtain samples for tests for heritable thrombophilia when the patient presents with deep vein thrombosis or pulmonary embolism. Testing is usually best delayed until at least a month after discontinuation of anticoagulation. Pregnancy and estrogen use reduce protein S levels significantly and increase resistance to APC. If possible, testing for heritable thrombophilia should be avoided during intercurrent illness, pregnancy, use

of a combined oral contraceptive or hormone replacement therapy. PCR-based tests for factor V Leiden and the prothrombin 20210A allele are unaffected by the above factors.

Effective use of internal quality assurance and participation in accredited external quality assessment schemes is essential. Internal quality control can ensure between-run precision but it is important to include both normal and borderline abnormal samples to control the assay at different levels of measurement. External quality assessment programs not only identify errors in individual laboratory performance but may also highlight methodologic errors and dilemmas in result interpretation.

Interpreting the results

Physiologic and pathologic variability

Many factors can affect the levels of the natural anticoagulants and other components of hemostasis. In adults, age and sex-related variations in antithrombin activity and antigen levels are minor so the reference ranges in healthy populations are narrow. Compared with adults and even older children, neonates have significantly different levels of many hemostasis components. Andrew et al., in a number of seminal publications, detailed reference ranges for many clotting factors and natural anticoagulants in both healthy full-term neonates[38] and in premature neonates.[39] Although still very useful as a guide, some of the ranges quoted would not necessarily transfer directly to currently used methods. Healthy newborns have about half of the normal adult antithrombin concentration and gradually reach the adult level by 6 months of age. Protein C activity levels appear to be related to age and sex but this is explained by blood lipid levels. Protein S levels are higher in males than in females and premenopausal women have lower levels than postmenopausal women. Overdiagnosis of protein S deficiency is therefore a risk in women. Because protein C and S are vitamin K-dependent, their concentrations are reduced in neonates. APC resistance is greater in females than in males.

Significant decreases in antithrombin activity are observed in patients on heparin treatment and in those with current thrombosis. Profound decreases in plasma antithrombin are seen in those with disseminated intravascular coagulation, liver disease and the nephrotic syndrome. Protein C activity is reduced by coumarins, in disseminated intravascular coagulation in severe liver disease, and in patients with sepsis. Measuring other vitamin K-dependent factors is often helpful in distinguishing heritable from acquired deficiency of protein C. Elevated levels of protein C have been reported in diabetic patients, in late pregnancy, during the puerperium and in patients using oral contraceptives or anabolic steroids. Protein S levels fall progressively during pregnancy, are reduced to lesser extent in women using estrogen-containing oral contraceptives or hormone replacement therapy and decrease during treatment with oral anticoagulants. Acquired protein S deficiency is seen in some patients with antiphospholipid antibodies and in disseminated intravascular coagulation and liver disease.

Reference ranges

Accurate and meaningful interpretation of individual test results is crucial. Attention to the validity of reference ranges for local methods and for the patient or population being studied is vital. Because so many preanalytical and analytical factors influence results, laboratories should determine their own local reference ranges for the tests that they offer. Ideally, for reference ranges for tests on adults, 120 "normal" healthy subjects should be included. The absolute minimum number needed is 40. The mean ±2 standard deviations may be employed for normal Gaussian distributions. As far as possible the sampling conditions applied to participants in the reference group should be applicable to the test population. Reference ranges must be constructed from samples handled in the same fashion as test samples. Reference ranges are applicable only to specific machine and reagent combinations and if any component of the "system" is changed new reference ranges should be established. In some circumstances the use of separate age and/or gender-specific reference ranges is necessary, e.g. in the neonate and during pregnancy.

It is appreciated that many laboratories find it increasingly difficult to recruit sufficient numbers of "normal" individuals to establish in-house reference ranges. Laboratories unable to establish a local reference range, or at least validate the manufacturer's quoted range, should consider whether they should be offering a thrombophilia testing service. The importance of locally determined reference ranges was seen in a retrospective survey of protein S assay results in 19 UK NEQAS exercises sent to participants between May 1998 and November 2002. In each of the groups of sample types, protein S deficient ($n = 4$), factor V Leiden ($n = 5$) and other defects ($n = 10$), protein S activity results varied between assay methods (Table 15.3). In this survey adoption of reference ranges provided from literature or manufacturers' data (without local validation) was shown to lead to errors in diagnosis.[22]

Patient-specific interpretative comment

Typically, thrombophilia test results are reported without patient-specific interpretive comment. Unfortunately, many requesting clinicians have little understanding of the vast number of factors that influence

Table 15.3 Inter-method variability for protein S activity assays. Data from the UK National External Quality Assessment Scheme (NEQAS) for Blood Coagulation, May 1998–November 2002.

Sample type	Protein S antigen (IU/dL)		Protein S activity (IU/dL)			
	Total PS	Free PS	All methods	Xa-based assay	Thromboplastin-based assay	Va-based assay
Protein S defect ($n = 4$)	47.8	18.4	27.6	39.6	29.2	21.5
No protein S defect						
FV Leiden ($n = 5$)	81.9	86.9	65.2	45.0	67.9	69.2
Other defect ($n = 10$)	88.2	80.0	87.0	79.1	83.5	82.3

thrombophilia test results and may interpret the results inappropriately – giving the patient possibly false reassurance if the tests are negative or overstating the risk associated with one of the more prevalent defects (e.g. factor V Leiden). In one large US academic medical center, physicians responded positively to the introduction of interpretive comments saying that they improved the diagnostic process and helped prevent misdiagnosis. In addition, interpretations appeared to improve ordering practices.[40]

Who should be tested?

A lengthy treatise on who should be tested and why is beyond the remit of this chapter. Suffice to say, where thrombophilia testing has been performed in the context of careful scientific studies it has led to greater understanding of the role of heritable thrombophilic defects in clinical disease, but it is often unclear what, if any, benefit accrues from testing individual patients in the clinical setting.

In general, screening of unselected patients in the hope of preventing venous thrombosis or pregnancy vascular complications is not cost effective. Identifying a thrombophilia seldom alters the management of an acute thrombotic event but, in a few cases, may lower the threshold for suggesting an extended period of anticoagulation. There is little evidence to support the use of thrombophilia testing to predict recurrence of thrombosis. Other measurements such as D-dimer levels have been shown to be of greater predictive value. Although finding a heritable thrombophilic defect usually has few implications for the patient with an acute venous thrombosis, it may be information viewed as useful to other family members. Affected women in symptomatic families may choose to avoid estrogen use for contraception or hormone replacement and may want to alert their antenatal care team to a potentially increased risk of a complicated pregnancy. However, clinicians and their patients should be aware that, although there is much published advice on the management of pregnant women with thrombophilia, with the exception of women with antiphospholipid syndrome, there is a lack of good evidence on which to base this advice.

Given the lack of evidence of clear benefit of thrombophilia testing in directing clinical management in most of the patients currently being tested and the potential for causing distress and possibly harm, clinicians should be advised that they should exercise restraint in ordering these tests and should consider carefully their reasons for testing individual patients.

References

1 Harper PLD. Screening for heparin binding variants of antithrombin. *J Clin Pathol* 1991; **44**: 1991.
2 Tollefsen DM, Majerus DW, Blank MK, Tollefsen DM, Majerus DW, Blank MK. Heparin cofactor II: purification and properties of a heparin-dependent inhibitor of thrombin in human plasma. *J Biol Chem* 1982; **257**: 2162–2169.
3 Corral J, Hernandez-Espinosa D, Soria JM, Gonzalez-Conejero R, Ordonez A, Gonzalez-Porras JR, *et al.* Antithrombin Cambridge II (A384S): an underestimated genetic risk factor for venous thrombosis. *Blood* 2007; **109**: 4258–4263.
4 Tait RC, Walker ID, Perry DJ, Islam SI, Daly ME, McCall F, *et al.* Prevalence of antithrombin deficiency in the healthy population. *Br J Haematol* 1994; **87**: 106–112.
5 Harper PL, Luddington RJ, Daly M, Bruce D, Williamson D, Edgar PF, *et al.* The incidence of dysfunctional antithrombin variants: four cases in 210 patients with thromboembolic disease. *Br J Haematol* 1991; **77**: 360–364.
6 Perry DJ, Daly ME, Tait RC, Walker ID, Brown K, Beauchamp NJ, *et al.* Antithrombin Cambridge II (Ala-384Ser): clinical, functional and haplotype analysis of 18 families. *Thromb Haemost* 1998; **79**: 249–253.
7 Jennings I, Kitchen S, Woods TA, Preston FE, Jennings I, Kitchen S, *et al.* Multilaboratory testing in thrombophilia through the United Kingdom National External Quality Assessment Scheme (Blood Coagulation) Quality Assurance Program. *Semin Thromb Hemost* 2005; **31**: 66–72.
8 Allaart CF, Poort SR, Rosendaal FR, Reitsma PH, Bertina RM, Briet E. Increased risk of venous thrombosis in carriers of hereditary protein C deficiency defect. *Lancet* 1993; **341**: 134–138.
9 Marlar RA, Mastovich S, Marlar RA, Mastovich S. Hereditary protein C deficiency: a review of the genetics, clinical presentation, diagnosis and treatment. [Review; 112 refs]. *Blood Coagul Fibrinolysis* 1990; **1**: 319–330.
10 Cooper PC, Cooper SM, Smith JM, Makris M. Chromogenic protein C assay: the importance of the blank. *Haemostasis* 2000; **30**: 46.

11 Marlar RA, Adcock DM, Madden RM, Marlar RA, Adcock DM, Madden RM. Hereditary dysfunctional protein C molecules (type II): assay characterization and proposed classification. *Thromb Haemost* 1990; 63: 375–379.

12 Faioni EM, Franchi F, Asti D, Mannucci PM, Faioni EM, Franchi F, et al. Resistance to activated protein C mimicking dysfunctional protein C: diagnostic approach [see comment]. *Blood Coagul Fibrinolysis* 1996; 7: 349–352.

13 Jennings I, Kitchen S, Cooper PC, Rimmer JE, Woods TA, Preston FE, et al. Further evidence that activated protein C resistance affects protein C coagulant activity assays. *Thromb Haemost* 2000; 83: 171–172.

14 de Moerloose P, Reber G, Bouviar CA. Spuriously low levels of protein C with a Protac activation clotting assay. *Thromb Haemost* 1988; 59: 543.

15 Simioni P, Lazzaro A, Zanardi S, Girolami A, Haire WD. Spurious protein C deficiency due to antiphospholipid antibodies. *Am J Hematol* 1991; 36: 299–301.

16 Sturk A, Morrien-Salomons WM, Huisman MV, Borm JJ, Buller HR, Ten Cate JW, et al. Analytical and clinical evaluation of commercial protein C assays. *Clin Chim Acta* 1987; 165: 263–270.

17 Mikami S, Tuddenham EG, Mikami S, Tuddenham EG. Studies on immunological assay of vitamin K dependent factors. II. Comparison of four immunoassay methods with functional activity of protein C in human plasma. *Br J Haematol* 1986; 62: 183–193.

18 Boyer C, Rothschild C, Wolf M, Amiral J, Meyer D, Larrieu MJ, et al. A new method for the estimation of protein C by ELISA. *Thromb Res* 1984; 36: 579–589.

19 Simmonds RE, Zoller B, Ireland H, Thompson E, de Frutos PG, Dahlback B, et al. Genetic and phenotypic analysis of a large (122-member) protein S-deficient kindred provides an explanation for the familial coexistence of type I and type III plasma phenotypes. *Blood* 1997; 89: 4364–4370.

20 Makris M, Leach M, Beauchamp NJ, Daly ME, Cooper PC, Hampton KK, et al. Genetic analysis, phenotypic diagnosis, and risk of venous thrombosis in families with inherited deficiencies of protein S. *Blood* 2000; 95: 1935–1941.

21 Tsuda T, Tsuda H, Yoshimura H, Hamasaki N, Tsuda T, Tsuda H, et al. Dynamic equilibrium between protein S and C4b binding protein is important for accurate determination of free protein S antigen. *Clin Chem Lab Med* 2002; 40: 563–567.

22 Jennings I, Kitchen S, Cooper P, Makris M, Preston FE, Jennings I, et al. Sensitivity of functional protein S assays to protein S deficiency: a comparative study of three commercial kits. *J Thromb Haemost* 2003; 1: 1112–1114.

23 Walker IDG. Investigation and management of heritable thrombophilia. *Br J Haematol* 2001; 114: 2001.

24 Bertina RM, Koeleman BPC, Koster T, Rosendaal FR, Dirven RJ, De Ronde H, et al. Mutation in blood coagulation factor V associated with resistance to activated protein C. *Nature* 1994; 369: 64–67.

25 Jorquera JI, Montoro JM, Fernandez MA, Aznar JA, Aznar J, Jorquera JI, et al. Modified test for activated protein C resistance [see comment]. *Lancet* 1994; 344: 1162–1163.

26 De Ronde H, Bertina RM, De Ronde H, Bertina RM. Careful selection of sample dilution and factor-V-deficient plasma makes the modified activated protein C resistance test highly specific for the factor V Leiden mutation. *Blood Coagul Fibrinolysis* 1999; 10: 7–17.

27 Samama MS, Gouin-Thibault I, Trossaert M, Van Dreden P, Combot C, Amiral J, et al. Low levels of protein S activity in factor V depleted plasma used in APC resistance test. *Thromb Haemost* 1998; 80: 715–716.

28 Benattar N, Schved JF, Biron-Andreani C, Benattar N, Schved JF, Biron-Andreani C. A new dilution for the modified APTT-based assay for activated protein C resistance: improvement of the reliability in patients with a lupus anticoagulant. *Thromb Haemost* 2000; 83: 967–968.

29 Martorell JR, Munoz-Castillo A, Gil JL, Martorell JR, Munoz-Castillo A, Gil JL. False positive activated protein C resistance test due to anti-phospholipid antibodies is corrected by platelet extract [see comment]. *Thromb Haemost* 1995; 74: 796–797.

30 Akhtar MS, Blair AJ, King TC, Sweeney JD, Akhtar MS, Blair AJ, et al. Whole blood screening test for factor V Leiden using a Russell viper venom time-based assay. *Am J Clin Pathol* 1998; 109: 387–391.

31 Bertina RM, Koeleman BP, Koster T, Rosendaal FR, Dirven RJ, De Ronde H, et al. Mutation in blood coagulation factor V associated with resistance to activated protein C [see comment]. *Nature* 1994; 369: 64–67.

32 Ledford M, Friedman KD, Hessner MJ, Moehlenkamp C, Williams TM, Larson RS, et al. A multi-site study for detection of the factor V (Leiden) mutation from genomic DNA using a homogeneous invader microtiter plate fluorescence resonance energy transfer (FRET) assay. *J Mol Diagn* 2000; 2: 97–104.

33 Poort SR, Rosendaal FR, Reitsma PH, et al. A common genetic variation in the 3'-untranslated region of the prothrombin gene is associated with elevated plasma prothrombin levels and an increase in venous thrombosis. *Blood* 1996; 88: 3698–3703.

34 Kratz A, Stanganelli N, Van Cott EM, Kratz A, Stanganelli N, Van Cott EM. A comparison of glass and plastic

blood collection tubes for routine and specialized coagulation assays: a comprehensive study [see comment]. *Arch Pathol Lab Med* 2006; **130**: 39–44.

35 De Ronde H, Bertina RM, De Ronde H, Bertina RM. Laboratory diagnosis of APC-resistance: a critical evaluation of the test and the development of diagnostic criteria. *Thromb Haemost* 1994; **72**: 880–886.

36 Luddington R, Peters J, Baker P, Baglin T, Luddington R, Peters J, *et al.* The effect of delayed analysis or freeze-thawing on the measurement of natural anticoagulants, resistance to activated protein C and markers of activation of the haemostatic system. *Thromb Res* 1997; **87**: 577–581.

37 Luddington R, Brown K, Baglin T. Effect of platelet phospholipid exposure on activated protein C resistance:

Implications for thrombophilia screening. *Br J Haematol* 1996; **92**: 744–746.

38 Andrew M, Paes B, Milner R, Johnston M, Mitchell L, Tollefsen DM, *et al.* Development of the human coagulation system in the full-term infant. *Blood* 1987; **70**: 165–172.

39 Andrew M, Paes B, Milner R, Johnston M, Mitchell L, Tollefsen DM, *et al.* Development of the human coagulation system in the healthy premature infant. *Blood* 1988; **72**: 1651–1657.

40 Laposata ME, Laposata M, Van Cott EM, Buchner DS, Kashalo MS, Dighe AS, *et al.* Physician survey of a laboratory medicine interpretive service and evaluation of the influence of interpretations on laboratory test ordering. *Arch Pathol Lab Med* 2004; **128**: 1424–1427.

16 Evaluation of antiphospholipid antibodies

M. Greaves

Antiphospholipid syndrome

Antiphospholipid syndrome is an important cause of thrombosis and pregnancy failure. Both are common in clinical practice and accurate diagnosis is essential to inform rational treatment decisions. Diagnosis is dependent upon recognition of the constellation of relevant clinical manifestations and confirmatory laboratory tests for antiphospholipid antibodies. Unfortunately, despite their widespread use, tests for antiphospholipid antibodies are not robust: there is no agreement on the most effective constellation of tests, standardization of methods is incomplete and reproducibility is poor. Because of these limitations the need for attention to quality assurance of tests for antiphospholipid antibodies and an awareness of their limitations are paramount if clinical management is to be optimal.

In this chapter the features of antiphospholipid syndrome are first reviewed, and the nature of antiphospholipid antibodies described, in order to set the context for a discussion of the important issues around the laboratory evaluation of antiphospholipid antibodies.

Definition of antiphospholipid syndrome

Antiphospholipid syndrome is an acquired thrombophilia with an immune pathogenesis. Diagnosis requires the coexistence of clinical manifestations,

thrombosis or pregnancy complications, and the presence of antiphospholipid antibodies. These include anticardiolipin antibodies, anti-β_2-lycoprotein I and lupus anticoagulant, which are described below. Internationally agreed diagnostic criteria for the syndrome have been established in order to improve diagnostic accuracy (Table 16.1).[1] There must be at least one clinical and at least one laboratory criterion present. The laboratory test must be consistently positive on at least two occasions 12 weeks apart as transient antibodies may occur, e.g. in infection, and such antibodies are not usually associated with clinical events.

The titer of anticardiolipin antibody must be moderate or high, as low titer antibodies are common and may not be clinically significant. The same applies to anti-β_2-glycoprotein I. The syndrome may occur against a background of systemic autoimmune disease, especially systemic lupus erythematosus (secondary antiphospholipid syndrome) or in isolation (primary antiphospholipid syndrome).

The common thrombotic events are venous thromboembolism and ischemic stroke but thrombosis in any vascular territory may occur. Some other clinical associations with antiphospholipid antibodies have been identified. These include thrombocytopenia, skin lesions including ulceration and livedo reticularis, and non-stroke neurologic conditions such as transverse myelopathy.

Antiphospholipid antibodies

The nomenclature of antiphospholipid antibodies can appear confusing as it is based on historical under-

Quality in Laboratory Hemostasis and Thrombosis, 1st edition. By Steve Kitchen, John D. Olson and F. Eric Preston. Published 2009 by Blackwell Publishing. ISBN: 978-1-4051-6803-8

Table 16.1 Clinical and laboratory criteria of antiphospholipid syndrome.

Clinical criteria	Laboratory criteria
Thrombosis: Arterial, venous or microvascular thrombosis in any tissue or organ	IgG and/or IgM anticardiolipin antibodies at moderate or high concentration and/or: IgG and/or IgM anti-β_2-glycoprotein I at moderate or high concentration and/or lupus anticoagulant
Pregnancy complications: Unexplained death of a morphologically normal fetus at or after 10 weeks Three or more unexplained consecutive abortions before 10 weeks Premature birth before 34 weeks due to severe pre-eclampsia or placental insufficiency	

standing which has been superceded without revision of the terminology. Antibodies that are apparently reactive with phospholipid have been recognized for many decades, in association with disease. The "serological false positive test for syphilis" is the earliest example. It was identified in some subjects with systemic lupus erythematosus (SLE) and was demonstrated to be brought about by antibodies in serum that bind to negatively charged phospholipid. Subsequently, cardiolipin, a phospholipid component of the mitochondrial membrane, was used routinely as the antigen in diagnostic assays in SLE and some other systemic autoimmune diseases. Eventually it was noted that tests for these anticardiolipin antibodies could identify patients with a prothrombotic state: antiphospholipid syndrome.

It was observed independently that the plasma of some subjects with SLE has a prolonged clotting time, especially the activated partial thromboplastin time (aPTT) or kaolin clotting time (KCT), in the absence of any clinical bleeding tendency. This was shown to be because of the presence of an *in vitro* inhibitor of coagulation; the term lupus anticoagulant was coined. This lupus anticoagulant coagulation inhibitor is an immunoglobulin. In SLE, both anticardiolipin antibodies and lupus anticoagulant may be present and, paradoxically, the presence of antiphospholipid antibodies, including lupus anticoagulant, is not only unaccompanied by clinical bleeding but is associated with an increased risk of thrombosis: antiphospholipid syndrome. Subsequently the link was made to recurrent pregnancy failure and other pregnancy complications.

In addition to the paradox of the association between lupus anticoagulant and thrombosis rather than bleeding there is a further complication in relation to terminology; recent observations have demonstrated clearly that, in relation to antiphospholipid antibodies, the relevant antigenic sites do not reside on phospholipid. In the early 1990s it was demonstrated that at least some antiphospholipid antibodies bind to a protein, β_2-glycoprotein I. This protein is present in high concentration in plasma. β_2-Glycoprotein I is a member of the family of complement control proteins (CCP). It binds avidly to anionic phospholipids and has a weak anticoagulant effect. Some other plasma proteins can also serve as target antigens for antiphospholipid antibodies. These include prothrombin, protein C and annexin V. They all have a propensity to bind to anionic phospholipid. The apparent binding of antiphospholipid antibodies to phospholipid is through the clustering of antigenic sites on the target phospholipid binding protein when the latter binds to a negatively charged phospholipid surface, facilitating bivalent antibody binding to epitopes on the bound protein. In the diagnostic laboratory this phenomenon is exploited for the detection of antiphospholipid antibodies by coating of plastic wells with phospholipid, β_2-glycoprotein I, prothrombin or other relevant protein in enzyme-linked immunosorbent assays (ELISA).

Lupus anticoagulants

Lupus anticoagulants are heterogeneous, an observation of some importance in relation to the need for the development of improved assays designed to detect clinically important lupus anticoagulant antibodies only. Both antiprothrombin and anti-β_2-glycoprotein I type antiphospholipid antibodies may have lupus anticoagulant activity. The likely explanation is that binding of such antibodies to their phospholipid-binding protein target interferes with the assembly of the prothrombinase complex on the template provided by anionic phospholipids. For example, antibodies to β_2-glycoprotein I enhance the binding of β_2-glycoprotein I to phospholipid *in vitro*. As a result thrombin generation is slowed, resulting in a prolonged time to clot formation in phospholipid-dependent coagulation tests, especially when available phospholipid is rate limiting such as in the KCT and the dilute Russell's viper venom time (DRVVT).

The pivotal role of β_2-glycoprotein I

Increased knowledge of the structure and properties of β_2-glycoprotein I has assisted in understanding of the nature and pathogenicity of antiphospholipid antibodies. β_2-Glycoprotein I has five domains characterized by CCP repeats. The first four are similar but the fifth is larger and includes a cluster of positively charged amino acids. This explains the anionic phospholipid-binding property. Antibodies may be directed against epitopes on any of the five domains. However, recent data indicate that it is only those that react with a specific epitope on domain I that have lupus anticoagulant activity. Furthermore, it is domain I antibodies that associate strongly with thrombotic manifestations.[2]

Observational studies suggest that positivity in tests for lupus anticoagulant is more strongly associated with thrombosis[3] and recurrent late fetal loss[4] than is the presence of anticardiolipin antibodies and the above observations relating to β_2-glycoprotein I indicate that clinical specificity may be improved by assay of anti-β_2-glycoprotein I rather than anticardiolipin antibodies. What is more, there is a potential to increase assay specificity still further by focusing on antibodies to domain I.

Lupus anticoagulant assays

All current tests for lupus anticoagulant are coagulation-based assays performed on citrated plasma. As such they are indirect tests and are not completely specific. For example, prolongation of clotting time can be obtained in the presence of other coagulation inhibitors or as a result of coagulation factor deficiency. However, the specificity can be improved through selection of reagents and conditions that increase sensitivity to lupus anticoagulant, by mixing studies to confirm inhibitory activity rather than factor deficiency, and by inclusion of additional steps to demonstrate the phospholipid-dependent nature of any inhibitor. There are numerous publications on the selection and performance of lupus anticoagulant assays, e.g. the guidelines on this topic prepared by the British Committee for Standards in Haematology.[5] The coagulation tests that are generally regarded to be most useful in the diagnostic laboratory are the aPTT, KCT and DRVVT. There is no test that is completely sensitive to and specific for lupus anticoagulant, so it is recommended that at least two tests are used together to improve sensitivity. Furthermore, the presence of anionic phospholipid in test plasma can potentially reduce assay sensitivity. The most likely source is blood cell membrane. To minimize this possibility plasma should be prepared as soon as possible after venepuncture, preferably within 1 hour, and subjected to further centrifugation or filtration to minimize phospholipid contamination.

Activated partial thromboplastin time

APTT reagents vary markedly in the composition and concentrations of phospholipid. This results in considerable heterogeneity in terms of sensitivity to lupus anticoagulant. Furthermore, the coagulation time in the aPTT test is influenced by the concentrations of all coagulation factors in the intrinsic and common pathways and this impacts on both sensitivity and specificity. For example, the shortening of the aPTT which is associated with an increased concentration of factor VIII, a common phenomenon in systemic disease, may mask any prolongation of the aPTT by a lupus inhibitor. The poor specificity caused by sensitivity to factor deficiency can be improved, however, by use of mixing tests with normal plasma to confirm the presence of an inhibitor. Some other modifications to the aPTT designed to improve specificity and/or sensitivity for lupus anticoagulant are performance of the test in duplicate using lupus anticoagulant sensitive and insensitive reagents and use of sensitive reagents in higher than usual dilution. In summary, when the aPTT is employed as a screening test for lupus anticoagulant it is essential that attention is paid to the limitations of the test for this purpose, optimal choice of reagents for maximum sensitivity and the pitfalls in interpretation of results.

Kaolin clotting time

In the KCT test there is no added phospholipid, clotting being dependent upon phospholipids in centrifuged plasma. This should render the test sensitive to lupus anticoagulant; however, the test suffers from the same problems as the aPTT test in relation to sensitivity and specificity for lupus anticoagulant because of the influence of other inhibitors and coagulation factor deficiencies on the clotting time. Specificity is improved through nullifying the effect of any factor deficiency by performing the test on a dilute mixture of test and normal plasma: a 1:4 mixture is recommended as this should guarantee correction of any factor deficiency while sensitivity to lupus anticoagulant is generally retained.

Dilute Russell's viper venom time

Russell's viper venom initiates clotting through activation of factor X. Because fewer coagulation factors are required for clotting to occur, use of the venom should result in a more specific test for lupus anticoagulant than the aPTT or KCT. In addition, sensitivity is increased by use of a high dilution of phospholipid. Specificity may be enhanced by demonstration of shortening of the clotting time of test plasma in a "platelet neutralization procedure." In this correction procedure anionic phospholipid is exposed on washed normal platelets by activation with calcium ionophore or through cell lysis induced by repeated freezing and thawing. The principle employed is that when such a preparation is added to lupus anticoagulant plasma the prolonged clotting time is corrected, but not if the prolongation is caused by factor deficiency. Alternative reagents have been employed, including platelet-derived microvesicles and a preparation containing hexagonal phase phospholipids. Numerous commercial assay kits based on the DRVVT are available. Several methods

for the calculation of the level of correction of prolonged DRVVT have been proposed. Unfortunately, there is no consensus on the most appropriate method, nor is there conformity in relation to the degree of correction that most reliably indicates positivity for lupus anticoagulant, despite evidence that this would improve reproducibility between DRVVT assays.[6]

In a survey carried out by the National External Quality Assurance Scheme (NEQAS) for Blood Coagulation in the UK[7] it was found that 98% of diagnostic laboratories employ the DRVVT for testing for lupus anticoagulant, 85% the aPTT and 34% the KCT. In addition, a small number of laboratories reported use of the tissue thromboplastin inhibition test/dilute prothrombin time. The principle of the test is that although thromboplastin contains very high concentrations of phospholipid, rendering the prothrombin time generally insensitive to lupus anticoagulant, when the thromboplastin reagent is diluted the phospholipid concentration is the rate limiting factor, and inhibition of prothrombinase reaction by lupus anticoagulant prolongs the clotting time. Thus, a progressive increase in clotting time with thromboplastin dilution is suggestive of lupus anticoagulant. Although the assay was found to be less sensitive than the KCT,[8] Arnout et al.[9] demonstrated subsequently that sensitivity and specificity for lupus anticoagulant could be improved markedly when a recombinant tissue thromboplastin (Innovin) was used in the assay, compared with results with a rabbit brain thromboplastin (Simplastin).

Numerous variations of the above assays have been recommended, and some other approaches to identification of lupus anticoagulant positive plasmas. This reflects the lack of a completely satisfactory test. For example, snake venom enzymes that activate prothrombin directly have been used in an attempt to improve specificity. Taipan venom and the venom of *Pseudonaja textilis* (Textarin) both activate prothrombin in a phospholipid and calcium-dependent manner, Textarin requiring the presence of factor V in addition. Tests employing these venoms are sensitive to lupus anticoagulant if the concentration of phospholipid employed is low. A modification of the Textarin-based assay that improves specificity employs a second venom-derived enzyme, Ecarin. Ecarin activates prothrombin in a phospholipid-independent manner and is therefore not sensitive to lupus anticoagulant. The Textarin : Ecarin ratio appears to have high sensitivity for lupus anticoagulant in some hands.[10]

Lupus anticoagulant assay performance

Because the tests for lupus anticoagulant are essentially indirect tests which may be influenced by the quality of the plasma sample, the presence of other inhibitors including anticoagulant drugs, coagulation factor deficiencies, and the choice of test, reagents and method of end-point detection, it is unsurprising that accuracy and reproducibility are not optimal. This has been revealed through external quality assurance programs. For example, in 1997 Jennings et al.[7] reported on the performance of lupus anticoagulant testing by 220 laboratories in the UK NEQAS for Blood Coagulation. Fewer than half of the laboratories identified a sample considered to be weakly positive for lupus anticoagulant correctly and around one-quarter of laboratories misinterpreted a sample mildly deficient in factor IX as lupus anticoagulant positive. In a follow-up study reported in 2002[11] there may have been some improvements but accurate identification of a weak lupus anticoagulant remained problematic for around one-third of participating laboratories. Unsurprisingly, similar results have been obtained in other countries.[12] Furthermore, Pengo et al.[13] demonstrated that when a comprehensive range of assays was applied by a reference laboratory around 25% of plasmas considered to be positive for lupus anticoagulant by participating specialized laboratories represented false positive results. Because lupus anticoagulant is the most informative marker of thrombosis risk in antiphospholipid syndrome, false negative and false positive results are likely to adversely affect therapeutic decisions resulting in poor clinical outcomes.

In recognition of the limitations of current assays for lupus anticoagulant, recommendations have been made in an attempt to improve assay performance. Attention to preanalytical variables has been referred to already. This also applies to control plasmas. In addition, local reference ranges using a minimum of 20 normal plasma samples should be established for each method and coagulometer. This applies equally to in-house methods and commercial kits. Pooled plasmas for calculation of clotting time ratios should be prepared from at least 12 individual normal plasma donations. In addition, when in-house assays are used, care must be taken to optimize assay conditions. For example, for the DRVVT, it is essential to titrate the venom reagent to determine the optimal clotting time for the coagulometer in use and to select the optimal dilution of phospholipid for maximal sensitivity and specificity.

Despite the recognition of these important variables and attention to them, in many diagnostic laboratories there remains a lack of conformity in lupus anticoagulant testing. This is reflected in variations in assay selection and the number of individual assays used to test each sample. Even the degree of correction required for maximal specificity in confirmatory tests has not been agreed. These are obvious areas for improvement.

Some other approaches to improvement in accuracy of lupus anticoagulant tests have been suggested. These include the development of widely available reference materials and standards, and new assays that better identify clinically important lupus anticoagulants. In relation to reference materials, the ideal would be well-characterized lupus anticoagulant positive plasmas from subjects with a firm diagnosis of antiphospholipid syndrome. However, a sufficient and regular supply of such materials for global use is not feasible. Alternative solutions have been sought, including the use of normal pooled plasma spiked with monoclonal antibodies to β_2-glycoprotein I or prothrombin. Although this approach appears to have some utility in assay standardization,[14] an obvious drawback is that the spiked plasmas may not adequately reflect the characteristics of clinically important antiphospholipid antibodies.

Whether the introduction of more specific tests for subtypes of lupus anticoagulants that are most closely linked to thrombosis and pregnancy failure might improve diagnostic accuracy is of interest but remains speculative. Research in this area has been led by the work of de Groot et al. Lupus anticoagulant activity is a feature of some antiprothrombin and some anti-β_2-glycoprotein I antibodies. They may occur alone or in combination in lupus anticoagulant positive plasmas.[15] Lupus anticoagulants that are prothrombin-dependent can be distinguished from the β_2-glycoprotein-I dependent antibodies by modified coagulation tests. Importantly, it appears that it is the latter antibodies that associate with thrombotic events in patients. Furthermore, in a landmark paper, de Laat *et al.*[2] demonstrated, in elegant experiments employing deletion mutants of β_2-glycoprotein I, that among anti-β_2-glycoprotein I antibodies it is the immunoglobulin G (IgG) antibodies that recognize the sequence Gly40-Arg43 of domain I that have lupus anticoagulant activity. This raises the possibility of the development of new, more specific tests for clinically important antibodies.

One such aPTT-based lupus anticoagulant assay which employs cardiolipin vesicles as a confirmatory reagent is deserving of further assessment.[16] Addition of cardiolipin vesicles shortened the prolonged clotting time caused by anti-β_2-glycoprotein I antibodies with lupus anticoagulant activity but further prolonged the clotting time in plasma with antiprothrombin antibodies with lupus anticoagulant activity. Pengo *et al.*[17] used a different approach. They found that a reduction in the final calcium concentration in a DRVVT and a dilute prothrombin time assay further prolonged the clotting time in the presence of β_2-glycoprotein I-dependent lupus anticoagulants whereas there was a shortening of clotting time in lupus anticoagulant positive, anti-β_2-glycoprotein I negative plasmas.

Such approaches could significantly improve the specificity of lupus anticoagulant assays for antiphospholipid syndrome. However, for now, there should be concerted efforts to standardize approaches to the use of coagulation assays for the diagnosis of antiphospholipid syndrome. Also, it is essential that diagnostic and research laboratories engaged in the identification of lupus anticoagulant positive plasmas use robust internal quality assurance measures and take part in external quality assurance programs in order to provide some reassurance on performance in this difficult area.

Assay of lupus anticoagulant in subjects treated with coumarin

The accurate identification of lupus anticoagulant in a patient with reduced concentrations of gamma-carboxylated coagulation factors because of treatment with coumarin is particularly challenging. Perhaps the simplest approach is to perform a lupus anticoagulant assay on a mixture of test and normal plasma on the assumption that the concentrations of vitamin K-dependent coagulation factors are increased to within the normal range in the plasma mix. However, inevitably this results in a dilution of the lupus anticoagulant immunoglobulin also, with consequential reduced assay sensitivity. Indeed, this dilution effect on the antibody has been demonstrated to significantly impair the detection of lupus anticoagulant, confirming the limitations of this method.[18]

Alternative approaches include the use of the Taipan snake venom time with a platelet neutralization procedure[19] and the Taipan snake venom time combined with the Ecarin time.[20] However, when one considers the poor performance of lupus anticoagulant assays performed without the added complication of reduced levels of vitamin K dependent coagulation factors it seems unlikely there can be confidence in the diagnosis of the presence of lupus anticoagulant in a subject under treatment with coumarin. As such, and in view of the implications of a diagnosis of antiphospholipid syndrome for duration of anticoagulant therapy, it would seem to be preferable to briefly interrupt anticoagulant treatment in order to perform lupus anticoagulant assays in those cases where a confident diagnosis is paramount.

There has been concern over the prolongation of the prothrombin time and/or International Normalized Ratio (INR) due to lupus anticoagulant and the possibility that this may result in insufficiently intensive anticoagulation in subjects with antiphospholipid syndrome who are treated with coumarin. However, in one large series only around 4% of lupus anticoagulant plasmas from non-anticoagulated patients had prolonged prothrombin time using a recombinant thromboplastin (Innovin).[21] In general, there appears to be little interference by lupus anticoagulants in the prothrombin time/INR if insensitive thromboplastin is employed with instrument-specific International Sensitivity Index.[22] (For further discussion of INR use in the presence of antiphospholipid antibodies see Chapter 18.)

Anticardiolipin assays

The solid phase assays employed for detection and quantitation of anticardiolipin antibodies have been refined over two decades. Commercial kits for the quantitation of IgG and IgM anticardiolipin antibodies are readily available. They carry theoretical advantages over lupus anticoagulant assays: testing in bulk is achievable, standards are readily available, coagulation factor deficiencies are irrelevant, immunoglobulin inhibitors of specific clotting factors do not interfere in the assay, and therapeutic anticoagulants have no impact on assay results. Unfortunately, anticardiolipin ELISAs cannot substitute for lupus anticoagulant assays for diagnostic purposes because in some subjects with antiphospholipid syndrome who are lupus anticoagulant positive, tests for anticardiolipin are negative.

The use of affinity purified standards is essential. They allow expression of IgG and IgM anticardiolipin antibodies in widely accepted antiphospholipid units: GPLU and MPLU, respectively. This is of great practical importance as the consensus guidelines for the firm diagnosis of antiphospholipid syndrome specify that as a diagnostic criterion anticardiolipin antibody must be present in medium or high titer, defined as >40 GPLU or MPLU or >99th percentile. This reflects the observation that low titer anticardiolipin antibodies are a frequent incidental finding. They are detected in up to 5% of tests and are often transient. Any relationship to thrombosis or pregnancy complications is weak or absent.

Although IgM anticardiolipin is included as a criterion in the consensus guideline, observational studies have generally suggested that the IgM isotype is only weakly associated with clinical events, if at all. Tests for IgA anticardiolipin are available but do not seem to be of diagnostic value and, as antibodies of IgA isotype do not form part of the consensus criteria for diagnosis, the use of IgA anticardiolipin ELISAs in the diagnostic laboratory cannot be recommended. There have been numerous descriptions of ELISAs employing alternative anionic phospholipids, e.g. phosphotidylserine. In general, such assays behave in a similar manner to anticardiolipin assays and their employment does not aid diagnosis of antiphospholipid syndrome.

Anticardiolipin assay performance

Despite the advantages of solid phase assays for detection of antiphospholipid antibodies, not least the ready availability of standards, assay performance is

disappointing. For example, in 1995 Reber et al.[23] compared the values obtained for six anticardiolipin standards in nine commercial anticardiolipin assay kits and an in-house method. Concordance was extremely poor, to the extent that the highest standard employed would not have been deemed even moderately positive according to the current consensus guideline for diagnosis of antiphospholipid syndrome in some assays. This implies that the attribution of a diagnosis of antiphospholipid syndrome in a particular patient may reflect the choice of anticardiolipin assay kit rather than the truth. A more recent report indicates that this unacceptable situation persists. In their analysis, in 2002, of results from 56 laboratories testing 12 samples for IgG and IgM anticardiolipin as part of an external quality assurance scheme, Favaloro and Silvestrini[24] reported an overall interlaboratory coefficient of variation of >50% in 74% of tests. Remarkably, they were led to conclude that "In the majority of cases laboratories could not decide on whether a sample was cardiolipin positive or negative." Unacceptable coefficients of variation between assays even when plasmas spiked with lyophilized, affinity purified immunoglobulin are used as test samples has been reported recently,[25] highlighting the lack of uniformity of assay reagents and methods currently employed.

Variables that have been identified to influence anticardiolipin assay performance include the quality of the cardiolipin used and the technique employed for coating plates. The use of uncoated wells/plates as blanks is essential in order to allow for non-specific binding.[26] An expert group has recommended four requirements for antiphospholipid ELISAs that may reduce interlaboratory variability:[27] performance of assays in duplicate; determination of the cut-off for positivity by analysis of at least 50 samples from normal subjects, preferably age and sex-matched with the typical clinic population; calculation of the cut-off level in percentiles; and employment of stable standards such as monoclonal anti-β_2-glycoprotein I antibodies. It seems unlikely that all of this advice is routinely followed by the majority of diagnostic laboratories at the present time.

Based on the nature of the putative pathogenic antibodies described above it is essential that anticardiolipin assays detect only those antibodies that are β_2-glycoprotein I-dependent. This can be provided in the fetal calf serum or adult bovine serum in the blocking agent that is used to reduce non-specific binding, or in the sample diluent. This requirement for diagnostic anticardiolipin assays to measure β_2-glycoprotein I-dependent antibodies and their generally poor performance has led to an ongoing debate regarding whether anticardiolipin assays should be replaced by anti-β_2-glycoprotein I ELISAs or whether they are complementary.[28]

Anti-β_2-glycoprotein I antibody assays

Improvements in our understanding of the nature of antiphospholipid antibodies led to the development of ELISAs for the quantitation of anti-β_2-glycoprotein I. Several commercial assay kits are routinely available for diagnostic use. In view of the observation that it is β_2-glycoprotein I-dependent lupus anticoagulants that are most strongly associated with clinical manifestations in antiphospholipid syndrome, and because the clinically relevant antibodies detected in anticardiolipin assays are β_2-glycoprotein I-dependent, it is reasonable to suppose that the assay of antibodies that bind specifically to β_2-glycoprotein I would provide improved diagnostic specificity. To some extent this may be true. Galli et al.[29] undertook a systematic review of the literature and reached the conclusion that anti-β_2-glycoprotein I antibodies are more strongly associated with thrombosis than anticardiolipin antibodies. Also, as indicated above, some anticardiolipin assays detect non-β_2-glycoprotein I-dependent antibodies. In some cases these antibodies are induced by infection and have no significance as far as risk of thrombosis is concerned. However, the situation is not completely straightforward. First, the anti-β_2-glycoprotein I assays are less well standardized at present than the long-established anticardiolipin assays. A titer in excess of the 99th centile is regarded as significant according to the international consensus criteria.[1] Second, the work of de Groot et al. already referred to indicates that it is only a subset of anti-β_2-glycoprotein I antibodies that have lupus anticoagulant activity (those recognizing Gly40-Arg43 on domain I) and it is lupus anticoagulant-type antibodies that associate most strongly with thrombosis. Third, anti-β_2-glycoprotein I antibodies have been reported to be present in association with infections; specifically syphilis, leptospirosis, visceral leishmaniasis and leprosy.[30] However, in a group of subjects with leprosy, Arvieux et al.[31] demonstrated that the anti-β_2-glycoprotein I antibodies which were present in a high proportion of subjects were distinct from those in antiphospholipid syndrome with respect to IgG subclass, avidity and epitope specificity. These observations provide further impetus to efforts to develop assays for antiphospholipid syndrome-specific anti-β_2-glycoprotein I antibodies.

Anti-β_2-glycoprotein I antibody assay performance

Disappointingly, anti-β_2-glycoprotein I assays appear to share the problems of inter-laboratory reproducibility exhibited by anticardiolipin assays. Reber et al.[32] reported on 28 test samples analyzed across 21 European centers. The proportion of results deemed to be positive ranged 50–93% for IgG isotype and 13–70% for IgM. Similarly, Favaloro et al.[33] reported poor performance of anti-β_2-glycoprotein I assays in an external quality assurance scheme. Interlaboratory coefficients of variation were more than 50% in 19 of 27 sera. The obvious implication, once again, is that whether a patient is deemed to have antiphospholipid syndrome varies depending upon the location of the diagnostic laboratory performing the assays. This is a most unsatisfactory situation as the risk of recurrent thrombosis in antiphospholipid syndrome is high and the principal treatment is anticoagulation with warfarin, an intervention that is associated with a significant rate of iatrogenic bleeding.

Antiprothrombin antibodies appear to be of low specificity for the diagnosis of antiphospholipid syndrome and assays for antiprothrombin antibodies are likely to suffer from the same issues of poor reproducibility as do anticardiolipin and anti-β_2-glycoprotein I assays. As such their use by diagnostic laboratories cannot be supported at the present time.

Summary and conclusions

Although the features of antiphospholipid syndrome and the diagnostic criteria are well defined, the serious deficiencies in the quality of the available laboratory tests for the condition have not been given adequate consideration in clinical practice. Assays for lupus anticoagulant, anticardiolipin and anti-β_2-glycoprotein I all perform poorly in quality assurance exercises. There is a need for consensus among laboratory scientists, clinicians and manufacturers of laboratory reagents and equipment on the most effective combination of assays and choice of reagents and methods for optimal sensitivity and specificity. At the same time research should concentrate on the development of assays for disease-specific antiphospholipid antibodies.

References

1 Miyakis S, Lockshin MD, Atsumi T, Branch DW, Brey RL, Cervera R, et al. International consensus statement on an update of the classification criteria for definite antiphospholipid syndrome (APS). *J Thromb Haemost* 2006; **4**: 295–306.

2 de Laat B, Derksen RH, Urbanus RT, de Groot PG. IgG antibodies that recognize epitope Gly40-Arg43 in domain I of beta 2-glycoprotein I cause LAC, and their presence correlates strongly with thrombosis. *Blood* 2005; **105**: 1540–1545.

3 Galli M, Luciani D, Bertolini G, Barbui T. Lupus anticoagulants are stronger risk factors for thrombosis than anticardiolipin antibodies in the antiphospholipid syndrome: a systematic review of the literature. *Blood* 2003; **101**: 1827–1832.

4 Opatrny L, David M, Kahn SR, Shrier I, Rey E. Association between antiphospholipid antibodies and recurrent fetal loss in women without autoimmune disease: a metaanalysis. *J Rheumatol* 2006; **33**: 2214–2221.

5 Greaves M, Cohen H, MacHin SJ, Mackie I. Guidelines on the investigation and management of the antiphospholipid syndrome. *Br J Haematol* 2000; **109**: 704–715.

6 Gardiner C, MacKie IJ, Malia RG, Jones DW, Winter M, Leeming D, et al. The importance of locally derived reference ranges and standardized calculation of dilute Russell's viper venom time results in screening for lupus anticoagulant. *Br J Haematol* 2000; **111**: 1230–1235.

7 Jennings I, Kitchen S, Woods TA, Preston FE, Greaves M. Potentially clinically important inaccuracies in testing for the lupus anticoagulant: an analysis of results from three surveys of the UK National External Quality Assessment Scheme (NEQAS) for Blood Coagulation. *Thromb Haemost* 1997; **77**: 934–937.

8 Exner T. Comparison of two simple tests for the lupus anticoagulant. *Am J Clin Pathol* 1985; **83**: 215–218.

9 Arnout J, Vanrusselt M, Huybrechts E, Vermylen J. Optimization of the dilute prothrombin time for the detection of the lupus anticoagulant by use of a recombinant tissue thromboplastin. *Br J Haematol* 1994; **87**: 94–99.

10 Forastiero RR, Cerrato GS, Carreras LO. Evaluation of recently described tests for detection of the lupus anticoagulant. *Thromb Haemost* 1994; **72**: 728–733.

11 Jennings I, Greaves M, Mackie IJ, Kitchen S, Woods TA, Preston FE, UK National External Quality Assessment Scheme for Blood Coagulation. Lupus anticoagulant testing: improvements in performance in a UK NEQAS proficiency testing exercise after dissemination of national guidelines on laboratory methods. *Br J Haematol* 2002; **119**: 364–369.

12 Tripodi A, Biasiolo A, Chantarangkul V, Pengo V. Lupus anticoagulant (LA) testing: performance of clinical laboratories assessed by a national survey using lyophilized affinity-purified immunoglobulin with LA activity. *Clin Chem* 2003; **49**: 1608–1614.

13 Pengo V, Biasiolo A, Bison E, Chantarangkul V, Tripodi A, Italian Federation of Anticoagulation Clinics (FCSA). Antiphospholipid antibody ELISAs: Survey on the performance of clinical laboratories assessed by using lyophilized affinity-purified IgG with anticardiolipin and anti-β_2-glycoprotein I activity. *Thromb Res* 2007; **120**: 127–133.

14 Jennings I, Mackie I, Arnout J, Preston FE, UK National External Quality Assessment Scheme for Blood Coagulation. Lupus anticoagulant testing using plasma spiked with monoclonal antibodies: performance in the UK NEQAS proficiency testing programme. *J Thromb Haemost* 2004; **2**: 2178–2184.

15 Horbach DA, van Oort E, Derksen RH, de Groot PG. The contribution of anti-prothrombin-antibodies to lupus anticoagulant activity: discrimination between functional and non-functional anti-prothrombin-antibodies. *Thromb Haemost* 1998; **79**: 790–795.

16 de Laat HB, Derksen RH, Urbanus RT, Roest M, de Groot PG. β_2-Glycoprotein I-dependent lupus anticoagulant highly correlates with thrombosis in the antiphospholipid syndrome. *Blood* 2004; **104**: 3598–35602.

17 Pengo V, Biasiolo A, Pegoraro C, Iliceto S. A two-step coagulation test to identify antibeta-glycoprotein I lupus anticoagulants. *J Thromb Haemost* 2004; **2**: 702–707.

18 Moore GW, Savidge GF. The dilution effect of equal volume mixing studies compromises confirmation of inhibition by lupus anticoagulants even when mixture specific reference ranges are applied. *Thromb Res* 2006; **118**: 523–528.

19 Rooney AM, McNally T, Mackie IJ, Machin SJ. The Taipan snake venom time: a new test for lupus anticoagulant. *J Clin Pathol* 1994; **47**: 497–501.

20 Moore GW, Smith MP, Savidge GF. The Ecarin time is an improved confirmatory test for the Taipan snake venom time in warfarinized patients with lupus anticoagulants. *Blood Coagul Fibrinolysis* 2003; **14**: 307–312.

21 Moore GW, Rangarajan S, Holland LJ, Henley A, Savidge GF. Low frequency of elevated prothrombin times in patients with lupus anticoagulants when using a recombinant thromboplastin reagent: implications for dosing and monitoring of oral anticoagulant therapy. *Br J Biomed Sci* 2005; **62**: 15, 8; quiz 47.

22 Tripodi A, Chantarangkul V, Clerici M, Negri B, Galli M, Mannucci PM. Laboratory control of oral anticoagulant treatment by the INR system in patients with the antiphospholipid syndrome and lupus anticoagulant: results of a collaborative study involving nine commercial thromboplastins. *Br J Haematol* 2001; **115**: 672–678.

23 Reber G, Arvieux J, Comby E, Degenne D, de Moerloose P, Sanmarco M, et al. Multicenter evaluation of nine commercial kits for the quantitation of anticardiolipin antibodies: the working group on methodologies in haemostasis from the GEHT (Groupe d'Etudes sur l'Hemostase et la Thrombose). *Thromb Haemost* 1995; **73**: 444–452.

24 Favaloro EJ, Silvestrini R. Assessing the usefulness of anticardiolipin antibody assays: a cautious approach is suggested by high variation and limited consensus in multilaboratory testing. *Am J Clin Pathol* 2002; **118**: 548–557.

25 Pengo V, Biasiolo A, Gresele P, Marongiu F, Erba N, Veschi F, et al., Participating Centers of Italian Federation of Thrombosis Centers (FCSA). Survey of lupus anticoagulant diagnosis by central evaluation of positive plasma samples. *J Thromb Haemost* 2007; **5**: 925–930.

26 de Moerloose P, Reber G, Vogel JJ. Anticardiolipin antibody determination: comparison of three ELISA assays. *Clin Exp Rheumatol* 1990; **8**: 575–577.

27 Tincani A, Allegri F, Balestrieri G, Reber G, Sanmarco M, Meroni P, et al. Minimal requirements for antiphospholipid antibodies ELISAs proposed by the European forum on antiphospholipid antibodies. *Thromb Res* 2004; **114**: 553–558.

28 de Moerloose P, Reber G. Antiphospholipid antibodies: do we still need to perform anticardiolipin ELISA assays? *J Thromb Haemost* 2004; **2**: 1071–1073.

29 Galli M, Luciani D, Bertolini G, Barbui T. Anti-β_2-glycoprotein I, antiprothrombin antibodies, and the risk of thrombosis in the antiphospholipid syndrome. *Blood* 2003; **102**: 2717–2123.

30 Santiago M, Martinelli R, Ko A, Reis EA, Fontes RD, Nascimento EG, et al. Anti-β_2 glycoprotein I and anti-cardiolipin antibodies in leptospirosis, syphilis and kala-azar. *Clin Exp Rheumatol* 2001; **19**: 425–430.

31 Arvieux J, Renaudineau Y, Mane I, Perraut R, Krilis SA, Youinou P. Distinguishing features of anti-β_2-glycoprotein I antibodies between patients with leprosy and the antiphospholipid syndrome. *Thromb Haemost* 2002; **87**: 599–605.

32 Reber G, Tincani A, Sanmarco M, de Moerloose P, Boffa MC, Standardization Group of the European Forum on Antiphospholipid Antibodies. Proposals for the measurement of anti-β_2-glycoprotein I antibodies. *J Thromb Haemost* 2004; **2**: 1860–1862.

33 Favaloro EJ, Wong RC, Jovanovich S, Roberts-Thomson P. A review of β_2-glycoprotein-I antibody testing results from a peer-driven multilaboratory quality assurance program. *Am J Clin Pathol* 2007; **127**: 441–448.

17 Monitoring heparin therapy

M. Johnston

Heparin

The discovery of heparin dates back to 1916. In that year, Jay McLean, a medical student at Johns Hopkins University, was searching for substances that caused clotting. Experimenting with homogenized dog liver, instead of finding a clotting material, McLean found a substance that prevented clotting. He named it heparin, from the Latin word for liver, *hepar*.[1] Heparin was first used in humans around 1940. It was prepared from extractions from porcine mucosa, and the procedure today is basically the same. Heparin, a sulfated glycosaminoglycan, has a mean size of 15,000 Da with a range of 3000–30,000 Da and is highly negatively charged.

This material is called unfractionated heparin (UFH), referring to the wide range of molecular weight products of which only one-third have anticoagulant properties.

Mechanism of action

The determination of the mechanism of action for heparin developed through studies carried out over several years by several researchers. In 1939, Brinkhous *et al.*[2] reported that heparin required a plasma cofactor in order for it to act as an anticoagulant. This cofactor was later identified by Abildgaard[3] as

antithrombin (AT). The mechanism for heparin–AT interaction was further studied by both Lindahl[4] and Rosenberg,[5] showing that heparin binds to AT through lysine residues. This produces a conformational change at the arginine reactive center, converting AT from a slow progressive inhibitor to a rapid-acting one. The AT is now able to bind via a covalent bond to the serine proteases of the coagulation pathway, irreversibly inhibiting their activity.

Subsequent work has shown that heparin binds to AT through a unique pentasaccharide sequence present in about one-third of UFH molecules.[6] Once bound, the heparin–AT complex can irreversibly inhibit the serine proteases of the coagulation pathway, but the strongest inhibition is against thrombin (IIa) and factor Xa (Xa). Thrombin is more readily inhibited than Xa by the heparin–AT complex (Fig. 17.1). Over years of *in vitro* experimentation with UFH, clinical use and clinical trials, heparin has been found to have a number of limitations.

Limitations of heparin

Pharmacokinetic

Heparin has been shown to bind non-specifically to proteins, endothelial cells and macrophages, thereby reducing its anticoagulant activity in a variable manner. Being negatively charged, heparin binds independent of the pentasaccharide to a variety of plasma proteins. These include histidine-rich glycoprotein, vitronectin, lipoproteins, fibronectin and fibrinogen. Many of these proteins are acute phase reactants and, when treating patients with venous thromboembo-

Quality in Laboratory Hemostasis and Thrombosis, 1st edition. By Steve Kitchen, John D. Olson and F. Eric Preston. Published 2009 by Blackwell Publishing. ISBN: 978-1-4051-6803-8

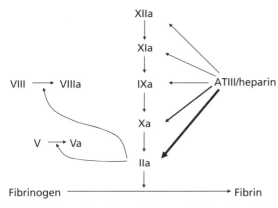

Fig. 17.1 Heparin/antithrombin irreversibly inactivates the serine proteases of the coagulation pathway with the strongest inhibition against Xa (Xa), and thrombin (IIa). After Hirsh, 2007.[13]

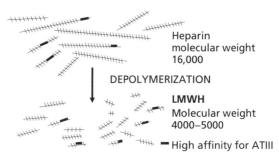

Fig. 17.2 Commerical grade heparin is chemically or enzymatically depolymerized to create low molecular weight heparin (LMWH) which contains the high-affinity pentasaccharide. After Hirsh, 2007.[13]

lism, post surgery and post myocardial infarction (MI), the variable levels of these proteins can lead to under-dosing heparin[7] as well as to a variable response of heparin from patient to patient. Heparin will also bind to platelet factor 4 (PF4)[8] and high molecular weight von Willebrand factor secreted from the activated platelet or endothelium.[9]

Clinical

Heparin can produce thrombocytopenia and osteoporosis.

Heparin-induced thrombocytopenia (HIT) is a result of heparin's high affinity for PF4. This binding results in a structural change in the PF4 so that it is recognized as a foreign protein and antibodies are therefore produced.[10] These IgG antibodies form complexes with PF4 and heparin on the platelet surface, triggering platelet activation through the Fc receptors on the platelet membrane.

Osteoporosis is a complication in approximately 2–3% of patients after 3 months of continuous heparin use. The mechanisms are well described in a paper by Shaughnessy et al.[11]

Low molecular weight heparins

In the early 1970s, researchers began experimenting with techniques to reduce the wide molecular weight range of heparin with a view to limiting the negative aspects of heparin treatment.

Johnson et al.[12] used gel filtration to separate heparin into four molecular weight groups. They found that as the molecular weight size decreased, the activated partial thromboplastin time (aPTT) became progressively shorter while the fractions still retained the ability to inhibit activated factor Xa. This observation has resulted in a plethora of research, the goal being to find an anticoagulant that provides protection from clot formation without the side effects of excessive bleeding.

Low molecular weight heparins (LMWHs) are prepared from UFH by chemical or enzymatic depolymerization and are, on average, one-third the molecular weight of the parent compound (Fig. 17.2).[13]

Because different methods of preparation are used, LMWHs are not equal, both when used clinically for a specific indication and in the laboratory, where the Xa : IIa ratios vary (Table 17.1). The LMWH preparations with the lower Xa : IIa ratios will have a greater effect on the activity assays of coagulation.

Inactivation of IIa by LMWH requires the simultaneous binding to the pentasaccharide and a minimum of an additional 13 saccharide units. Inactivation of factor Xa requires only the pentasaccharide unit (Fig. 17.3).[14]

Heparin-induced thrombocytopenia

HIT has been defined by Warkentin et al.[15] as a 50% or greater decrease in platelet count beginning on or after day 5 of heparin therapy, without any other apparent cause and recovering once heparin therapy is stopped. For patients on UFH, the risk of developing this immunologic disorder is 3% but, of those, the mortality rate can be as high as 20%. Patients receiving LMWH have a <1% risk of developing HIT, and with fondaparinux an even lesser risk. The greater the heparin chain length and charge of the glycosoaminogylcans, the greater the risk of developing HIT.

Clinical suspicion of HIT requires laboratory testing to identify if the auto-antibodies are present. Because of the high incidence of thrombosis, treatment should be changed to other anticoagulant therapies, usually direct thrombin inhibitors. Testing should be carried out as soon as possible.[16]

Table 17.1 Characteristics of low molecular weight heparin (LMWH) preparations.

	Anti-Xa:anti-IIa ratio	MW range
Dalteparin	2.7:1	2000–9000
Enoxaparin	3.8:1	3000–8000
Tinzaparin	1.9:1	3000–6000
Reviparin	3.5:1	Mean MW 4000
Nadroparin	3.6:1	Median MW 4500
Ardepari	1.9:1	Mean MW 6000

MW, molecular weight.

This testing typically consists of either serologic or functional assays. Two commerical enzyme-linked immunosorbent assays (ELISAs) are available and detect IgG antibodies as well as IgA and IgM to the heparin–PF4 (polyanion–PF4) complexes. The serotonin release method is a functional assay and is considered the gold standard. However, the assay is laborious and requires donor platelets. Both the serologic (ELISA) and functional serotonin release assay have high sensitivity to HIT of ≥97%; however, only the serotonin assay has high specificity (95–97%). The ELISA has specificity ranges from 74–86% when tested only for the IgG autoantibody, but worsened when IgA and IgM are added. Because of the low specificity, this test may detect antibodies in patients without HIT.[15] Therefore, a positive test should be interpreted with caution. Conversely, negative test results provide a high level of confidence that the patient's thrombocytopenia may be due to another cause.

In a recent survey of North American specialized laboratories, 88% of 44 reporting laboratories used the commercial ELISAs to identify HIT.[17]

Current techniques used to measure heparin in plasma

- Activated partial thromboplastin time (aPTT).
- Protamine sulfate neutralization (PS).

Pentasaccharide-containing fractions with less than 18 saccharide units 50–75%

Pentasaccharide-containing fractions with 18 or more saccharide units 25–50%

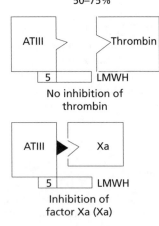

No inhibition of thrombin

Inhibition of factor Xa (Xa)

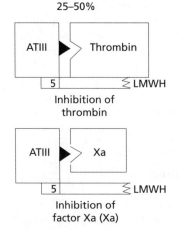

Inhibition of thrombin

Inhibition of factor Xa (Xa)

Fig. 17.3 Low molecular weight activity. Approximately 25–50% of the low molecular weight heparin (LMWH) molecules of different commercial preparations contain at least 18 saccharide units; these molecules inhibit both thrombin and factor Xa. The remaining 50–75% of LMWH molecules contain fewer than 18 saccharide units and only inhibit factor Xa. After Hirsh, 2007.[13]

- Xa inhibition, chromogenic and clotting.
- IIa inhibition, chromogenic and clotting.

Of these, the Xa inhibition chromogenic method is the most widely used for LMWH, fondaparinux and the newer inhibitors of Xa (Chapter 19).

The aPTT test still remains the procedure of choice for monitoring UFH. It is a simple, rapid and inexpensive assay providing results within 30 minutes of blood collection. However, the method is difficult to standardize. The aPTT test requires the entire cascade of coagulation proteins to be intact for the accurate measurement of heparin levels. Patients with lupus anticoagulant or antiphospholipid syndrome generally have elevated aPTTs and must be monitored using heparin assays.

Besides levels of the various coagulation factors, reagents and instrumentation will affect the sensitivity to heparin and can result in a fourfold difference in results between reagents, making the results from one laboratory to another difficult to correlate.[18] A study by Bates et al. assayed six different aPTT reagents on five instrument platforms and compared the results to the anti-Xa heparin levels.[18] The conclusion was that, for the reagents studied and presuming the therapeutic interval to be 0.3–0.7 IU/mL heparin, using a ratio of 2.0 : 3.5 more closely represented the therapeutic heparin level than the reported 1.5–2.5 times control plasma.

Studies have been carried out by the International Society on Thrombosis and Haemostasis Scientific and Standardization Committee (ISTH SSC) in an attempt to standardize the method by applying a correction factor similar to the use of an International Sensitivity Index (ISI) for prothrombin time testing.[19] Because of the wide variety of phospholipids, activators and instruments, there was limited success and further work has not been initiated. It is recommended that each aPTT method be calibrated against anti-Xa heparin assays. The following is an accepted method for standardization.[20]

Recommended protocol

1 Blood is collected from patients (ideally 50 patients) being treated with continuous intravenous heparin. These samples are taken at least 4–6 hours after a heparin bolus but less than 24 hours after the first dose of oral anticoagulant.

2 Blood samples are centrifuged at a minimum of 1700 g for 15 minutes. The plasma is transferred to a clean tube and recentrifuged for 5 minutes at 1700 g. The plasma is carefully transferred to a storage tube and frozen at −35°C or lower until testing is performed.

3 The plasma is thawed to 37°C for 5 minutes and the aPTT and heparin levels measured.

4 The relationship between aPTT and heparin level is plotted using linear regression analysis. The heparin level is plotted on the x axis and the aPTT values on the y axis. The line of best fit is calculated from the regression equation.

An alternate procedure and one that is less onerous is to freeze platelet-poor plasma from heparinized patients with known anti-Xa heparin levels at −70°C. Before retiring one lot number of aPTT reagent, aPTT measurements with the current reagent lot number and the new reagent lot number are performed side by side. If the values are within the tolerance of the assay, no further work is required. If the aPTT results are different, a regression analysis is performed using the anti-Xa values previously established, or the full procedure as described above is repeated.

Split samples may also be used. Once the laboratory has narrowed down the possible replacement aPTT reagent then split samples may be measured with the new and old reagents. The comparison data are plotted with the old reagent on the x axis and the new on the y axis. Regression analysis or simply visual analysis is performed to discrepant results. A difference of 5 seconds between pairs is considered acceptable. The means and standard deviations for each set of data are calculated and recorded for use in charting the cumulative summation of difference over time.[21] By doing this, the cumulative shift in the reagent performance in the presence of heparin can be determined. A cumulative change of 5–7 seconds is reason for concern while a cumulative change of more than 7 seconds requires action. This may require looking at different reagents to choose one with a similar pattern as the previous reagent with an acceptable level of variation, or performing the aPTT, Xa heparin levels as in the full protocol for establishing a therapeuptic range or informing the physicians of the change in the aPTT therapeutic range. Spiking heparin into normal pooled plasma is not an acceptable procedure for determining the aPTT therapeutic range for heparin. The *in vitro* spiked plasma invariably give a much steeper aPTT–heparin response curve than *ex vivo* samples. This is due, in part, to the normal levels of coagulation proteins in the spiked normal plasma.

The therapeutic range for UFH levels is 0.2–0.4 IU/mL using protamine sulfate neutralization assay method[22] or 0.30–0.70 IU/mL using anti-Xa assays.[23]

Protamine sulfate assay

The assay is based on the neutralization of UFH, a highly negatively charged molecule, by PS, a positively charged protein. A series of concentrations of PS are prepared and added to plasma. Thrombin is added and the clotting times measured. The concentration of PS to normalize the IIa clotting time is considered the heparin concentration. This procedure can only be used for UFH.[24]

Chromogenic Xa inhibition heparin assays

The chromogenic assay was introduced in the late 1970s and still remains the assay of choice for monitoring LMWH and other direct Xa inhibitors. LMWH does not require constant monitoring. The drug is provided as weight-adjusted doses and monitoring is generally not required except in patients who are very obese; very thin patients; patients with renal disease; patients with malignancy; women in the third trimester of pregnancy; and pediatric patients.[25] The clinical condition of the patient dictates the frequency of testing in these groups. Patients with renal disease should be monitored closely at the beginning of their treatment and then less often.

There are a number of different assays available to the laboratory; these include one-stage, two-stage and hybrid assays. The chromogenic assays are all based on the original description by Teien *et al.*[26]

A generic chromogenic factor Xa heparin assay

The principle of all chromogenic heparin assays is the same: heparin in the sample binds with AT forming heparin–AT complexes. The heparin–AT complex inhibits factor Xa which has been added in excess. The residual Xa activity is measured by its action on a specific substrate, sensitive and highly specific for Xa. The resulting release of paranitroaniline (pNA) is measured at 405 nm, and the reaction is inversely proportional to the concentration of heparin in the plasma.

$$\text{Heparin} + \text{AT(plasma and exogenous)} \rightarrow [\text{Hep-AT}]$$
$$[\text{Hep-AT}] + [\text{FXa(excess)}] \rightarrow [\text{FXa-AT-Hep}] + [\text{residual FXa}]$$
$$[\text{residual FXa}] + \text{Substrate} \rightarrow \text{Peptide} + \text{pNA}$$

The differences among assays are the incubation time of the reaction, the buffer used to dilute the plasma, the substrate and the addition of exogenous AT. The presence of dextran sulfate in the buffer reduces the influence of PF4.[27] The assays may be one or two-stage procedures and may be used for measurement of LMWH or UFH with the appropriate calibration line. Assays are available that have been validated to use a single calibration line for both LMWH and UFH.[28]

Interfering substances

One should be aware of the limitations of concentrations of interfering substances. The manufacturer for each assay provides maximum allowable levels of bilirubin, hemoglobin and triglycerides.

One-stage assays

One-stage methods for measuring heparin have been developed to simplify the assay and improve turnaround time. These assays do not add exogenous AT.

The assay is based on the principle of competitive inhibition. Xa is added to a plasma substrate mix resulting in two simultaneous reactions: hydrolysis of substrate by Xa and inhibition of Xa by the heparin–AT complex. Once the reaction reaches equilibrium, the quantity of PNA released from the substrate is inversely proportional to the concentration of heparin in the test plasma.

$$\text{Heparin} + \text{AT}_{(\text{plasma})} + \text{Substrate} + \text{Xa} \rightarrow \text{pNA}$$

There are differing opinions on whether exogenous AT should be added to a heparin assay. One opinion is that the AT should not be added so one would rely on the level of AT in the patient's plasma. This would represent the functional response within the patient. Others believe AT should not be a rate-limiting protein and should be added to the test procedure to ensure 100% levels are present. This allows for the absolute drug concentration within the patient.

In patients with AT levels between 35% and 130%, the addition of exogenous AT has no effect on the resulting heparin concentration.[29]

Hybrid assays

A two-stage anti-Xa assay that incorporates a single calibration curve enabling the measurement of UFH or LMWH has been developed.[30]

Xa inhibition clotting assays

Assays are commercially available that are based on the principle of the ability of heparin to complex with antithrombin resulting in the inhibition of factor Xa.

An example of such an assay[31] uses undiluted plasma mixed with an equal volume of Xa and is incubated for a fixed period of time. This mix is then recalcified by the addition of a recalmix consisting of calcium chloride, brain cephalin, factor V and fibrinogen. The clotting time is measured and interpolated from a previously constructed calibration curve. Exogenous AT is not added in this assay, and the manufacturer recommends diluting the test plasma in normal pooled plasma if the patient is known to be AT deficient, or a newborn. Patients treated with warfarin should have their plasma diluted in normal plasma to correct for the low factor II levels in their plasma. Xa concentration used in the assay is not given.

Another example of such an assay incorporates bovine AT into the procedure. In this assay the patient plasma is diluted 1:3 (UFH) and 1:5 (LMWH) in saline and an equal volume of AT is added. The concentration of AT is not given. The mix is allowed to incubate, followed by the addition of an excess of bovine Xa. Again, the concentration is not given. The mix is further incubated followed by the addition of a specially treated substrate plasma. Details are not given. After a short incubation, 0.025 mol CaCl$_2$ is added and the clotting time measured.

In these assays, calibration curves are prepared using the heparin preparation used for treatment, or a commercial secondary standard referenced against the World Health Organization (WHO) second

International LMWH Standard or the WHO fifth International UFH Standard. The concentrations of heparin are plotted on the x axis of semi-log or log–log graph paper and the time in seconds for each respective point plotted on the y axis. As with the chromogenic assays, the question of the calibration material and control plasmas is an issue and is described below.

IIa inhibition assays

Available assays use bovine IIa and human AT. Because the inhibition of IIa by LMWH is variable, the assays available also vary in their ability to quantify LMWH. The assay principles are the same as for the factor Xa inhibition assays except the Xa is replaced by IIa in the assay.

Heparin + AT → [Hep-AT]

[Hep-AT] + [excess IIa] → [FIIa-Hep-AT] + [residual IIa]

[IIa (residual)] + IIa-Substrate → Peptide + pNA

Quality control and assurance

Preanalytical variables

Specimen collection

Careful venipuncture technique must be used when collecting blood for all coagulation testing, including heparin assays. The tourniquet should be applied for a minimal period of time and the venipuncture must be clean with a good flow of blood into the collection tube. Difficult venipunctures may result in platelet activation and subsequent release of PF4. PF4 readily binds UFH, resulting in an underestimation of the drug. The affinity for LMWH to PF4 is less but still careful venipuncture is essential. The needle gauge also will contribute to platelet activation and a 21 gauge needle or less is recommended.

The blood (9 volumes) is collected into 0.109 mol buffered citrate anticoagulant (1 volume). Changing citrate concentrations will result in different aPTT times, effecting a change in the therapeutic range for UFH.

There are special tubes available to minimize platelet activation: CTAD (citrate, theophylline, adenosine and dipyridamole) are available from Becton Dickinson.

Blood processing

Within 1 hour of collection, blood must be centrifuged at a minimum of 1700 *g* for 15 minutes at 22°C (room temperature). The plasma is carefully removed from the collection tube using a plastic pipette and placed in a plastic tube or container.

To assure platelet-free plasma, two procedures may be used:

1 Filtration, using a 0.22 µm filter (Gelman, Sciences, Ann Arbor, MI, USA).

2 Double centrifugation technique. After the first centrifugation, the plasma is removed from the tube as above and the plasma centrifuged again for 5 minutes at the same speed. The plasma from this tube is carefully removed and placed in a clean plastic tube ready for freezing or assay. It is strongly advised that one of these procedures be used if the plasma is to be frozen.[32]

Heparin calibration curves

The WHO provides biologic reference preparation for a number of coagulation proteins including heparin. The current primary heparin standards available are:

• Fifth International Standard, 1998, for UFH is available in lyophilized form at a concentration 2031 IU/ampoule.

• Second International Standard, 2003, for LMWH is available in lyophilized form at a concentration of 1097 IU/mL anti-Xa units and 326 IU anti-IIa per ampoule.

Many manufacturers have available UFH and LMWH calibration material. This material is a secondary standard and should always be referenced by the manufacturer against the primary WHO standard. The type of LMWH used to spike the secondary plasma standard should also be made available to the laboratory by the manufacturer.

In a 2004 College of American Pathologists (CAP) survey an UFH heparin sample was sent to 82 laboratories. The results among laboratories and among methodologies when read off a calibration curve prepared with UFH demonstrated reasonable correlation among methods, but still a wide range among laboratories, 0.2–0.64 anti-Xa units/mL. The imprecision was marked among methodologies and laboratories when the sample values were read off a LMWH calibration curve. In both instances the one-stage assay measured lower levels of heparin. These findings dem-

onstrate the need for two calibrators, one for UFH and one for LMWH. It remains to be seen if the assays incorporating the two heparins in the reference line will result in improved precision.

It has also been recommended that a calibration line specific for the type of LMWH being used in patient treatment be established. Two publications, both in abstract form, have demonstrated that this may not be required.[33,34] The slopes and intercepts of plasma spiked with different LMWHs showed similar slopes and intercepts and, although different, the differences were not clinically significant. This is reassuring and adds confidence in using a commercially prepared calibration material even though it may be a different LMWH from that being used in the hospital.

If using a commercial or generic calibrator, it is recommended that a control plasma be prepared with the heparin product used for patient treatment.

Control plasmas

Control plasmas may be purchased from the kit manufacturer; however, it is preferable, at least at the validation stage of the assay, to prepare in-house controls. This is especially true if a laboratory is using a commercial calibration material to establish the calibration line. At least two levels of heparin controls are necessary, with one level just at the lower part of the reference line and one level close to the upper end.

This may be achieved by preparing a pool of normal plasma that has been rendered platelet-free (see above). A commercial plasma may be used but it must be a plasma that has been prepared for this specific use, i.e. it *must* be free of platelets before freezing and lypholization. Any residual PF4 resulting from inadequate preparation will result in falsely low heparin levels.

The heparin used to spike the plasma, when possible, should be the same heparin used for patient treatment.

Summary

Monitoring unfractionated heparin

The aPTT remains the most commonly used method for monitoring UFH in spite of all its known standardization issues. Although it is a functional assay, it has many limitations including variable levels of clotting factors, masking the heparin anticoagulant effect. Anti-IIa and anti-Xa chromogenic assays could be used but, because of the costs, these assays have not become mainstream for monitoring UFH. Rosborough[35] addressed the question of cost by monitoring 268 patients treated with UFH with both aPTT and anti-Xa assays. He found that those patients monitored with the anti-Xa assay had fewer dose adjustments and fewer tests in a 24-hour period, and that in a 96-hour period, the anti-Xa assay cost $4.37 more than the aPTT assay.

Monitoring low molecular weight heparin

Anti-Xa chromogenic assays do not have the incumbent problem of the variable clotting factors from one patient sample to another, masking the true biologic activity of the measurement. Standardization is possible through the use of international standards. All commercial reference plasmas should be traceable to these standards. This will lead to better precision and accuracy between laboratories. Evidence of this has been demonstrated in recent CAP surveys and in the 2003 collaborative study to calibrate the WHO second International Standard where the coefficients of variation between laboratories was approximately 5% despite different kits and methods being used.[36]

Anti-IIa clotting assays are more difficult to standardize and are not widely used. It has been reported that one of these assays consistently underestimates the heparin level.[37] LMWHs have high ratios of anti-Xa : anti-IIa concentrations and the low concentrations of anti-IIa found in therapeutic treatment levels make anti-IIa assays difficult to use. These assays can be reliably used in monitoring UFH.

Fondaparinux, a synthetic pentasaccharide based on the chemical structure of the natural pentasaccharide of heparin, is a direct Xa inhibitor and requires a specific calibration line. Varying concentrations of fondaparinux are added to normal platelet poor plasma and a calibration line is constructed. The therapeutic range for treatment with fondaparinux is 0.6–1.5 µg/mL.

The future

The current assays for measuring heparin have been criticized for not adequately measuring the biologic effect of the drug. The endogenous thrombin potential assay has the possibility of fulfilling this requirement but, at the present time, it remains primarily a research test.

References

1 McLean J. The thromboplastic action of cehalin. *Am J Physiol* 1916; **41**: 250–257.

2 Brinkhous KM, Smith HP, Warner ED, *et al*. The inhibition of blood clotting: an unidentified substance which acts in conjunction with heparin to prevent the conversion of prothrombin into thrombin. *Am J Physiol* 1939; **125**: 683–687.

3 Abildgaard U. Highly purified antithrombin III with heparin cofactor activity prepared by disc electrophoresis. *Scand J Clin Lab Invest* 1968; **21**: 89–91.

4 Lindahl U, Backstrom G, Hook M, *et al*. Structure of the antithrombin-binding site of heparin. *Proc Natl Acad Sci U S A* 1979; **6**: 3198–3202.

5 Rosenberg RD, Lam L. Correlation between structure and function of heparin. *Proc Natl Acad Sci U S A* 1979; **76**: 1218–1222.

6 Casu B, Oreste P, Torri G, *et al*. The structure of heparin oligosaccharide fragments with high anti- (factor Xa) activity containing the minimal antithrombin III-binding sequence. *Biochem J* 1981; **97**: 599–609.

7 Hirsh J, van Aken WG, Gallus AS, *et al*. Heparin kinetics in venous thrombosis and pulmonary embolism. *Circulation* 1976; **53**: 691–695.

8 Amiral J, Bridey F, Dreyfus M, *et al*. Platelet factor 4 complexed to heparin is the target for antibodies generated in heparin-induced thrombocytopenia. *Thromb Haemost* 1992; **68**: 95–96.

9 Sobel M, McNeill PM, Carlson PL, *et al*. Heparin inhibition of von Willebrand factor-dependent platelet function *in vitro* and *in vivo*. *J Clin Invest* 1991; **87**: 1787–1793.

10 Kelton JG, Smith JW, Warkentin TE, Hayward CP, Denomme GA, Horsewood P. Immunoglobulin G from patients with heparin-induced thrombocytopenia binds to a complex of heparin and platelet factor 4. *Blood* 1994; **83**: 3232–3239.

11 Shaughnessy SG, Young E, Deschamps P, Hirsh J. The effects of low molecular weight and standard heparin on calcium loss from fetal rat calvaris. *Blood* 1995; **86**: 1368–1373.

12 Johnson EA, Kirkwood TB, Stirling Y, *et al*. Four heparin preparations: anti-Xa potentiating effect of heparin after subcutaneous injection. *Thromb Haemost* 1976; **35**: 586–591.

13 Hirsh J. *Low Molecular Weight Heparins*, 4th edn. Hamilton, Canada: B.C. Decker, 2007.

14 Casu B, Oreste P, Torri G, *et al*. The structure of heparin oligosaccharide fragments with high anti- (factor Xa) activity containing the minimal antithrombin III-binding sequence. *Biochem J* 1981; **97**: 599–609.

15 Warkentin T, Sheppard J, Moore J, *et al*. Laboratory testing for the antibodies that cause heparin-induced thrombocytopenia: how much class do we need? *J Lab Clin Med* 2005; **146**: 341–346.

16 Arnold D, Kelton J. Testing for heparin-induced thrombocytopenia: are we there yet? *J Thromb Haemost* 2007; **5**: 1371–1372.

17 Price E, Hayward C, Moffat K, Moore J, *et al*. Laboratory testing for heparin-induced thrombocytopenia is inconsistent in North America: a survey of North American specialized coagulation laboratories. *Thromb Haemost* 2007; **98**: 1357–1361.

18 Bates SM, Weitz JI, Johnston M, Hirsh J, Ginsberg JS. Use of a fixed activated partial thromboplastin time ratio to establish a therapeutic range for unfractionated heparin. *Arch Intern Med* 2001; **161**: 385–391.

19 Van der Veld EA, Poller L. The aPTT monitoring of heparin: the ISTH/ICSH collaborative study. *Thromb Haemost* 1995; **73**: 73–81.

20 Brill-Edwards P, Ginsberg JS, Johnston M, Hirsh J. Establishing a therapeutic range for heparin therapy. *Ann Intern Med* 1993; **1193**: 104–109.

21 Olson JD, Arkin CH, Brandt JT, Cunningham MT, Giles A, Koepke JA, *et al*. Laboratory monitoring of unfractionated heparin therapy. *Arch Pathol Lab Med* 1998; **122**: 782–798.

22 Chiu HM, Hirsh J, Yung WL, Regoeczi E, Gent M. Relationship between anticoagulant and antithrombotic effects of heparin in experimental venous thrombosis. *Blood* 1977; **49**: 171–184.

23 Hirsh J, Fruster V. Guide to anticoagulant therapy. I. Heparin. *Circulation* 1994; **89**: 1449–1468.

24 Refn I, Vestergaa L. The titration of heparin with protamine. *Scand J Clin Lab Invest* 1954; **6**: 284.

25 Laposata M, Green D, van Cott ENM, Barrowcliffe TW, Goodnight SH, Soslik RC. The clinical use and laboratory monitoring of low molecular weight heparin, danaparoid, hirudin and related compounds, and argatroban. College of American Pathologist Conference XXXI on Laboratory Monitoring of Anticoagulant Therapy. *Arch Pathol Lab Med* 1998; **122**: 799–807.

26 Teien AN, Lie M. Evaluation of an amidolytic heparin assay method: increased sensitivity by adding purified antithrombin III. *Thromb Res* 1977; **10**: 399–410.

27 Lyons SG, Lasser EC, Stein R. Modification of an amidolytic heparin assay to express protein-bound heparin and to correct for the effect of antithrombin III concentration. *Thromb Haemost* 1987; **58**: 884–887.

28 Diapharma web site: www.diapharma.com/support /product. Accessed Nov. 2007.

29 Aniara Corporation. Biophen Heparin Technical file. Ref.A221003/A221006.

30 Diapharma web site: www.diapharma.com. Chromogenix – Heparin Monograph. Accessed Dec. 2007.

31 Yin ET, Wessler S, Butler JV. Plasma heparin: A unique, practical submicrogram sensitive assay. *J Clin Lab Med* 1973; **81**: 298–310.

32 NCCLS (CLSI) document H21-A3. (1998) *Collection, Transport and Processing of Blood S for Coagulation Testing and General Performance of Coagulation Assays: Approved Guideline*, 3rd edn.

33 Chan AKC, Black L, Ing C, Williams S, Brandao L. Do we need different standard curves for measuring different low molecular weight heparins? *J Thromb Haemost* 2007; 5 (Suppl 2): P-S-128.

34 McGrath J, Johnston M, Angeloni F, Ginsberg J. Does monitoring patients on low molecular weight heparin (LMWH) require type specific reference lines for antifactor Xa heparin assays. *J Thromb Haemost* 2001; Supplement, P-S-2239.

35 Rosborough TK. Monitoring unfractionated heparin therapy with antifactor Xa activity results in few monitoring tests and dosage changes the monitoring with the activated partial throboplastin time. *Pharmacotherapy* 1999; **19**: 760–766.

36 Barrowcliffe TW. Laboratory monitoring of low molecular-weight heparin therapy. Part II. *J Thromb Haemost* 2005; **3**: 575–576.

37 Boneu B. Laboratory monitoring of low-molecular-weight-heparin therapy. Part II. *J Thromb Haemost* 2005; **3**: 573–574.

18 Monitoring oral anticoagulant therapy

A. Tripodi

Vitamin K antagonists (VKA) are widely used as oral anticoagulants for the treatment of venous thromboembolism and for the prevention of systemic embolism in patients with atrial fibrillation or prosthetic heart valves.[1] VKA exert their anticoagulant effect by interfering with the cyclic conversion of vitamin K, thus inhibiting the carboxylation of glutamate residues to γ-carboxyglutamate at the N-terminal domains of the procoagulant factors IX, VII, X and II, and of the naturally occurring anticoagulants, proteins C, S and Z.[1] The process of γ-carboxylation which takes place in the hepatocytes is mediated by the enzyme carboxylase with vitamin K acting as a cofactor. As a consequence of the antagonizing effect of oral anticoagulants, vitamin K-dependent coagulation factors are synthesized as a-carboxylated or partially carboxylated forms that do not bind phospholipid surfaces, thus leading to defective coagulation *in vivo* and *in vitro*.[1] The dose–response effect of VKA is variable and their dosage must be monitored closely to prevent undesirable over- or under-anticoagulation. Assessing the effect directly through the measurement of their plasmatic concentration, although feasible,[2] would be of little value and difficult in practice.[1] Interaction of VKA with other drugs, dependency from diet, seasonal variation and age, suggest that assessing plasma coagulability by means of laboratory tests may be the most appropriate method for drug dosage.[1] The establishment of therapeutic intervals (i.e. optimal level of anticoagulation to prevent thrombosis, but still sufficient to minimizing the hemorrhagic risk) has in fact been achieved by dosing VKA through a coagulation test.[1]

The prothrombin time (PT) is the logical choice because it is a global test sensitive to most of the coagulation factors depressed by VKA intake, it is also easy to perform and relatively inexpensive. However, an important limitation of the PT soon becomes evident. Thromboplastin preparations extracted from different tissues show different responsiveness to the coagulation defect induced by VKA intake, thus making PT results obtained with different thromboplastins in different laboratories not comparable.[3] As a consequence, patients had to refer to the same laboratory for monitoring and the adoption of "universal" therapeutic intervals established by clinical trials was not possible. This situation has limited for many years the use of oral anticoagulants despite the fact that early clinical trials of treatment and prophylaxis showed promising results.

During the last decades of the 20th century many attempts were made to make PT results comparable (for review see Poller[3]), which culminated in the adoption of the system elaborated by Kirkwood[4] and later endorsed by the World Health Organization (WHO).[5,6] This system is based on the expression of PT results by means of the International Normalized Ratio (INR).[6] Commercial thromboplastins are calibrated against an International Reference Preparation (IRP) for thromboplastin held by WHO by

Quality in Laboratory Hemostasis and Thrombosis, 1st edition. By Steve Kitchen, John D. Olson and F. Eric Preston. Published 2009 by Blackwell Publishing. ISBN: 978-1-4051-6803-8

measuring paired PTs with both reagents for plasmas from healthy individuals and from patients stabilized on VKA.[6] The procedure allows the determination of the International Sensitivity Index (ISI), which is an index of the responsiveness of the reagent to be calibrated (working thromboplastin) to the coagulation defect induced by VKA, relatively to the IRP.[6] By definition, an ISI equal to 1.00 means the same responsiveness as the IRP, whereas an ISI greater or smaller than 1.00 means a smaller or greater responsiveness, respectively.[6] Knowledge of the ISI value permits the conversion of PT results obtained with any given working reagent into the INR.[6] The following paragraphs are devoted to discussing how the system works, what are its limits and future directions.

Thromboplastin calibration

There are two models of calibration: full calibration according to WHO and local calibration. The two models are interrelated with the second a simplification of the first. The relative merits and shortcomings of the two models are discussed below. For more details, the reader may refer to van den Besselaar *et al.*[6,7]

WHO calibration

The ISI value is determined by parallel testing for PT of the plasmas from 20 healthy subjects and 60 patients stabilized on VKA treatment with an IRP and with the thromboplastin to be calibrated. Patients must be chosen from those who are in good health and on long-term treatment (at least 6 months). As additional requirements they must not be on heparin therapy and should not have undergone major dose changes during the last two visits. Healthy individuals must be chosen from those who do not have a personal or family history of hemorrhagic or thrombotic diseases, or other diseases known to alter hemostasis. The calibration procedure may be conveniently performed over 10 working sessions (not necessarily consecutive), each including two healthy individuals and six patients. In principle, the plasmas should be fresh, but frozen plasmas can also be used especially for batch–batch calibration of the same thromboplastin. Plasmas are intended as single donations, but

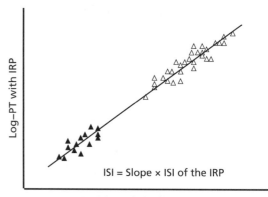

Fig. 18.1 Calibration of prothrombin time (PT) measuring systems according to the World Health Organization (WHO) model. IRP, International Reference Preparation for thromboplastin. ISI, International Sensitivity Index. Closed and open symbols, PT values from healthy individuals and patients on vitamin K antagonist (VKA) treatment, respectively.

pooled plasmas may also be suitable. Testing is usually performed as single determinations by using the manual (tilt tube) technique or automated coagulometers for clot detection. The manual technique for clot detection is mandatory for testing with the IRP.[6]

As shown in Fig. 18.1, paired PT values are plotted as coagulation times (seconds) on a double-log scale (IRP on the vertical axis) and the best-fit orthogonal regression line is drawn through the data points. The slope of the line represents the responsiveness of the working reagent to the defect induced by VKA relative to that of the IRP. The ISI is calculated as the product of the slope times the ISI value of the IRP. The final ISI will be assigned after identification and removal of data points whose INR, as determined with both the IRP and the working thromboplastin, is outside the interval 1.5–4.5. Likewise, data points lying at a perpendicular distance of 3 or more standard deviations from the line must also be identified and discarded before the final calculation of the ISI.[6]

The precision of the calibration is acceptable if the coefficient of variation (CV) of the slope is 3% or less. The CV depends on the precision of the measurements obtained with the IRP and the working thromboplastin, but also on the numbers and distribution of plasmas from the normal donors and patients on VKA used for calibration. Another important requisite to judge the calibration is to test whether the orthogonal regression line drawn through the patient-only data points passes through the mean of the data points obtained for the healthy subjects.[6] Statistical analyses specifically designed for this requirement are available,[8] but in practice it may suffice to test whether the values of the INR determined with the ISI calculated for the patient-only line deviates from the INR determined with the ISI calculated for the controls plus patients line.[6] If this difference is >10%, alternative calculation of the INR may be required,[8] but this does not occur often.

Hierarchy of WHO International Reference Preparations

IRPs are crucial for the model of WHO calibration. As shown in Fig. 18.2, two different IRPs are currently available from WHO and an additional one from the Institute for Reference Materials and Measurements (IRMM) of the European Commission. rTF/95 is a human recombinant relipidated tissue factor;[9] RBT/05[10] and CRM 149 S[11] are from rabbit brain. All have been indirectly calibrated against the primary IRP coded 67/40 to which an arbitrary ISI equal to 1.00 had been assigned. Between the current

IRPs and 67/40 there have been other preparations (Fig. 18.2) whose stocks are now exhausted. All of them have been directly or indirectly calibrated against 67/40, so that continuity of the system is ensured. The reasons to maintain at least two IRPs is twofold:

1 The assumption that the calibration is more precise when performed against an IRP of the same species of the working thromboplastin. This would require an additional IRP from bovine origin, which was in fact available until recently,[12] but it was dismissed on the ground that very few commercial thromboplastins from bovine origin are available.[13] Furthermore, evidence has been provided that bovine thromboplastins can be reliably calibrated by using IRPs from rabbit origin.[13]

2 To maintain more than one IRP rests on the fact that these preparations, although stable, may deteriorate over time. The presence of at least two IRPs permits occasional checking of their relative stability by cross-calibration.[14]

When stocks of any of the IRPs is close to exhaustion or shows signs of deterioration, a replacement preparation is selected and calibrated by large international collaborative studies against all the existing IRPs. The assigned ISI is the average of all the individual values obtained with each IRP.[6,15] Established IRPs are distributed upon request to manufacturers and national control laboratories along with protocols to be used for calibration of commercial thromboplastins and national secondary standards.

Local calibration

The responsibility to determine the ISI usually rests on the manufacturer as the above full calibration according to WHO recommendation would be beyond the expertise of most clinical laboratories. However, in recent years it has become evident that the ISI of commercial thromboplastins depends not only on reagents, but also on the coagulometers used for testing.[16–18] The effect of the coagulometer on the ISI may be minimized by two alternative procedures:

1 To calibrate commercial thromboplastins on specific coagulometers. This can be achieved by testing plasmas with the IRP by the manual technique and the working thromboplastin with the coagulometer.

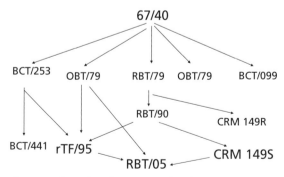

Fig. 18.2 Hierarchy of International Reference Preparation (IRP) for thromboplastin. IRPs coded as small font have already been dismissed.

This gives an instrument-specific ISI value. It is the best solution, but difficult to put into practice because of the many possible thromboplastin–coagulometer combinations.

2 The calibration is performed locally by the user. Two different systems of local calibration have been devised over the last 15 years and are now available.

Local ISI determination
This system requires a set of lyophilized plasmas certified in terms of PT by using an IRP and the manual technique.[19] These calibration plasmas can then be tested locally by means of the thromboplastin–coagulometer combination and the value plotted against the certified PT value with the IRP.[19] The slope of the best-fit orthogonal regression line can eventually be used to calculate the local ISI in a manner analogous to that of the WHO recommended procedure (Fig. 18.3).

"Direct" INR determination
This system requires a set of lyophilized calibration plasmas certified directly in terms of the INR

by means of an IRP.[20] These calibration plasmas are then tested locally and their coagulation times plotted against the certified INR values to draw a local calibration curve that may ultimately serve to convert patient coagulation times into INR (Fig. 18.4).

Advantages and disadvantages of local calibration
The advantages of these procedures are that they do not require expertise with the manual technique to record coagulation times, do not need the IRP nor the availability of considerable numbers of fresh plasmas from healthy individuals and patients on VKA treatment. Furthermore, the "direct" INR determination does not require knowledge of the ISI nor that of the mean normal PT (see p. 183).

The disadvantages are that they use lyophilized plasmas that do not necessarily mimic their fresh counterpart. Numerous surveys carried out over the last 15 years have shown light and shadows associated with the use of these simplified procedures for local calibration.[21-24]

In general, the two procedures proved effective in improving the between-laboratory agreement of the

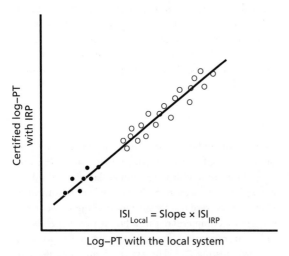

Fig. 18.3 Local calibration of prothrombin time (PT) measuring system by means of lyophilized plasmas certified in terms of PT with an International Reference Preparation (IRP) for thromboplastin. ISI, International Sensitivity Index. Closed and open symbols, PT values from healthy individuals and patients on vitamin K antagonist (VKA) treatment, respectively.

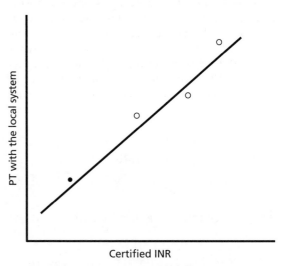

Fig. 18.4 Local calibration of prothrombin time (PT) measuring system by means of lyophilized plasmas certified in terms of International Normalized Ratio (INR) with an International Reference Preparation (IRP) for thromboplastin. Closed and open symbols, PT values from healthy individuals and patients on vitamin K antagonist (VKA) treatment, respectively.

INR,[21,22] although doubts may remain about the efficacy to maintain the accuracy of the INR measurement.[25] The most important shortcoming associated with these procedures is that the INR determined for the calibration plasmas is often dependent on the type of thromboplastin or IRP used for testing.[26] The above mentioned differences, which vary with different sets of plasmas, are often greater than those recorded for fresh plasmas[26] and this probably means that the process of lyophilization (protein denaturation, addition of preservatives, buffers and stabilizers) make those plasmas somewhat different from their fresh counterpart which they are supposed to be compared with. Furthermore, the source of those plasmas may also have a role.[26]

Artificially depleted plasmas obtained by selective absorption of vitamin K dependent coagulation factors mimic the prolongation of the coagulation times recorded for plasmas from patients on VKA, but their composition is different for obvious reasons. Plasmas from patients on VKA (coumarin plasmas) would be more suitable, but are more difficult to obtain in large amounts and with the range of INR required to cover the whole spectrum of anticoagulation.

The working party of the International Society on Thrombosis and Haemostasis (ISTH) has recently issued guidelines on how to prepare and use calibration plasmas, to which the reader may refer for more details.[7] The most important recommendation stemming from the guidelines is that each set of calibration plasmas must be validated before it can be used for local calibration. The validation requires that 10 or more fresh plasmas from patients on VKA be tested for the INR by using the local combination of thromboplastin–coagulometer previously calibrated by the set of calibration plasmas. The INR for the same plasmas will then be determined by the same combination of thromboplastin–coagulometer calibrated as recommended by WHO (fresh plasmas and the IRP). If the mean values of the two determinations do not differ by more than 10%, the set of plasmas may be used for local calibration of subsequent lots of the same thromboplastin when used in combination with the same coagulometer.

Practical experience made with several sets of lyophilized calibration plasmas showed that generalization on the use of these plasmas for all types of thromboplastins may prove unfeasible.[23] The reasons are presently unknown and probably rest on the interaction between thromboplastins and lyophilized plasmas. The (theoretical) argument that coumarin plasmas work better than artificially depleted plasmas in the above respect has been disputed[27] and this emphasizes the need to validate calibration plasmas before use with a particular combination of thromboplastin–coagulometer.

Conversion of PT into INR and issues affecting results

Conversion of PT into INR

Once a combination of thromboplastin–coagulometer has been calibrated, the conversion of the coagulation time (seconds) into INR is straightforward. If the ISI of the thromboplastin–coagulometer is known, the patient coagulation time is converted into ratio (patient : normal coagulation time) and this is raised to a power equal to the ISI of thromboplastin–coagulometer combination according to the equation:[6]

$$INR = (PT_{patient}/MNPT)^{ISI}$$

where the MNPT is the geometrical mean normal PT obtained by testing plasmas from 20 or more healthy individuals.

If the system ISI is not known, the patient coagulation time may be converted into INR by "direct" interpolation by means of a locally determined calibration curve relating coagulation times for the calibration plasmas versus the respective certified INR values.[7] By definition, the INR value for any given patient is the PT ratio that would have been obtained had the patient's plasma been tested with the IRP instead of the working thromboplastin.[6]

Issues affecting results

Looking at the equation that defines the INR one can easily realize how and to what extent any of the parameters needed for its calculation may affect the final result.

Patient's prothrombin time
The variables that may influence this parameter are both preanalytical and analytical. Among the first

the most important are the quality of venepuncture; the effect brought about by the blood collection system; the type and concentration of the anticoagulant; the centrifugation; and the type and time of storage before analysis. The analytical variables are concerned with the type of thromboplastin and coagulometers and the concentration of calcium chloride.

As for any other coagulation test, blood for the PT test should be obtained by clean venepuncture with minimum stasis to avoid undesirable activation of blood coagulation. Blood must be transferred rapidly into the tube containing the appropriate proportion of anticoagulant and mixed gently by repeated inversion to prevent onset of coagulation activation. The use of evacuated tubes for blood collection is recommended as it ensures a more standardized procedure of blood drawing than the syringe technique. The anticoagulant of choice for blood coagulation testing is trisodium citrate at a concentration of 109 mmol/L (corresponding to 3.2%),[6] although concentrations ranging from 105 to 109 mmol/L may be acceptable.[28] In many countries the concentration of 129 mmol/L (or 3.8%) is still used, but this should be urgently replaced as the concentration of citrate may considerably influence the determination of the ISI and therefore of the INR. Evidence has been provided that the low concentration of the anticoagulant (in the face of a standard concentration of calcium chloride) results in shorter coagulation times. However, this shortening does not affect normal and anticoagulated plasmas to the same extent and therefore has considerable effect on the ISI of any thromboplastin–coagulometer combination.[29]

The correct proportion of blood:anticoagulant is 9:1. In evacuated tubes this proportion is ensured by the vacuum if sufficient time is allowed for the blood to flow. However, visual inspection of the correct level of the blood in the tube is highly recommended. Citrate does not cross cell membranes; therefore, its concentration is higher in plasmas from patients with high hematocrit and lower in plasma from patients with low hematocrit. This translates in longer or shorter coagulation times, respectively. However, correction for the proportion of blood:anticoagulant is not strictly needed unless the patient's hematocrit is very low (<0.20) or very high (>0.60). Whenever needed, a correction chart proposed by Ingram and Hills[30] can be used to determine the appropriate amounts of citrate to be used in combination with the abnormal hematocrit.

Tubes for blood collection can considerably influence the PT, especially for patients on VKA. This holds true even when the concentration of the anticoagulant is maintained constant.[28,31] The main reasons for those differences rest on the type of plastic (or siliconized glass), and the effect of buffers or contaminants.[32] Users should be aware of those differences and should check new brands of tubes to ascertain whether they are comparable to the old brands.[33] Whenever needed, new values for the ISI and mean normal PT must be established and applied to the calculation of the INR.

Centrifugation should be carried out at a speed sufficient to obtain platelet-poor plasma. Residual platelets do not affect the PT greatly and therefore centrifugation for 15 minutes at 2000 g is adequate. To avoid deterioration of coagulation factors it is advised to carry out centrifugation at (controlled) room temperature. Prior to the analyses, plasma samples must be stored at room temperature (20–24°C) to avoid cold activation of factor VII which might considerably shorten the PT especially for patients on VKA. Although storage times up to 24 hours have been advocated as safe,[34] occasional changes may occur in individual patients and it is therefore strongly recommended to complete the analyses not later than 4 hours from blood collection. Frozen plasmas may be used provided that they have been stored in capped plastic tubes, rapidly frozen (liquid nitrogen) and stored at a temperature lower than −30°C. Thawing before analysis should be performed rapidly (immersion of tubes in a water bath at 37°C for 1–2 minutes) to avoid the formation of cryoprecipitate.

Mean normal prothrombin time
The guidelines issued by WHO state that the value to be used as denominator in the equation to calculate the INR should be the geometric mean of the PT values for 20 or more healthy individuals.[6] This value must be determined locally with the combination of thromboplastin–coagulometer used for testing patient plasmas. The value is valid for that particular batch of thromboplastin and must be recalculated whenever changes of thromboplastin and/or coagulometer occur.

As an alternative to the mean normal PT (MNPT), the PT value of a pooled normal plasma, stored frozen and tested along with the patients' plasmas may be also appropriate, provided that the material has been prepared by pooling a sufficient number of individual donations to ensure an average value close to the MNPT. Likewise, commercial lyophilized normal pooled plasmas may also be suitable if they have been prepared as above and their clotting times are close to the MNPT.[35]

International Sensitivity Index

Being exponential, the effect of the ISI on the INR calculation may be considerable especially with relatively unresponsive thromboplastins (ISI > 1.00). The WHO guidelines recommend using thromboplastins with ISI values close to 1.00, although ISI ranging from 0.90 to 1.70 (determined by manual technique) may be acceptable.[6]

Limits of the INR

General limits

It should be realized that the INR is an average approximate scale and therefore occasional between-system differences can occur even in the face of well-calibrated thromboplastin–coagulometer combinations. The PT test, which forms the basis for the INR scale, is a global test responsive to many coagulation factors (VII, X, V, II and fibrinogen). Some of these factors are vitamin K dependent (VII, X and II) and therefore taken into consideration by the calibration procedure. However, the relative responsiveness of different thromboplastins to the activity of individual vitamin K dependent coagulation factors may vary. Furthermore, other coagulation factors to which the PT is responsive (V and fibrinogen) are vitamin K independent and therefore escape the calibration procedure.[36] It is therefore not surprising that small variations in the above coagulation factors may give rise to variation in the INR value measured with different thromboplastins even when they are accurately calibrated. However, the above differences are not great enough to hamper the use of the INR in the clinical practice of dose prescription of VKA treatment, as demonstrated by the relatively low rate of adverse events recorded in a large field inception cohort study carried out

recently in oral anticoagulation clinics using the INR.[37]

Specific limits

In addition to the above general limitations, clinicians using the INR scale for dose prescription should be aware of other specific limitations of this scale.

Patients not yet stabilized on VKA treatment

Strictly speaking, the scale is valid only for patients stabilized on VKA. In fact, the ISI is determined by using plasmas from patients who are in the stable phase of VKA treatment.[6] This has two important implications:

1 The responsiveness of the thromboplastin to the defect induced by VKA intake is calculated when vitamin K dependent coagulation factors are stably depressed. During the induction phase, the coagulation factors are depressed at a different rate depending on the relative half-life of the individual factors, with factor VII being the first and factor II the last to be reduced. Obviously, those thromboplastins that are more responsive to factor VII will give INR values greater than those that are less responsive. Notwithstanding this limit the INR scale can be safely used even during the induction phase.[38]

2 The scale is (at least in principle) not valid for patients other than those treated with VKA. For instance, recent evidence highlighted this fact showing that the INR is unable to harmonize results obtained for patients with cirrhosis.[39] The most likely explanation is that the defect induced by VKA intake (similar though it may seem) is qualitatively different from that induced by cirrhosis. The lack of harmonization of the INR in the setting of cirrhosis is disturbing as the PT-INR has long been (and it is still) used as a parameter to assess survival in patients with chronic liver disease[40] and ultimately to calculate the "model for end-stage liver disease (MELD)" score, which is ostensibly used to prioritize patients for liver transplantation.[41] If one considers that the INRs for patients with cirrhosis are not harmonized in different laboratories, the practical implication is that there is no parity of organ allocation as it depends on the responsiveness of the thromboplastin used for testing by a particular laboratory. This translates in the undesirable

situation where those patients who refer for INR measurement to laboratories using relatively more responsive thromboplastins may achieve priority for liver transplantation. The possible solution would be to calibrate the INR measuring system by determining the ISI for patients with chronic liver disease in a manner analogous to that for patients on VKA, whereby plasmas from the latter are replaced with plasmas from the former.[39] This system of alternative calibration proved feasible,[39,42] but implies that manufacturers should provide for each of their reagents two different ISI (i.e. the ISI_{vka} and the ISI_{liver}).

INR values outside the interval of anticoagulation corresponding to 1.5–4.5

Strictly speaking, the INR is valid within the interval of anticoagulation corresponding to 1.5–4.5. This is because plasmas from patients selected for calibration lay within this interval, therefore the linearity of relationship and the ensuing validity of the ISI cannot be checked outside this interval. This implies that INR values >4.5 are not very accurate and should be interpreted with caution.

Heparin

The treatment of acute venous thromboembolism requires imbrication of heparin with VKA at least until the patient INR is within the therapeutic interval.[1] During this phase the PT is prolonged as a function of VKA intake, but (although to a lesser extent) also as a function of heparin. Therefore, the prescribing physician might be induced to withdraw heparin before the INR has reached the real therapeutic interval. Most of the commercial thromboplastins contain antiheparin substances (polybrene or heparinases) in their formulation which are able to quench heparin up to 1 IU/mL activity. It is recommended to check the package insert of the thromboplastin for more details.

Lupus anticoagulant

Patients with lupus anticoagulant (LA) may occasionally present with prolonged PT. This means that when they are treated with VKA because of a thrombotic event their INR reflects the combined effects of anticoagulation and LA and this may make the assessment of the degree of anticoagulation uncertain. Numerous studies have addressed this issue and

although results are somewhat contrasting the conclusion is that there is no massive influence of LA on the INR.[43–45] However, there are thromboplastins and patients for whom an effect has been shown.[44,45] Whenever possible, the PT should be measured before starting treatment with VKA. In case of prolongation there is an indication to switch to an insensitive thromboplastin.

Alternatively, other less sensitive or insensitive methods of laboratory control may be used. For instance, combined thromboplastins (brain extracts added with optimal amounts of factor V and fibrinogen) require a plasma:thromboplastin ratio lower than that of conventional thromboplastins. Such thromboplastins are apparently less sensitive to the LA because the effect of the anticoagulant would be diluted out.[46] Another option would be monitoring the treatment through the measurement of an individual coagulation factor. The preferred candidate would be factor X for which there are methods based on amidolytic measurement not influenced by LA.[45] However, it should be realized that no validated therapeutic intervals based on such measurements are available.

Implementation of the INR

The full implementation of the INR requires combined efforts and partnership from the industry, national control laboratories, laboratory workers and clinicians.

According to WHO recommendations, manufacturers of commercial thromboplastins should determine the ISI of their reagents and state the value together with the coagulometer(s) for which they are valid on the package insert. Batch–batch consistency cannot be taken for granted and the ISI should be checked for each production lot. Manufacturers should also state clearly the IRP (or secondary standard) and the procedure adopted for calibration.

WHO strongly encourages health authorities to establish one or more National Control Laboratories.[6] These laboratories should supervise the correct implementation of the INR, monitor the performance of clinical laboratories through the organization of regular external quality control surveys specifically designed for the INR, check of the validity of the ISI of commercial thromboplastins, establish national secondary standards where required and provide assistance/advice to manufacturers for calibration of thromboplastins.

Laboratory workers are instrumental for the implementation of the INR. Besides being responsible for the correct measurement they also have a key role in disseminating the relevant information to clinicians to whom the system of calibration and its limit should be explained.

Conclusions and future directions

The PT test was first described more than 70 years ago to investigate the coagulability of plasmas from patients with liver disease.[47] Since then it has been extensively used as a laboratory tool to investigate congenital and acquired coagulopathies and for the laboratory control of oral anticoagulant therapy. Because of the increasing numbers of patients who benefit from oral anticoagulation, the PT is probably the most frequently requested coagulation test.

Attempts have been made to replace the PT with other tests such as single factor measurements[48] or biochemical markers of coagulation activation,[49,50] but these attempts have not gone beyond the publication of reports in scientific journals. It is predicted that the PT will stay in place at least until new direct antithrombin or anti-factor Xa drugs,[51] which (allegedly) do not require laboratory monitoring, enter the scene of treatment and prophylaxis of venous and arterial thromboembolism.

However, in spite of its popularity, PT has many shortcomings when used to monitor patients on VKA, some of them not entirely resolved. An adequate and robust system of local calibration is the most urgent to be tackled and resolved. Certified calibration plasmas are the way to go, but their quality should be improved to make them more similar to fresh plasmas. Preliminary experience showed that fresh frozen plasma may be more suitable than lyophilized plasma for local calibration,[26] but shipment to distant locations (although possible) is problematic. There is therefore an urgent need to explore new venues for lyophilization with the aim of maintaining unaltered the properties of fresh coumarin plasmas.

References

1 Ansell J, Hirsh J, Poller L, Bussey H, Jacobson A, Hylek E. The pharmacology and management of the vitamin K antagonists: the Seventh ACCP Conference on Antithrombotic and Thrombolytic Therapy. *Chest* 2004; **126** (3 Suppl): 204S–233S. Erratum in: *Chest* 2005; **127**: 415–416 (dosage error in text).

2 Lombardi R, Chantarangkul V, Cattaneo M, Tripodi A. Measurement of warfarin in plasma by high performance liquid chromatography (HPLC) and its correlation with the international normalized ratio. *Thromb Res* 2003; **111**: 281–284.

3 Poller L. International Normalized Ratios (INR): the first 20 years. *J Thromb Haemost* 2004; **2**: 849–860.

4 Kirkwood TB. Calibration of reference thromboplastins and standardisation of the prothrombin time ratio. *Thromb Haemost* 1983; **49**: 238–244.

5 WHO Expert Committee on Biological Standardization. Thirty-third report. *World Health Organ Tech Rep Ser* 1983; **687**: 81–105.

6 van den Besselaar AMHP, Poller L, Tripodi A. WHO Expert Committee on Biological Standardization. Forty-eighth report. Guidelines for thromboplastins and plasma used to control oral anticoagulant therapy. *WHO Technical Report Series* 1999; **889**: 64–93.

7 van den Besselaar AMHP, Barrowcliffe TW, Houbouyan-Réveillard LL, Jespersen J, Johnston M, Poller L, *et al.*, on behalf of the Subcommittee on Control of Anticoagulation of the Scientific and Standardization Committee of the ISTH. Guidelines on preparation, certification and use of certified plasmas for ISI calibration and INR determination. *J Thromb Haemost* 2004; **2**: 1946–1953.

8 Tomenson JA. A statistician's independent evaluation. In *Thromboplastin Calibration and Oral Anticoagulant Control*, van den Besselaar AMHP, Lewis SM, Gralnick HR, eds. Boston: Martinus Nijhoff, 1984: 87–108.

9 Tripodi A, Chantarangkul V, Negri B, Clerici M, Mannucci PM, on behalf of the Subcommittee on Control of Anticoagulation. International collaborative study for the calibration of a proposed reference preparation for thromboplastin, human recombinant, plain. *Thromb Haemost* 1998; **79**: 439–443.

10 Chantarangkul V, van den Besselaar AMHP, Witteveen E, Tripodi A. International collaborative study for the calibration of a proposed international standard for thromboplastin, rabbit, plain. *J Thromb Haemost* 2006; **4**: 1339–1345.

11 van den Besselaar AMHP. Multi-center calibration of the third BCR reference material for thromboplastin, rabbit, plain, coded CRM 149S: long-term stability of previous BCR reference materials. *Thromb Haemost* 1995; **74**: 1465–1467.

12 Hermans J, van den Besselaar AM, Loeliger EA, van der Velde EA. A collaborative calibration study of reference materials for thromboplastins. *Thromb Haemost* 1983; **50**: 712–717.

13 van den Besselaar AM, Tripodi A. Is there a need for replacement of the International Reference Preparation for Thromboplastin, Bovine, Combined (OBT/79)? *J Thromb Haemost* 2005; **3**: 2365–2366.

14 Linsinger TP, van den Besselaar AMHP, Tripodi A. Long-term stability of relationships between reference materials for thromboplastins. *Thromb Haemost* 2006; **96**: 210–214.

15 Tripodi A, Poller L, van den Besselaar AMHP, Mannucci PM, on behalf of the Subcommittee on Control of Anti-coagulation. A proposed scheme for calibration of international reference preparations of thromboplastin for the prothrombin time. *Thromb Haemost* 1995; **74**: 1368–1369.

16 Poggio M, van den Besselaar AMHP, van der Velde EA, Bertina RM. The effect of some instruments for pro-thrombin time testing on the International Sensitivity Index (ISI) of two rabbit tissue thromboplastin reagents. *Thromb Haemost* 1989; **62**: 868–874.

17 Chantarangkul V, Tripodi A, Mannucci PM. The effect of instrumentation on thromboplastin calibration. *Thromb Haemost* 1992; **67**: 588–589.

18 van den Besselaar AMHP, Houbouyan LL, Aillaud MF, Denson KW, Johnston M, Kitchen S, *et al.* Influence of three types of automated coagulometers on the International Sensitivity Index (ISI) of rabbit, human, and recombinant human tissue factor preparations: a multi-center study. *Thromb Haemost* 1999; **81**: 66–70.

19 Poller L, Triplett DA, Hirsh J, Carroll J, Clarke K. A comparison of lyophilized artificially depleted plasmas and lyophilized plasmas from patients receiving warfarin in correcting for coagulometer effects on international normalized ratios. *Am J Clin Pathol* 1995; **103**: 366–371.

20 Houbouyan LL, Goguel AF. Long-term French experi-ence in INR standardization by a procedure using plasma calibrants. *Am J Clin Pathol* 1997; **108**: 83–89.

21 Chantarangkul V, Tripodi A, Cesana BM, Mannucci PM. Calibration of local systems with lyophilized calibrant plasmas improves the interlaboratory variability of the INR in the Italian external quality assessment scheme. *Thromb Haemost* 1999; **82**: 1621–1626. Erratum in: *Thromb Haemost* 2000; **83**: VIII.

22 Kitchen S, Jennings I, Woods TA, Preston FE. Local cali-bration of international normalised ratio improves between laboratory agreement: results from the UK National External Quality Assessment Scheme. UK NEQAS (Blood Coagulation) Steering Committee. *Thromb Haemost* 1999; **81**: 60–65.

23 van den Besselaar AMHP, Houbouyan-Reveillard LL. Field study of lyophilized calibrant plasmas for fresh plasma INR determination. *Thromb Haemost* 2002; **87**: 277–281.

24 Poller L, Keown M, Ibrahim S, van den Besselaar AMHP, Roberts C, Stevenson K, *et al.*, European Concerted Action on Anticoagulation. Comparison of local Inter-national Sensitivity Index calibration and 'direct INR' methods in correction of locally reported International Normalized Ratios: an international study. *J Thromb Haemost* 2007; **5**: 1002–1009.

25 van den Besselaar AMHP. International Normalized Ratio: towards improved accuracy. *Thromb Haemost* 1999; **82**: 1562–1563.

26 van den Besselaar AM, Houbouyan-Reveillard LL, Aillaud MF, Denson KW, Droulle C, Johnston M, *et al.* Multicenter evaluation of lyophilized and deep-frozen plasmas for assignment of the International Normalized Ratio. *Thromb Haemost* 1999; **82**: 1451–1455.

27 Poller L, van den Besselaar AMHP, Jespersen J, Tripodi A, Houghton D. A comparison of artificially depleted, lyophilized coumarin and fresh coumarin plasmas in thromboplastin calibration. European Concerted Action on Anticoagulation. *Br J Haematol* 1998; **101**: 462–467.

28 van den Besselaar AMHP, Chantarangkul V, Tripodi A. A comparison of two sodium citrate concentrations in two evacuated blood collection systems for prothrombin time and ISI determination. *Thromb Haemost* 2000; **84**: 664–667.

29 Chantarangkul V, Tripodi A, Clerici M, Negri B, Man-nucci PM. Assessment of the influence of citrate concen-tration on the International Normalized Ratio (INR) determined with twelve reagent–instrument combina-tions. *Thromb Haemost* 1998; **80**: 258–262.

30 Ingram GI, Hills M. The prothrombin time test: effect of varying citrate concentration. *Thromb Haemost* 1976; **36**: 230–236.

31 van den Besselaar AMHP, Bertina RM, van der Meer FJ, den Hartig J. Different sensitivities of various throm-boplastins to two blood collection systems for monitor-ing oral anticoagulant therapy. *Thromb Haemost* 1999; **82**: 153–154.

32 van den Besselaar AM, Witteveen E, Meeuwisse-Braun J, van der Meer FJ. The influence of exogenous magne-sium chloride on the apparent INR determined with human, rabbit, and bovine thromboplastin reagents. *Thromb Haemost* 2003; **89**: 43–47.

33 Tripodi A, Chantarangkul V, Bressi C, Mannucci PM. How to evaluate the influence of blood collection systems on the international sensitivity index: protocol applied to two new evacuated tubes and eight coagulometer–

thromboplastin combinations. *Thromb Res* 2002; **108**: 85–89.

34 Rao LV, Okorodudu AO, Petersen JR, Elghetany MT. Stability of prothrombin time and activated partial thromboplastin time tests under different storage conditions. *Clin Chim Acta* 2000; **300**: 13–21.

35 Peters RH, van den Besselaar AM, Olthuis FM. Determination of the mean normal prothrombin time for assessment of international normalized ratios: usefulness of lyophilized plasma. *Thromb Haemost* 1991; **66**: 442–445.

36 Tripodi A, Chantarangkul V, Akkawat B, Clerici M, Mannucci PM. A partial factor V deficiency in anticoagulated lyophilized plasmas has been identified as a cause of the international normalized ratio discrepancy in the external quality assessment scheme. *Thromb Res* 1995; **78**: 283–292.

37 Palareti G, Leali N, Coccheri S, Poggi M, Manotti C, D'Angelo A, *et al*. Bleeding complications of oral anticoagulant treatment: an inception-cohort, prospective collaborative study (ISCOAT). Italian Study on Complications of Oral Anticoagulant Therapy. *Lancet* 1996; **348**: 423–428.

38 Johnston M, Harrison L, Moffat K, Willan A, Hirsh J. Reliability of the international normalized ratio for monitoring the induction phase of warfarin: comparison with the prothrombin time ratio. *J Lab Clin Med* 1996; **128**: 214–217.

39 Tripodi A, Chantarangkul V, Primignani M, Fabris F, Dell'Era A, Sei C, *et al*. The International Normalized Ratio calibrated for cirrhosis (INR$_{liver}$) normalizes PT results for MELD calculation. *Hepatology* 2007; **46**: 520–527.

40 Malinchoc M, Kamath PS, Gordon FD, Peine CJ, Rank J, ter Borg PC. A model to predict poor survival in patients undergoing transjugular intrahepatic portosystemic shunts. *Hepatology* 2000; **31**: 864–871.

41 Wiesner R, Edwards E, Freeman R, Harper A, Kim R, Kamath P, *et al*. United Network for Organ Sharing Liver Disease Severity Score Committee. Model for end-stage liver disease (MELD) and allocation of donor liver. *Gastroenterology* 2003; **124**: 91–96.

42 Bellest L, Eschwege V, Poupon R, Chazoullieres O, Robert A. A modified International Normalized Ratio as an effective way of prothrombin time standardization in hepatology. *Hepatology* 2007; **46**: 528–534.

43 Moll S, Ortel TL. Monitoring warfarin therapy in patients with lupus anticoagulants. *Ann Intern Med* 1997; **127**: 177–185.

44 Robert A, Le Querrec A, Delahousse B, Caron C, Houbouyan L, Boutiere B, *et al*. Control of oral anticoagulation in patients with the antiphospholipid syndrome: influence of the lupus anticoagulant on International Normalized Ratio. Groupe Methodologie en Hemostase du Groupe d'Etudes sur l'Hemostases et la Thrombose. *Thromb Haemost* 1998; **80**: 99–103.

45 Tripodi A, Chantarangkul V, Clerici M, Negri B, Galli M, Mannucci PM. Laboratory control of oral anticoagulant treatment by the INR system in patients with the antiphospholipid syndrome and lupus anticoagulant: results of a collaborative study involving nine commercial thromboplastins. *Br J Haematol* 2001; **115**: 672–678.

46 Rapaport SI, Le DT. Thrombosis in the antiphospholipid antibody syndrome. *New Engl J Med* 1995; **333**: 665.

47 Quick AJ. The prothrombin time in hemophilia and obstructive jaundice. *J Biol Chem* 1935; **109**: 73–74.

48 Furie B, Diuguid CF, Jacobs M, Diuguid DL, Furie BC. Randomized prospective trial comparing the native prothrombin antigen with the prothrombin time for monitoring oral anticoagulant therapy. *Blood* 1990; **75**: 344–349.

49 Millenson MM, Bauer KA, Kistler JP, Barzegar S, Tulin L, Rosenberg RD. Monitoring "mini-intensity" anticoagulation with warfarin: comparison of the prothrombin time using a sensitive thromboplastin with prothrombin fragment F1+2 levels. *Blood* 1992; **79**: 2034–2038.

50 Tripodi A, Cattaneo M, Molteni A, Cesana BM, Mannucci PM. Changes of prothrombin fragment 1+2 (F 1+2) as a function of increasing intensity of oral anticoagulation: considerations on the suitability of F 1+2 to monitor oral anticoagulant treatment. *Thromb Haemost* 1998; **79**: 571–573.

51 Ansell J. New anticoagulants and their potential impact on the treatment of thromboembolic disease. *Curr Hematol Rep* 2004; **3**: 357–362.

Monitoring new anticoagulants

E. Gray & T. W. Barrowcliffe

Unfractionated heparin and warfarin have been in use as therapeutic anticoagulants since the 1930s and 1950s, respectively. While these two anticoagulants are effective in the prevention and treatment of thrombosis, there are drawbacks in their use. These include unpredictability in dosage required for therapeutic effect, the need for continuous monitoring and, in the case of unfractionated heparin, the development of antibodies that can lead to heparin-induced thrombocytopenia. Low molecular weight heparins, derivatives of unfractionated heparin, were first described in 1976[1] and have been in clinical use since the 1980s. The clinical advantages of low molecular weight heparins include greater predictability, dose-dependent plasma levels, a long half-life and less bleeding for a given antithrombotic effect.[2] Low molecular weight heparins are administered in fixed doses for prophylaxis and body weight adjusted doses for treatment of thrombosis. Laboratory monitoring is not generally necessary.[3] However, dose-finding trials have not been carried out in special populations, such as patients with renal failure or severe obesity. It has been suggested that monitoring should be considered in such patients.[4-6] Several laboratory assays have been proposed for this purpose, including the anti-factor Xa assay, and more global clotting tests, such as the Heptest.[6,7] Anti-factor Xa chromogenic assay kits are now widely available, and the anti-factor Xa assay is the test currently recommended by the College of American Pathologists for the monitoring of low molecular weight heparins.[8]

New anticoagulants

In the past decade, development of new anticoagulants has focused on two major drug classes that have high specificity for either factor Xa or thrombin. These new generation anticoagulants are small molecules, either produced by chemical synthesis or recombinant technology. Their pharmacokinetics and pharmacodynamics are more predictable than warfarin, unfractionated heparin and low molecular weight heparins. Indirect FXa inhibitors such as fondaparinux and idraparinux bind specifically to antithrombin and are reported to have 100% bioavailability following subcutaneous injection. Coagulation monitoring has not been recommended for these therapeutics.[9] However, it is prudent to have appropriate and sensitive methods that will detect the concentration and activity of these anticoagulants in case of overdose or for monitoring specific patient groups. Table 19.1 shows examples of these new anticoagulants. The indirect FXa inhibitors are antithrombin dependent and inhibit only free FXa, while the direct FXa inhibitors are antithrombin independent and inhibit both free FXa and FXa bound in the prothrombinase complex. While FXa inhibitors inhibit FXa, which then leads to inhibition of the process of thrombin formation, the direct thrombin inhibitors target thrombin, the enzyme that converts fibrinogen to fibrin. Although the net effect of FXa and thrombin

Quality in Laboratory Hemostasis and Thrombosis, 1st edition. By Steve Kitchen, John D. Olson and F. Eric Preston. Published 2009 by Blackwell Publishing. ISBN: 978-1-4051-6803-8

Table 19.1 Indirect, direct FXa inhibitors and thrombin inhibitors that are in clinical use or in clinical trials.

Indirect FXa inhibitors	Direct FXa inhibitors	FXa and thrombin inhibitor	Direct thrombin inhibitors
Fondaparinux	Otamixaban	BIBT 986	Dabigatran etexilate
Idraparinux	DX-9065a		Lepirudin
Biotinylated idraparinux	Rivaroxaban		Bivalirudin
	Apixaban		Argatroban
	LY517717		
	YM150		
	DU-176b		
	PRT-054021		

inhibitors is the suppression of coagulation, the mechanisms by which these inhibitors exert their action differ and therefore different laboratory monitoring methods will vary in their sensitivities to these inhibitors.

Calibration for accuracy of measurement

Unlike unfractionated heparin and low molecular weight heparins which are heterogeneous and polydisperse polysaccharides, these new anticoagulants are mostly chemically synthesized and homogeneous entities. However, their mechanisms of action are complex and therefore they behave more like a biological than a chemically defined drug. The measurement of these anticoagulants should therefore follow the principle of bioassay, i.e. "like versus like."[10] Regardless of assay methods used, each product should be used to construct calibration curves for the estimation of *ex vivo* plasma concentrations or activities of that product. The activity of these products should be expressed in either mass or molar concentration rather than units. Figure 19.1 shows standard curves for two direct thrombin inhibitors, argatroban and hirudin, in an anti-IIa chromogenic assay. Although both anticoagulants inhibit thrombin, they yielded calibration curves with significantly different slopes and hence are not interchangeable for the accurate estimation of plasma concentrations of either thrombin inhibitors. Similar examples can be provided for other anticoagulants and other assay

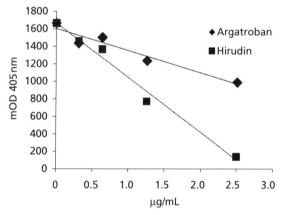

Fig. 19.1 Anti-IIa chromogenic assay: standard curves for argatroban and hirudin.

methods. Therefore, at the present time, the recommendation is that the calibrator of the assay must be the same as the drug being assayed.

Methods for monitoring indirect FXa inhibitors

Indirect FXa inhibitors such as fondaparinux and idraparinux potentiate the inactivation of free FXa by antithrombin. The routine prothrombin time (PT) and activated partial thromboplastin time (aPTT) are not sensitive to this class of inhibitors. Walenga and Hoppensteadt[11] found that within the therapeutic range aPTT was insensitive to fondaparinux. The

College of American Pathologists proficiency test results in 2006 showed that prophylactic or therapeutic concentrations of fondaparinux prolonged the PT by approximately 1 s and the aPTT by 4–5 s.[12] The anti-Xa clot-based or chromogenic assays are the most sensitive method for monitoring this class of inhibitors. Heptest is a commercially available clot-based anti-Xa assay, while there are a number of anti-Xa chromogenic kits, all of which are designed for low molecular weight heparins rather than for small synthetic indirect FXa inhibitors. The principle of Heptest is based on the ability of heparin and similar compounds to catalyse the inhibition of exogenous FXa by antithrombin in plasma. The residual FXa is determined by the addition of phospholipid and calcium to the plasma and the endpoint of the assay is the measurement of the clotting times. The resultant clotting times may also be influenced by inhibition of prothrombin activation and thrombin inhibition. Therefore, the clot-based Heptest is less specific than the chromogenic methods. The chromogenic assays have the same principle as the Heptest, but residual FXa is estimated by addition of a peptide substrate specific for FXa. Upon cleavage by FXa, the peptide substrate releases p-nitroaniline which can be monitored by optical density (OD) at 405 nm. For fondaparinux, variability in results using different anti-Xa kits calibrated with different low molecular weight heparins indicated that there is a need to use a fondaparinux preparation as the reference standard and that the concentration of fondaparinux should be estimated in µg/mL.[13–16] Concerns were also raised over the presence or absence of exogenous antithrombin in these kits. It has been suggested that at high doses the monitoring anti-Xa assay may need to be supplemented with antithrombin to obtain the total amount of pentasaccharide in circulation.[11] However, results from a number of studies have shown that there were no significant differences between the amount of fondaparinux detected using anti-Xa methods with or without exogeneous antithrombin.[13–15]

Recently, a prothrombinase-induced clotting time (PiCT) assay has been introduced[17] and found to be useful for monitoring unfractionated heparin, low molecular weight heparin, indirect and direct FXa inhibitors and direct thrombin inhibitors. This is a two-step assay, appears to have a wide dynamic range and is able to detect high concentrations of

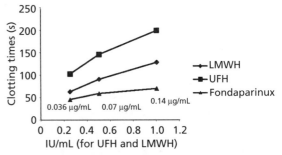

Fig. 19.2 Prothrombinase-induced clotting time (PiCT): calibration curves for unfractionated heparin (UFH), low molecular weight heparin (LMWH) and fondaparinux. Concentrations of UFH and LMWH in IU/mL were as stated on the axis, while the concentration of fondaparinux in µg/mL is next to the data points

anticoagulants. In this test, the plasma sample containing the anticoagulant is mixed with a reagent containing a combination of a defined amount of FXa, phospholipids and Russell's viper venom V (RVV-V), an enzyme from venom of the snake *Daboia russelli* that directly activates FV. After 180-s incubation, the amount of prothrombinase complex formed is related to the residual FXa. The clotting time is recorded following the addition of calcium. Figure 19.2 shows an example of standard curves produced by an unfractionated heparin, a low molecular weight heparin and fondaparinux. The results from the PiCT assay correlate well with Heptest and chromogenic FXa assays.[18,19] A one-step modification of this assay is also available and has been found to be more sensitive to certain types of anticoagulants.

Methods for monitoring direct FXa inhibitors

The logical choice of monitoring methods for direct FXa inhibitors is anti-Xa-based assays. Pharmacokinetics and pharmacodynamic studies of direct Xa inhibitors such as otamixaban and DX 9065a indicated that clot-based assays may also be employed for monitoring of this class of anticoagulants.[20–26] In these studies, increases in anti-Xa activity as assessed by anti-Xa chromogenic assay, prolongation of clotting times in the Heptest, aPTT, PT, dilute PT (dPT), Russell's viper venom clotting time (RVVT), dilute Russell's viper venom clotting time (dRVVT) were found to correlate well with plasma concentrations of the FXa inhibitors as measured by liquid chromatography/tandem mass spectrometry (LC/MS/MS). aPTT and PT reagents vary in their sensitivity to different FXa inhibitors and local validation of these methods is necessary before the use of these reagents for monitoring of therapy.[26–28] It should be noted that therapeutic aPTT ratios and PT International Normalized Ratios (INR) established for unfractionated heparin, low molecular weight heparins and warfarin should not be used as guidance for safety and efficacy of these drugs. The PiCT test has also been investigated for monitoring of DX 9065a, but was only found to be sensitive to this inhibitor when the modified one-step method (omission of the 180-s pre-incubation step) was used.[29]

Methods for monitoring dual inhibitor of FXa and thrombin

BIBT 986, a synthetic anticoagulant, inhibits both FXa and thrombin. Theoretically, both FXa and thrombin-based assays would be suitable methods for monitoring this inhibitor. Pharmacokinetic and pharmacodynamic studies[30,31] in humans have shown that there is a linear relationship between plasma concentrations of the drug and pharmacodynamic responses assessed by changes in clotting times of routine coagulation tests such as the aPTT, thrombin time (TT) and ecarin clotting time (ECT). Similar to other thrombin inhibitors, BIBT 986 is also able to prolong the PT, but the sensitivity is poor by comparison with aPTT, TT and ECT.

Methods for monitoring direct thrombin inhibitors

Direct thrombin inhibitors are now used clinically for the prophylaxis and treatment of thrombosis and related cardiovascular diseases. Although all these inhibitors bind to thrombin and inhibit its activity, their chemical structures, binding affinities and modes of action are different and, accordingly, their behavior in various monitoring tests are different. Routine anticoagulant monitoring tests such as the aPTT have been used to estimate the activity of these inhibitors.[8] Other tests such as the ECT, anti-IIa chromogenic assays and point-of-care ECT have also been used for monitoring.[32–34]

Gray and Harenberg[35] evaluated the robustness and the sensitivity of these different monitoring methods in an international collaborative study utilizing a panel of plasmas spiked with lepirudin and argatroban. This study found that the aPTT (when expressed as a ratio to normal plasma) and the ECT tests gave the lowest interlaboratory variability. The aPTT and anti-IIa chromogenic assays showed similar sensitivity to lepirudin and argatroban, but all three ECT kits (wet ECT, dry ECT, thrombin inhibitor management [TIM]) were more sensitive to argatroban than to lepirudin (Fig. 19.3). These findings were confirmed by Gosselin et al.[36] The two-step PiCT test was found to yield more reproducible results, but a

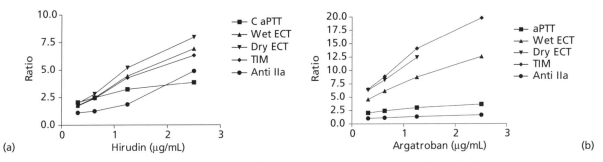

Fig. 19.3 (a) Geometric mean ratios of responses of lepirudin spiked plasmas to normal plasma. (b) Geometric mean ratios of responses of argatroban spiked plasmas to normal plasma.

linear dose–response relationship was not obtained within the therapeutic ranges of all the thrombin inhibitors.[37]

Monitoring anticoagulants using global tests

Global tests such as the aPTT and the PT only provide a snapshot of the coagulation status and do not take into account the dynamics of the hemostatic pathways. Because of the recent availability of automated and semi-automated instruments for other global methods such as the thrombin generation test and thromboelastography, there is now an increased interest in these informative but laborious tests for monitoring of procoagulant and anticoagulant therapies.

The thrombin generation test measures thrombin production over time and can be quantified by calculating the area under the thrombin generation curve. This area under the curve is commonly referred to as the endogenous thrombin potential (ETP). Other parameters such the lag time, peak thrombin and the overall shape of the curves also provide useful information on the activity of the therapeutics. Anticoagulants that give similar prolongation of aPTT and PT may have different behavior in the thrombin generation test. Figure 19.4 shows thrombin generation curves of plasma spiked with hirudin or argatroban. With increasing concentration, hirudin delayed thrombin generation without decreasing the overall amount of thrombin generated, while argatroban delayed thrombin generation as well as reducing the amount of thrombin generated (Table 19.2). The interlaboratory reproducibility of thrombin generation tests results is poor even when the same concentrations of tissue factor and phospholipid were used.[38,39] Standardization of methods is required before a useful clinical correlation can be drawn.

The point-of-care based thromboelastography (TEG) or thromboelastometry (ROTEM) measure the mechanics of clot formation and lysis.[40] Preliminary studies on anticoagulants are being made by research

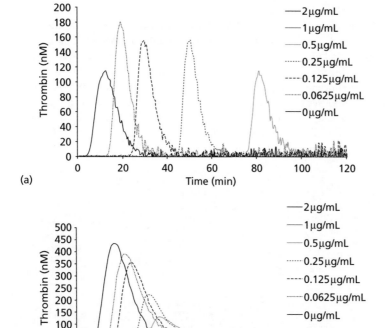

Fig. 19.4 (a) Thrombin generation curves of plasma spiked with different concentrations of hirudin. Results are obtained from the Thrombinoscope. Thrombin was not detected with plasmas spiked with 1 or 2 µg/mL of hirudin. (b) Thrombin generation curves of plasma spiked with different concentrations of argatroban. Results are obtained from the Thrombinoscope. Thrombin was not detected with plasma sample spiked with 2 µg/mL of argatroban.

Table 19.2 Inhibition of thrombin generation by hirudin and argatroban, measured by the Thrombinoscope, using 1 pM tissue factor/4 µM phospholipid in normal platelet-poor plasma.

	Thrombin inhibitors	Concentration (µg/mL)						
		0	0.0625	0.125	0.25	0.5	1	2
Lag time (min)	Hirudin	5.83	14.35	24.88	43.83	76.36	NC	NC
	Argatroban	3.89	6.22	7.67	11.44	12.89	16.22	25.11
ETP (min*nM)	Hirudin	1303	1498	1399	1312	1132	NC	NC
	Argatroban	3084	3017	2698	1933	1737	NC	NC

ETP, endogenous thrombin potential; NC, not calculated.

laboratories.[41,42] However, the interlaboratory reproducibility of these tests is difficult to assess as whole blood samples are normally used for testing. External quality assessment providers are recognizing the need for standardization of these tests and currently the UK National External Quality Assessment Scheme (NEQAS) is organizing proficiency tests for these techniques.[43]

Conclusions

The new anticoagulants can be broadly classified into FXa and thrombin inhibitors. The FXa inhibitors can be monitored by anti-Xa chromogenic or clot-based methods, while the aPTT and ECT are useful for thrombin inhibitors. The PiCT tests appear to be sensitive to a wide range of anticoagulants. As new therapeutics have different mechanisms than the traditional anticoagulants such as heparin and warfarin and there are no international standards available, product specific reference material should be used to standardize each method used for monitoring.

References

1 Johnson EA, Kirkwood TB, Stirling Y, Perez-Requejo JL, Ingram GI, Bangham DR, et al. Four heparin preparations: anti-Xa potentiating effect of heparin after subcutaneous injection. Thromb Haemost 1976; 35: 586–591.

2 Warkentin TE, Levine MN, Hirsch J, Horsewood P, Roberts RS, Gent M, et al. Heparin-induced thrombocytopenia in patients treated with low-molecular weight heparin or unfractionated heparin. N Engl J Med 1995; 332: 1330–1335.

3 Hirsh J, Raschke R. Heparin and low-molecular weight heparin. The seventh ACCP Conference on Antithrombotic and Thrombolytic Therapy. Chest 2004; 126: 188S–203S.

4 Kessler CM. Low molecular weight heparins: practical considerations. Semin Hematol 1997; 34: 35–42.

5 Abbate R, Gori AM, Farsi A, Attansio M, Pepe G. Monitoring of low-molecular-weight heparins in cardiovascular disease. Am J Cardiol 1998; 82: 33L–36L.

6 Samama MM. Contemporary laboratory monitoring of low molecular weight heparins. Clin Lab Med 1995; 15: 119–123.

7 Kessler CM, Esparraguera IM, Jacobs HM, Druy E, Fortune WP, Holloway DS, et al. Monitoring the anticoagulant effects of a low molecular weight heparin preparation. Am J Clin Pathol 1995; 103; 642–648.

8 Laposata M, Green K, Elizabeth MVC, et al. College of American Pathologists Conference XXXI on Laboratory Monitoring of Anticoagulant Therapy: the clinical use and laboratory monitoring of low-molecular-weight heparin, danaparoid, hirudin and related compounds, and argatroban. Arch Pathol Lab Med 1998; 122: 799–807.

9 Gross PL, Weitz JI. New anticoagulants for treatment of venous thromboembolism. Arterioscler Thromb Vasc Biol 2008; 28: 380–386.

10 Barrowcliffe TW. Heparin assays and standardisation. In Heparin: Chemical and Biological Properties, Clinical Applications. Lane DA, Lindahl U, (eds). Edward Arnold, 1989.

11 Walenga JM, Hoppensteadt DA. Monitoring the new antithrombotic drugs. Semin Thromb Hemost 2004; 30: 683–695.

12 Smogorzewska A. Effect of fondaparinux on coagulation assays: Results of College of American Pathologists Proficiency Testing. *Arch Pathol Lab Med* 2006; **130**: 1605–1611.

13 Depasse F, Gerotziafas GT, Busson J, van Dreden P, Samama MM. Assessment of three chromogenic and one clotting assays for the measurement of synthetic pentasaccharide fondaparinux (Arixtra®) anti-Xa activity. *J Thromb Haemost* 2004; **2**: 346–348.

14 Klaeffling C, Piechottka G, Daemgen-von Brevern G, Mosch G, Mani H, Luxembourg B, *et al*. Development and clinical evaluation of two chromogenic substrate methods for monitoring fondaparinux sodium. *Ther Drug Monit* 2006; **28**: 375–381.

15 Paolucci F, Frasa H, Van Aarle F, Capdevla A, Clavies MC, van Dinther T, *et al*. Two sensitive and rapid chromogenic assays of fondaparinux sodium (Arixtra) in human plasma and other biological matrices. *Clin Lab* 2003; **49**: 451–60.

16 Dämgen-von Brevern G, Kläffling C, Lindhoff-Last E. Monitoring anticoagulation by fondaparinux: determination of anti-factor Xa-level. *Hamostaseologie* 2005; **25**: 281–285.

17 Calatzis A, Spannagl M, Gempeler-Messina P, Kolde HJ, Schramm W, Haas S. The prothrombinase induced clotting test: A new technique for the monitoring of anticoagulants. *Haemostasis* 2000; **30** (Suppl. 2): 172–174.

18 Harenberg J, Giese C, Hagedorn A, Traeger I, Fenyvesi T. Determination of antithrombin-dependent factor Xa inhibitors by prothrombin-induced clotting time. *Semin Thromb Hemost* 2007; **33**: 503–507.

19 Graff J, Picard-Willems B, Harder S. Monitoring effects of direct FXa-inhibitors with a new one-step prothrombinase-induced clotting time (PiCT) assay: Comparative *in vitro* investigation with heparin, enoxaparin, fondaparinux and DX 9065a. *Int J Clin Pharmacol Ther* 2007; **45**: 237–243.

20 Gerbutavicius R, Iqbal O, Messmore HL, Wehrmacher WH, Hoppensteadt DA, Gerbutaviciene R, *et al*. Differential effects of DX-9065a, argatroban, and synthetic pentasaccharide on tissue thromboplastin inhibition test and dilute Russell's viper venom test. *Clin Appl Thromb Hemost* 2003; **9**: 317–323.

21 Tobu M, Iqbal O, Ma Q, Schultz C, Jeske W, Hoppensteadt D, *et al*. Global anticoagulant effects of a synthetic anti-factor Xa inhibitor (DX-9065a): Implications for interventional use. *Clin Appl Thromb Hemost* 2003; **9**: 1–17.

22 Rezaie AR. DX-9065a inhibition of factor Xa and the prothrombinase complex: Mechanism of inhibition and comparison with therapeutic heparins. *Thromb Haemost* 2003; **89**: 112–121.

23 Paccaly A, Ozoux ML, Chu V, Simcox K, Marks V, Freyburger G, *et al*. Pharmacodynamic markers in the early clinical assessment of otamixaban, a direct factor Xa inhibitor. *Thromb Haemost* 2005; **94**: 1156–1163.

24 Paccaly A, Frick A, Ozoux ML, Chu V, Rosenburg R, Hinder M, *et al*. Pharmacokinetic/pharmacodynamic relationships for otamixaban, a direct factor Xa inhibitor, in healthy subjects. *J Clin Pharmacol* 2006; **46**: 45–51.

25 Hinder M, Frick A, Jordaan P, Hesse G, Gebauer A, Maas J, *et al*. Direct and rapid inhibition of factor Xa by otamixaban: a pharmacokinetic and pharmacodynamic investigation in patients with coronary artery disease. *Clin Pharmacol Ther* 2006; **80**: 691–702.

26 Mueck W, Becka M, Kubitza D, Voith B, Zuehisdorf M. Population model of the pharmacokinetics and pharmacodynamics of rivaroxaban – an oral, direct factor Xa inhibitor – in healthy subjects. *Int J Clin Pharmacol Ther* 2007; **45**: 335–344.

27 Tobu M, Iqbal O, Hoppensteadt DA, Shultz C, Jeske W, Fareed J. Effects of a synthetic factor Xa inhibitor (JTV-803) on various laboratory tests. *Clin Appl Thromb Hemost* 2002; **8**: 325–336.

28 Laux V, Perzborn E, Kubitza D, Misselwitz F. Preclinical and clinical characteristics of rivaroxaban: a novel, oral, direct factor Xa inhibitor. *Semin Thromb Hemost* 2007; **33**: 515–523.

29 Graff J, Picard-Willems B, Harder S. Monitoring effects of direct FXa-inhibitors with a new one-step prothrombinase-induced clotting time (PiCT) assay: Comparative *in vitro* investigation with heparin, enoxaparin, fondaparinux and DX 9065a. *Int J Clin Pharmacol Ther* 2007; **45**: 237–243.

30 Leitner JM, Jilma B, Mayr FB, Cardona F, Spiel AO, Firbas C, *et al*. Pharmacokinetics and pharmacodynamics of the dual FII/FX inhibitor BIBT 986 in endotoxin-induced coagulation. *Clin Pharmacol Ther* 2007; **81**: 858–866.

31 Graefe-Mody EU, Schühly U, Rathgen K, Stähle H, Leitner JM, Jilma B. Pharmacokinetics and pharmacodynamics of BIBT 986, a novel small molecule dual inhibitor of thrombin and factor Xa. *J Thromb Haemost* 2006; **4**: 1502–1509.

32 Nowak G, Bucha E. Quantitative determination of hirudin in blood and body fluids. *Semin Thromb Hemost* 1996; **22**: 197–202.

33 Hafner G, Fickenscher K, Friesen HJ, Konheiser U, Ehrenthal W, Lotz J, *et al*. Evaluation of an automated chromogenic substrate assay for the rapid determination of hirudin in plasma. *Thromb Res* 1995; **77**: 165–173.

34 Koster A, Hansen R, Grauhan O, Hausmann H, Bauer M, Hetzer R, et al. Hirudin monitoring using the TSA ecarin clotting time in patients with heparin-induced-thrombocytopenia type II. *J Cardiothorac Vasc Anesth* 2000; **14**: 249–252.

35 Gray E, Harenberg J; ISTH Control of Anticoagulation SSC Working Group on Thrombin Inhibitors. Collaborative study on monitoring methods to determine direct thrombin inhibitors lepirudin and argatroban. *J Thromb Haemost* 2005; **3**: 2096–2097.

36 Gosselin RC, King JH, Janatpour KA, Dager WE, Larkin EC, Owings JT. Comparing direct thrombin inhibitors using aPTT, ecarin clotting times, and thrombin inhibitor management testing. *Ann Pharmacother* 2004; **38**: 1383–1388.

37 Fenyvesi T, Jörg I, Harenberg J. Monitoring of anticoagulant effects of direct thrombin inhibitors. *Semin Thromb Hemost* 2002; **28**: 361–368.

38 Lawrie AS, Gray E, Leeming D, Davidson SJ, Purdy G, Iampietro R, et al. A multicentre assessment of the endogenous thrombin potential using a continuous monitoring amidolytic technique. *Br J Haematol* 2003; **123**: 335–341.

39 Dargaud Y, Luddington R, Gray E, Negrier C, Lecompte T, Petros S, et al. Effect of standardization and normalization on imprecision of calibrated automated thrombography: An international multicentre study. *Br J Haematol* 2007; **139**: 303–309.

40 Luddington RJ. Thromboelastography/thromboelastometry. *Clin Lab Haematol* 2005; **27**: 81–90.

41 Demir M, Iqbal O, Hoppensteadt DA, Piccolo P, Ahmad S, Schultz CL, et al. Anticoagulant and antiprotease profiles of a novel natural heparinomimetic mannopentaose phosphate sulfate (PI-88). *Semin Thromb Hemost* 2000; **26** (Suppl 1): 39–46.

42 Mousa SA. Comparative efficacy of different low-molecular-weight heparins (LMWHs) and drug interactions with LMWH: implications for management of vascular disorders. *Clin Appl Thromb Hemost* 2001; **7**: 131–140.

43 Jennings I, Kitchen DP, Woods TA, Kitchen S, Walker ID. Emerging technologies and quality assurance: the United Kingdom National External Quality Assessment Scheme perspective. *Semin Thromb Hemost* 2007; **33**: 243–249.

20 Detecting and quantifying functional inhibitors in hemostasis

B. Verbruggen, I. Nováková & W. van Heerde

Functional inhibitors of hemostasis are immunoglobulins that interfere with blood coagulation. Two different classes of inhibitors can be recognized. Most frequent are lupus anticoagulants, a subgroup of antiphospholipid antibodies, which bind to a complex of phosphoplipids and phospholipid-binding proteins (β_2-glycoprotein 1, prothrombin and others) resulting in prolongation of clotting times.[1] Antiphospholipid antibodies, especially the lupus positive ones, are well-recognized risk factors for venous and arterial thrombosis. However, occasionally patients with lupus anticoagulants present with hemorrhagic diathesis when one or more coagulation factors are decreased. The latter may be caused by elevated clearance of coagulation proteins–phospholipids complexes that are bound to non-neutralizing lupus antibodies.[2] Lupus inhibitors are outside the scope of this chapter and are discussed elsewhere (Chapter 16).

The other class of inhibitors recognizes functional epitopes of one of the individual coagulation proteins thereby inhibiting the functionality of that specific protein. Two different subclasses have been described: autologous and allogenic inhibitors.

Autologous inhibitors may develop in patients with previously normal hemostasis by a deregulation of the immune system. The most frequent spontaneous autologous inhibitor is directed against factor

VIII (FVIII). The reported incidence is 1 in 1.48 million/year.[3] Autologous FVIII inhibitors, mostly affecting elderly people, are in a minority of cases associated with an autoimmune disease or with malignancy but frequently have no underlying associated disease. It is a serious complication because of bleeding problems with a mortality of about 10%.[3]

Autologous inhibitors against each of the clotting factors V, XI, XII, XIII and the vitamin K dependent proteins are described but are very rare.[4]

Allogenic inhibitors against individual coagulation factors may develop in patients with congenital factor deficiency because of treatment with the missing coagulation factor or in patients otherwise treated with clotting products. Among these inhibitors, FVIII inhibitors in hemophilia A patients who are treated with FVIII products are most frequent. The overall inhibitor incidence is 25–30% with the highest reported incidence in severely affected patients with genotypes that completely lack FVIII. The lowest incidence is reported in mild hemophiliacs.[5] The development of FVIII inhibitors usually occurs early after the beginning of therapy (less than 30 exposure days) and for this reason generally occurs during childhood.

Factor IX (FIX) inhibitors in patients with hemophilia B are much less common (1.5–3%) than FVIII inhibitors.[6] Because of the low incidence little is known about its risk factors and immunologic processes associated with development.

Factor XI (FXI) inhibitors may occur in severe FXI deficiency (FXI:C <0.01 IU/mL) which is almost exclusively described in Azkenazi and Iraqi Jews. The

Quality in Laboratory Hemostasis and Thrombosis, 1st edition. By Steve Kitchen, John D. Olson and F. Eric Preston. Published 2009 by Blackwell Publishing. ISBN: 978-1-4051-6803-8

frequency of inhibitors in patients with severe disease following plasma infusion is >30%;[7] most cases are detected at routine screening because most patients do not bleed spontaneously.

Allogenic inhibitors against other hemostasis factors have a low to very low frequency.

Clinical manifestations of hemostasis inhibitors

Autologous inhibitors in individuals with previously normal hemostasis manifest themselves clinically by an unexpected moderate to severe bleeding tendency. Especially in the case of FVIII autoantibodies the disease may be life-threatening and the appropriate medical intervention is a prerequisite for survival.

Allogenic inhibitors in patients with a pre-existing hemorrhagic disorder who are treated preventively or therapeutically for bleeding complications manifest themselves by excessive bleeding, bleeding in unusual parts of the body or a low recovery and/or half-life of infused hemostatic products. However, the latter findings are not pathognomonic of the presence of an inhibitor. Antibodies without inhibitor activity may also decrease clotting factor concentrations as a result of an increased clearance rate of the antigen–antibody complex.[8] Additionally, increased clearance of infused FVIII concentrate may be caused by low von Willebrand factor (VWF) concentrations[9] and additional unknown factors may contribute to low recoveries.[10] Therefore, the clinical suspicion of an inhibitor has to be confirmed by objective laboratory tests. Laboratory investigation of inhibitors always starts with screening tests followed, if necessary, by more specific tests to identify the exact nature of the inhibitor.

Screening tests for inhibitor detection

Inhibitors of the classic hemostasis pathway invariably are detected by use of one or more prolonged basic clotting tests such as activated partial thromboplastin time (aPTT), prothrombin time (PT) and thrombin time (TT). Prolonged clotting times may be an accidental find when screening a patient for a bleeding problem. However, these tests are the first to be performed when a patient presents with the suspicion of an inhibitor.

In order to discriminate between true factor deficiencies, which also prolong clotting tests, and inhibitors, it is necessary to perform mixing tests with normal pooled plasma, preferably in a ratio of 1:1. A prolonged clotting time that is not corrected in the mixing study is an indication for the presence of an inhibitor provided that the presence of heparin has been excluded. Most coagulation factor inhibitors have a progressive mode of action. This means that inhibitors can only be detected with a prolonged incubation time of the mixture (≥60 minutes). Ideally, mixing studies should be performed both with short (≤1 minute) and long incubation times in order to discriminate between fast-acting inhibitors and slow-acting ones. However, this does not give additional information on the nature of the inhibitor because both types are described for lupus anticoagulants and individual clotting factor inhibitors.[11]

A lupus anticoagulant is suspected in cases of failure to correct a prolonged aPTT in a 1:1 mixture within 5 seconds of normal pooled plasma.[12] However, such a general agreement neither exists for the other basic coagulation tests for detecting lupus anticoagulant, nor for other types of inhibitors such as FVIII inhibitors. Therefore, each laboratory has to build up its own experience and include appropriate control samples in the assay in order to draw conclusions on mixing tests.

The presence of an inhibitor can be confirmed by treating the plasma with sepharose-bound protein A, protein G or 2-mercaptopyridine. Proteins A and G are surface proteins of streptococci that bind the Fc-part of IgG immunoglobulins, whereas it has been suggested that the interaction of IgM and 2-mercaptopyridine results from combined electron donating and accepting action of the ligand or, alternatively, a mixed mode hydrophilic–hydrophobic interaction. In our laboratory, HiTrap™ Protein A HP, HiTrap™ Protein G HP and HiTrap™ IgM Purification HP columns from Amersham Biosciences are used to remove from plasma immunoglobulins IgG (protein A and G) or IgM and additionally purify the immune inhibitor. Purified plasma samples result in normal mixing studies when immunoglobulins are responsible for the abnormal mixing study. Eventually, the purified immunoglobulins may be used to confirm inhibitor activity.

Inhibitors against individual coagulation factors

Assay principle

All functional assays to confirm and quantify inhibitors of individual coagulation factors are based on a universal method of measuring the decrease of clotting factor activity in a mixture of an exogenous source of the clotting factor (e.g. normal pooled plasma) and the putative inhibitor plasma in a certain time period. A reference measurement needs to be performed with the same method substituting the patient plasma by a control plasma sample that does not contain an inhibitor. Residual factor activities in the assay mixtures are measured by one-stage clotting assays (mostly aPTT) or chromogenic ones.

Immunologic assays are not suitable for inhibitor detection because they do not discriminate between antibodies with and without inhibitor activity.[13–15] However, in FVIII inhibitor-positive samples good correlations were found between enzyme-linked immunosorbent assay (ELISA) methods and inhibitor methods but variable results have been reported on specificity and sensitivity of the immunologic methods compared to inhibitor activity assays.[16–18]

Available methods

Initially all inhibitor assays were focused on the measurement of FVIII inhibitors. The first assay to measure FVIII inhibitor activity was described by Biggs and Macfarlane[19] using the thromboplastin generation test followed by the Oxford method[20] using bovine FVIII concentrate (cryoprecipitate) in a mixing test with patient plasma. Later, Kasper et al.[21] described the Bethesda assay and introduced a more uniform measurement of FVIII inhibitors by using normal pooled plasma as FVIII source in a 1:1 mix with patient plasma and imidazole buffer as control sample. The sensitivity and specificity of the assay was further improved in the Nijmegen assay by buffering the normal pooled plasma and replacing the imidazole buffer by inhibitor-free deficient plasma.[22] This method focuses on FVIII but can also be used

for measuring other clotting factor inhibitors by replacing FVIII-deficient plasma by the appropriate factor-deficient plasma and assaying the residual activity of the appropriate factor. The method is recommended by the International Society on Thrombosis and Haemostasis Factor VIII/IX Scientific Subcommittee[23] for FVIII inhibitor testing. For this reason the main points of this assay are described here in detail.

Reagents

- aPTT reagent.
- Inhibitor-free plasma deficient for the factor to be measured (factor activity <0.01 IU/mL).
- Normal pooled plasma with an assigned factor level of 1 IU/mL.
- 0.1 mol/L imidazole buffered normal pooled plasma. Preparation: add one volume of buffered 4 mol/L imidazole pH 7.4 to 39 volumes of a pool of citrated plasma of 50 healthy blood donors. Adjust pH to 7.4.
- 33 mmol/L calcium chloride.

Equipment

- Plastic tubes, pipettes and normal medical laboratory equipment.
- Citrate-containing vacuum blood collection tubes.
- Incubator or water bath of 37°C.
- Coagulometer.

The assay can be carried out using semi-automated or manual techniques. However, in order to obtain more reliable results it is advisable to use fully automated devices to measure clotting times.

Method

The method is shown schematically in Fig. 20.1. To inactivate residual factor activity before testing, patient and factor deficient control plasma samples are heated at 58°C for at least 1.5 hours. In order to remove any debris caused by the heating process, the samples have to be centrifuged at 4000 g for 2 minutes (Eppendorf centrifuge). Heated test plasma as well as factor-deficient control plasma are mixed with equal volumes of imidazole buffered normal pooled plasma pH 7.4 and incubated for 2 hours at 37°C. Subsequently, the remaining factor activity in both test and

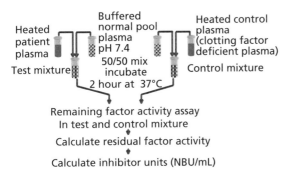

Fig. 20.1 Schematic methodology of the Nijmegen–Bethesda assay for quantification of inhibitors.

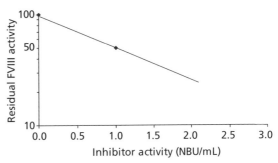

Fig. 20.2 Calibration curve for quantification of inhibitors. On the y axis the residual factor activity expressed as the relative percentage factor activity of the test mixture compared to the control mixture (logarithmic). On the x axis is the inhibitor activity in Nijmegen–Bethesda unit/mL (linear).

control mixtures is determined by an one-stage factor assay or a chromogenic factor assay.

Evaluation of test results

The "residual factor activity" is defined as the relative percentage factor activity of the test mixture compared to the control mixture. One Nijmegen Bethesda unit (NBU) is defined as the amount of inhibitor that results in 50% residual factor activity. Inhibitor activity of patient samples is read in NBU/mL from a semi-logarithmic plot representing the correlation between residual factor activity (logarithmic) and inhibitor activity (linear).[21] The regression line is fully defined by 100% residual factor activity with 0 NBU/mL inhibitor and 50% residual activity with 1 NBU/mL inhibitor (Fig. 20.2). Dose–response curves of test plasma needs to show parallellism with this calibration curve. If not, inhibitor data are not reliable and an alternative strategy needs to be followed (e.g. type 2 FVIII inhibitors).

When the residual factor activity of undiluted sample is below 25%, retesting of more diluted samples is recommended because of non-linearity of inhibitor concentration and residual activity with high inhibitor titers. Dilutions have to be made with deficient plasma.

Expected values

Until now only data on FVIII inhibitor assays have been published. In most reference laboratories 0.6 NBU/mL is used as the cut-off value. This value has been derived from results with the classic Bethesda

assay and is a reflection of the low specificity of this method. However, the sensitivity and specificity, including the cut-off value, have been improved in the Nijmegen assay.[23] In fact, every individual laboratory has to assign the laboratory-specific cut-off value by assaying positive and negative inhibitor samples from hemophilia patients. This may be difficult to perform as most laboratories do not have these samples available. An alternative is to dilute one or more inhibitor-positive samples with inhibitor-free FVIII deficient plasma to low and very low inhibitor levels, compare the data of the inhibitor assays of these dilutions with a set of inhibitor-negative plasma samples and establish the methodologic cut-off value.

Clinical validation studies comparing inhibitor titers and kinetic parameters still have to be performed in order to establish the clinical significance of (low) inhibitor titers.

Assay characteristics

A number of variables can influence the assay and may contribute to an undesirably high intra- and inter-laboratory coefficient of variation of the results.

Buffered normal pooled plasma is used as a clotting factor source in the incubation mixture with patient and reference sample. As an example, increased FVIII content of the pooled plasma will need more inhibitor to inactivate a certain percentage of FVIII and thus will lower the inhibitor titer. However, decreased FVIII content of the pooled plasma will need less inhibitor to inactivate a certain percentage of FVIII and will increase the inhibitor titer. Thus, increased factor activity in the pooled plasma will undernote the inhibitor activity when compared with a pooled plasma of lower factor activity. A plasma pool of at least 50 healthy donors is necessary to guarantee a level as close as possible to 1 IU FVIII/mL. Yet it is advisable to calibrate the FVIII content of the pool against an international standard for FVIII to ensure the potency.[24] Less than 50 donors in the pool may result in more deviation from 1 IU/mL and calibration with an external standard is then essential. A pool of at least 20 donors is needed to guarantee acceptable levels for the other clotting factors.

The residual factor activity measurements will only be minimally influenced by aberrations in the factor content of the pool for this is a relative measure that is not influenced by factor variations.

The *pH stability* of the incubation mixtures is an essential feature of the Nijmegen assay. During incubation at 37°C the pH in non-buffered mixtures increases resulting in uncontrolled and non-specific inactivation of labile coagulation factors.[22] pH stabilization of the incubation mixture by buffering the normal pooled plasma will overcome this problem and increase the specificity and sensitivity of the method.

Residual factor VIII activity in the patient plasma can interfere with the inhibitor assay by increasing the remaining factor activity after incubation with normal pooled plasma leading to falsely low inhibitor titers. This problem can be overcome by heating the test and control plasma at 58°C for 90 minutes. This will destroy all the clotting factors (Table 20.1); immunoglobulins are heat resistant leaving the inhibitor data unchanged.

An *incubation time* of 2 hours is sufficient to bind all the inhibitors to the active site of the protein. However, there is a special group of inhibitors that inactivate the protein by proteolytic cleavage of the active site. These so-called proteolytic inhibitors can also be measured with the Nijmegen assay but need an incubation time that must be extended in order to fully exhibit the inhibitory action.[25] However, there is no simple test available to discriminate between proteolytic and neutralizing antibodies. Time dependency of the inhibitor titer may be useful but is only described for purified anti-FVIII IgG.[25]

Table 20.1 Activity of clotting factors in normal pooled plasma before and after heating at 58°C for 90 minutes.

Factor	Native activity	Activity after heating
II	1 IU/mL	0.008 IU/mL
V	1 IU/mL	0.009 IU/mL
VII	1 IU/mL	0.009 IU/mL
X	1 IU/mL	0.008 IU/mL
VIII	1 IU/mL	0.007 IU/mL
IX	1 IU/mL	0.009 IU/mL
XI	1 IU/mL	0.004 IU/mL

Pitfalls and limitations of the inhibitor assay

Quality assessment of inhibitor assays is still a problem for individual laboratories because *standard and control samples* are not (yet) available. Intra-laboratory day-to-day quality assessment can be performed by assaying negative and positive inhibitor samples which are stored at −80°C. Concerning intra-laboratory reproducibility, special attention has to be given to the process of liquid handling as at a workshop of the National Institute for Biological Standards and Control (NIBSC) it was shown that the main determinant of the test variability was between-operator variations in liquid handling (e.g. pipetting, preparation of dilutions) (S. Raut, personal communication). Moreover, it was found that the variability of the inhibitor assay was mainly caused by variations in the FVIII activity assays brought about by aberrant liquid handling.

Inter-laboratory surveys of FVIII inhibitor assays have been organized since 2005 by the European Concerted Action on Thrombophilia Foundation (ECAT) and by the UK National External Quality Assessment Scheme (NEQAS). The results of the ECAT surveys show a rather high inter-laboratory coefficient of variation of about 30% for the Nijmegen assay and more than 40% for the original Bethesda method. Further standardization of the methods is needed to improve these figures.

Differentiation between *lupus anticoagulants* (LA) and inhibitors against coagulation factors is of clinical relevance because of the different therapeutic strategies for the two abnormalities (i.e. antithrombotic agents for LA and hemostatic agents for the factor inhibitors).[26] However, the presence of LA in plasma may prolong the aPTT clotting times and may therefore interfere with factor inhibitor assays and result in falsely positive inhibitor titers.[27] Alternatively, inhibitors against individual coagulation factors can interfere with lupus testing and may cause falsely positive lupus confirmation tests.[28,29] Unfortunately, tests that fully discriminate between LA and coagulation factor inhibitors are still lacking. In order to ascertain the presence or absence of LA it is strongly advised to use at least two tests of different design.[27] The diluted Russell viper venom test should be included as it is hardly influenced by inhibitors of the intrinsic factors (e.g. FVIII, FIX).[27] Alternatively, the interference of LA in the measurement of factor inhibitors, especially FVIII inhibitors, can be bypassed by measuring the residual activity in the Nijmegen assay with chromogenic substrates. Chromogenic substrate assays are not influenced by LA and are therefore more specific than aPTT-based assays.[11,30,31]

FVIII inhibitors can be characterized as either *type I or II* according to their kinetic behaviour. Type 1 inhibitors mostly occur as alloantibodies in FVIII-treated hemophiliacs and have second order inactivation kinetics resulting in complete inhibition of FVIII activity at high plasma concentrations.

Type II inhibitors, mostly autologous antibodies, are defined as being unable to inactivate FVIII:C completely, even at maximum antibody concentration, and the lack of linearity between the logarithm of residual FVIII activity and the antibody concen-

tration.[32] How to define inhibitors as type I or II can best be investigated by measuring the effect of varying concentrations of the inhibitor on the FVIII inactivation.[18]

The lack of linearity between FVIII residual activity and inhibitor concentration with type II in the inhibitor test will result in dilution-dependent inhibitor data. Therefore, in order to obtain reliable results when monitoring a patient with type II FVIII inhibitor, typical dilutions of the patient plasma have to be used that give residual activities that are as close to 50% as possible.

The *type of deficient plasma* used as control sample and as substrate plasma in the residual activity assay greatly influences the FVIII inhibitor test results. As VWF is the natural carrier protein for FVIII, the VWF concentration is essential for its stability during the incubation process. It was shown by our group[33] that inhibitor titers, derived from assays with VWF-free immune-depleted FVIII-deficient plasma as control sample and as substrate in the FVIII activity assay were 30–50% lower than titers of assays using VWF containing deficient plasma (Table 20.2).

Aberrant results were also found when using heterogeneous systems with chemically depleted plasma (CDP) as control sample and immune-depleted or congenital deficient plasma as substrate plasma. The production process can generate activated factor V in the CDP, caused shortening of the clotting times in the control mixture and thus overestimation of the inhibitor titer.[33]

Finally, during the process of immune-depletion anti-FVIII may be co-eluted from the column into the FVIII-deficient plasma resulting in falsely low inhibitor titers.[33]

Table 20.2 Factor VIII inhibitor activities of an inhibitor-positive sample (1 NBU/mL) analyzed with different combinations of deficient plasma in the control mixture and as substrate plasma in the FVIII assay.

Type of control sample	Type of substrate plasma in factor VIII assay		
	Chemically depleted plasma	Immune-depleted	Congenital deficient plasma
Chemically depleted plasma	0.94	1.66	1.66
Immune-depleted	0.97	0.58	1.10
Congenital deficient plasma	0.99	0.87	1.16

In conclusion, it is strongly recommended that VWF containing FVIII deficient plasma is used, either congenital or immune-depleted, in a homogenous system and to check each commercial immune-depleted FVIII deficient plasma for FVIII antibodies before use.

In order to decrease the costs of the assay, albumin can also be used as a control sample in combination with von Willebrand containing substrate plasma.[34]

Inhibitors against other clotting factors

Probably the most frequently occurring coagulation inhibitor besides FVIII and FIX inhibitors are *inhibitors against factor V*. Until 2002, 126 cases have been reported in literature of which 87 have been reported in the decade before 2002.[35] An annual incidence of 0.29 cases per million was reported in an Australian region,[36] confirming the relatively high incidence.

In two-thirds of the patients described by Streiff,[35] the FV inhibitors were caused by exposure to bovine thrombin. This thrombin, which is widely used for hemostatic control in surgery patients, is contaminated with factor V and this may induce antibodies to bovine factor V that cross-react with human factor V.[37] Patients will present with both an abnormal PT and aPTT and low or very low factor V activity. Mixing studies have to be used to confirm the presence of the inhibitor which can be quantified using the Nijmegen assay.

Thrombin inhibitors are reported much less frequently than factor V inhibitors although most of them also arise, like FV antibodies, from treatment with bovine thrombin products.[38] Thrombin inhibitors are extremely rare in patients without an underlying disease and are mostly related to autoimmune diseases.

Thrombin inhibitors cause a broad window of abnormal clotting assays both in native plasma and in mixing studies including abnormal PT, aPTT, TT, fibrinogen assays and clotting factor assays because thrombin is the final protease activity in all assays.[39] These inhibitors may be difficult to distinguish from lupus anticoagulants which exhibit similar abnormal results except for the TT which is normal in lupus plasma. Furthermore, one has to be aware of the fact that acquired abnormal fibrinogen molecules with increased sialylation of carbohydrate side chains may also present with abnormal TT mixing studies.[40]

These abnormal molecules, usually synthesized in diseases of the liver or the biliary tract, inhibit fibrin clot formation of normal fibrinogen. The TT of these plasma samples mixed with normal plasma normalizes after defibrination at 56°C. Confirmation of the presence of an inhibitor can be performed by treating the plasma with protein A and/or protein G which will result in normal TT in immune-mediated TT prolongation.

There are rare publications on *inhibitors of fibrinogen function*. The mechanisms of these inhibitors include direct inhibition of fibrin monomer aggregation due to paraproteins,[41,42] delay of fibrinopeptide B release[43] and of fibrinopeptide A release.[44] Most commonly, these patients have a prolonged TT both in the native patient plasma and in a 1:1 mixture with normal plasma. The presence of acquired abnormal fibrinogen protein, as described in the previous paragraph, can be excluded by normalization of TT of a mix of defibrinated patient plasma with normal plasma. Confirmation of the presence of an inhibitor can be performed by treating the plasma with protein A and/or protein G which will result in normal TT in immune-mediated TT prolongation and, when possible, characterization of the immunoglobulin.[43]

Acquired deficiencies and *inhibitors of factor XIII* have been described in association with drugs, chronic renal failure, hepatic cirrhosis and lymphoproliferative disorders.[45] Rarely, serious hemorrhagic complications can be caused by factor XIII inhibitors. Inhibitors to factor XIII cannot be detected with baseline coagulation screening tests such as aPTT, PT or TT, as these tests are not factor XIII sensitive. Factor XIII inhibitors are classified into three types:

1 Inhibitors that interfere with factor XIII activity by preventing activation of factor XIII.
2 Inhibitors that interfere with the function of factor XIIIa.
3 Inhibitors altering the reactivity of the fibrin substrate.[46]

All types of inhibitors strongly interfere with activity assays and can be diagnosed by mixing studies with normal plasma using quantitative photometric assays.

Patients with *ADAMTS 13 deficiency* present with life-threatening microvascular thrombotic complications and the syndrome is known as thrombotic thrombocytopenic purpura (TTP). In most cases the deficiency is caused by a functional inhibitor to

ADAMTS 13.[47] The inhibitor cannot be detected with usual baseline tests and so for detection of these inhibitors mixing tests have to be performed. Of the four tests that are currently available (multimeric analysis, collagen binding assay, FRETS-vWF 73 and GST-vWF 73 assay), the FRETS-vWF 73 assay appears to be superior in detecting and quantifying auto-inhibitors to the cleaving protease.[48] The test is based on cleavage of a 73-aminoacid protein fragment derived from VWF containing the substrate for ADAMTS 13. This results in increased fluorescence over time with normal plasma while ADAMTS 13 deficient plasma and/or inhibitor plasma has no effect.[48]

Acquired von Willebrand factor deficiency (AVWD) is a heterogeneous syndrome with clinical features similar to congenital von Willebrand disease but no prior history of personal or familiar bleeding tendency.[49] It is mainly associated with lymphoproliferative and myeloproliferative disorders, solid tumors and immunologic and cardiovascular disorders. Three main mechanisms can be differentiated:

1 The presence of circulating antibodies.
2 Selective adsorption of VWF to abnormal cells.
3 Increased VWF proteolysis.

The syndrome is characterized by decreased VWF activity and antigen, decreased collagen binding capacity, low FVIII activity, mostly type 2-like multimeric patterns because of loss of high multimers and increased aPTT. Unlike the congenital form, the plasma VWF–propeptide concentration is normal but the VWF clearance from circulation after DDAVP treatment is increased. FVIII inhibitors cannot be detected in these patients and only in 30% of patients can inhibitors to VWF be shown in a mixing assay.[50,51] Quantification of inhibitors can be performed by a modified Nijmegen inhibitor assay using the ristocetin cofactor activity assay to measure the residual VWF activity in a mixture with normal plasma. An ELISA assay may be more sensitive but may also detect non-inhibiting antibodies.[52] Confirmation of the presence of an inhibitor can be obtained by investigation of inhibitory effect of patient IgG on the binding of ^{125}I–VWF to platelets.[50]

Conclusions

Functional inhibitors to proteins involved in the coagulation process must always be considered when a patient presents with unexpected bleeding, thrombotic complications or with abnormal clotting assays. Although mixing studies with patient and normal plasma are the first choice of laboratory investigation, they will not always result in the detection of the inhibitor or render an explanation for the coagulation abnormality. Specific tests have to be performed to identify the nature of the putative inhibitor. Sometimes non-inhibiting antibodies, analyzed with immunologic assays, are the cause of the underlying abnormality. The ultimate confirmation of the presence of an inhibitor usually needs advanced methods (e.g. IgG purification, radiolabeling of proteins) which unfortunately are usually not available in standard diagnostic laboratories.

References

1 Arnout J. Antiphospholipid antibody syndrome: diagnostic aspects of lupus anticoagulants. *Thromb Haemost* 2001; **86**: 75–82.

2 Urbanus RT, Derksen RH, de Groot PG. Current insight into diagnostics and pathophysiology of the antiphospholipid syndrome. *Blood Rev* 2008; **22**: 93–105.

3 Collins PW, Hirsch S, Baglin TP, Dolan G, Hanley J, Makris M, *et al.*, UK Haemophilia Centre Doctors' Organisation. Acquired hemophilia A in the United Kingdom: a 2-year national surveillance study by the United Kingdom Haemophilia Centre Doctors' Organisation. *Blood* 2007; **109**: 1870–1877.

4 Scott-Timperley LJ, Haire WD. Autoimmune coagulation disorders. *Rheum Dis Clin North Am* 1997; **23**: 411–423.

5 Oldenburg J, El-Maarri O, Schwaab R. Inhibitor development in correlation to factor VIII genotypes. *Haemophilia* 2002; **8** (Suppl 2): 23–29.

6 DiMichele D. Inhibitor development in haemophilia B: an orphan disease in need of attention. *Br J Haematol* 2007; **138**: 305–315.

7 Salomon O, Zivelin A, Livnat T, Dardik R, Loewenthal R, Avishai O, *et al.* Prevalence, causes, and characterization of factor XI inhibitors in patients with inherited factor XI deficiency. *Blood* 2003; **101**: 4783–4788.

8 Dazzi F, Tison T, Vianello F, Radossi P, Zerbinati P, Carraro P, *et al.* High incidence of anti-FVIII antibodies against non-coagulant epitopes in haemophilia A patients: a possible role for the half-life of transfused FVIII. *Br J Haematol* 1996; **93**: 688–693.

9 Vlot AJ, Mauser-Bunschoten EP, Zarkova AG, Haan E, Kruitwagen CL, Sixma JJ, *et al.* The half-life of infused

factor VIII is shorter in hemophiliac patients with blood group O than in those with blood group A. *Thromb Haemost* 2000; 83: 65–69.

10 Mondorf W, Klinge J, Luban NL, Bray G, Saenko E, Scandella D, Recombinate PUP Study Group. Low factor VIII recovery in haemophilia A patients without inhibitor titre is not due to the presence of anti-factor VIII antibodies undetectable by the Bethesda assay. *Haemophilia* 2001; 7: 13–19.

11 Blanco AN, Alcira Peirano A, Grosso SH, Gennari LC, Pérez Bianco R, Lazzari MA. A chromogenic substrate method for detecting and titrating anti-factor VIII antibodies in the presence of lupus anticoagulant. *Haematologica* 2002; 87: 271–278.

12 Brandt JT, Barna LK, Triplett DA. Laboratory identification of lupus anticoagulants: results of the Second International Workshop for Identification of Lupus Anticoagulants. On behalf of the Subcommittee on Lupus Anticoagulants/Antiphospholipid Antibodies of the ISTH. *Thromb Haemost* 1995; 74: 1597–1603.

13 Klinge J, Auerswald G, Budde U, Klose H, Kreuz W, Lenk H, Scandella D, Paediatric Inhibitor Study Group of the German Society on Thrombosis and Haemostasis. Detection of all anti-factor VIII antibodies in haemophilia A patients by the Bethesda assay and a more sensitive immunoprecipitation assay. *Haemophilia* 2001; 7: 26–32.

14 Martin PG, Sukhu K, Chambers E, Giangrande PL. Evaluation of a novel ELISA screening test for detection of factor VIII inhibitory antibodies in haemophiliacs. *Clin Lab Haematol* 1999; 21: 125–128.

15 Blanco AN, Peirano AA, Grosso SH, Gennari LC, Bianco RP, Lazzari MA. An ELISA system to detect anti-factor VIII antibodies without interference by lupus anticoagulants: preliminary data in hemophilia A patients. *Haematologica* 2000; 85: 1045–1050.

16 Sahud MA, Pratt KP, Zhukov O, Qu K, Thompson AR. ELISA system for detection of immune responses to FVIII: a study of 246 samples and correlation with the Bethesda assay. *Haemophilia* 2007; 13: 317–322.

17 Shetty S, Ghosh K, Mohanty D. An ELISA assay for the detection of factor VIII antibodies: comparison with the conventional Bethesda assay in a large cohort of haemophilia samples. *Acta Haematol* 2003; 109: 18–22.

18 Ling M, Duncan EM, Rodgers SE, Somogyi AA, Crabb GA, Street AM, *et al.* Classification of the kinetics of factor VIII inhibitors in haemophilia A: plasma dilution studies are more discriminatory than time-course studies. *Br J Haematol* 2001; 114: 861–867.

19 Biggs R, Macfarlane RG. *Human Blood Coagulation and its Disorders*, 2nd edn. Oxford: Blackwell Scientific Publications, 1962.

20 Biggs R, Bidwell E. A method for the study of antihaemophilic globulin inhibitors with reference to six cases. *Br J Haematol* 1959; 5: 379–395.

21 Kasper C, Aledort L, Counts R, Edson J, Fratantone J, Green D, *et al.* A more uniform measurement of factor VIII-inhibitors. *Thromb Diath Haemorrh* 1975; 34: 869–872.

22 Verbruggen B, Novakova I, Wessels H, *et al.* The Nijmegen modification of the Bethesda assay for factor VIII:C inhibitors: improved specificity and reliability. *Thromb Haemost* 1995; 73: 247–251.

23 Giles AR, Verbruggen B, Rivard GE, Teitel J, Walker I, and the Association of Hemophilia Center Directors of Canada. A detailed comparison of the performance of the standard versus the Nijmegen modification of the Bethesda assay in detecting factor VIII:C inhibitors in the haemophilia A population of Canada. *Thromb Haemost* 1998; 79: 872–875.

24 Mannucci PM, Tripodi A. Factor VIII clotting activity. *Laboratory Techniques in Thrombosis. A Manual.* 2nd edition of ECAT Assay Procedures. 1999; 107–113.

25 Lacroix-Desmazes S, Wootla B, Dasgupta S, Delignat S, Bayry J, Reinbolt J, *et al.* Catalytic IgG from patients with hemophilia A inactivate therapeutic factor VIII. *J Immunol* 2006; 177: 1355–1363.

26 Triplett DA. Simultaneous occurrence of lupus anticoagulant and factor VIII inhibitors. *Am J Hematol* 1997; 56: 195–196.

27 Tripodi A, Mancuso ME, Chantarangkul V, Clerici M, Bader R, Meroni PL, *et al.* Lupus anticoagulants and their relationship with the inhibitors against coagulation factor VIII: considerations on the differentiation between the two circulating anticoagulants. *Clin Chem* 2005; 51: 1883–1885.

28 Favaloro EJ, Bonar R, Duncan E, Earl G, Low J, Aboud M, *et al.*, RCPA QAP in Haematology Haemostasis Committee. Identification of factor inhibitors by diagnostic haemostasis laboratories: a large multi-centre evaluation. *Thromb Haemost* 2006; 96: 73–78.

29 Favaloro EJ, Bonar R, Duncan E, Earl G, Low J, Aboud M, *et al.* Misidentification of factor inhibitors by diagnostic haemostasis laboratories: recognition of pitfalls and elucidation of strategies: a follow-up to a large multicentre evaluation. *Pathology* 2007; 39: 504–511.

30 Chandler WL, Ferrell C, Lee J, Tun T, Kha H. Comparison of three methods for measuring factor VIII levels in plasma. *Am J Clin Pathol* 2003; 120: 34–39.

31 Blanco AN, Cardozo MA, Candela M, Santarelli MT, Pérez Bianco R, Lazzari MA. Anti-factor VIII inhibitors and lupus anticoagulants in haemophilia A patients. *Thromb Haemost* 1997; 77: 656–659.

32 Gawryl MS, Hoyer LW. Inactivation of factor VIII coagulant activity by two different types of human antibodies. *Blood* 1982; **60**: 1103–1109.

33 Verbruggen B, Giles A, Samis J, Verbeek K, Mensink E, Novákovà I. The type of factor VIII deficient plasma used influences the performance of the Nijmegen modification of the Bethesda assay for factor VIII inhibitors. *Thromb Haemost* 2001; **86**: 1435–1439.

34 Verbruggen B, van Heerde W, Novákovà I, Lillicrap D, Giles A. A 4% solution of bovine serum albumin may be used in place of factor VIII:C deficient plasma in the control sample in the Nijmegen modification of the Bethesda factor VIII:C inhibitor assay. *Thromb Haemost* 2002; **88**: 362–364.

35 Streiff MB, Ness PM. Acquired FV inhibitors: a needless iatrogenic complication of bovine thrombin exposure. *Transfusion* 2002; **42**: 18–26.

36 Favaloro EJ, Posen J, Ramakrishna R, Soltani S, McRae S, Just S, *et al*. Factor V inhibitors: rare or not so uncommon? A multi-laboratory investigation. *Blood Coagul Fibrinolysis* 2004; **15**: 637–647.

37 Ortel TL, Mercer MC, Thames EH, Moore KD, Lawson JH. Immunologic impact and clinical outcomes after surgical exposure to bovine thrombin. *Ann Surg* 2001; **233**: 88–96.

38 Savage WJ, Kickler TS, Takemoto CMA. Acquired coagulation factor inhibitors in children after topical bovine thrombin exposure. *Pediatr Blood Cancer* 2007; **49**: 1025–1029.

39 La Spada AR, Skålhegg BS, Henderson R, Schmer G, Pierce R, Chandler W. Brief report: fatal hemorrhage in a patient with an acquired inhibitor of human thrombin. *New Engl J Med* 1995; **333**: 494–497.

40 Cunningham MT, Brandt JT, Laposata M, Olson JD. Laboratory diagnosis of dysfibrinogenemia. *Arch Pathol Lab Med* 2002; **126**: 499–505. Review.

41 Dear A, Brennan SO, Sheat MJ, Faed JM, George PM. Acquired dysfibrinogenemia caused by monoclonal production of immunoglobulin lambda light chain. *Haematologica* 2007; **92**: e111–117.

42 Saif MW, Allegra CJ, Greenberg B. Bleeding diathesis in multiple myeloma. *J Hematother Stem Cell Res* 2001; **10**: 657–660.

43 Llobet D, Borrell M, Vila L, Vallvé C, Felices R, Fontcuberta J. An acquired inhibitor that produced a delay of fibrinopeptide B release in an asymptomatic patient. *Haematologica* 2007; **92** (Suppl): ECR09.

44 Gris JC, Schved JF, Branger B, Aguilar-Martinez P, Vécina F, Oulès R, *et al*. Autoantibody to plasma fibrinopeptide A in a patient with a severe acquired haemorrhagic syndrome. *Blood Coagul Fibrinolysis* 1992; **3**: 519–529.

45 Nijenhuis AV, van Bergeijk L, Huijgens PC, Zweegman S. Acquired factor XIII deficiency due to an inhibitor: a case report and review of the literature. *Haematologica* 2004; **89**: ECR14.

46 Gregory TF, Cooper B. Case report of an acquired factor XIII inhibitor: diagnosis and management. *Proc Bayl Univ Med Cent* 2006; **19**: 221–223.

47 Furlan M, Robles R, Galbusera M, Remuzzi G, Kyrle PA, Brenner B, *et al*. von Willebrand factor-cleaving protease in thrombotic thrombocytopenic purpura and the hemolytic-uremic syndrome. *New Engl J Med* 1998; **339**: 1578–1584.

48 Shelat SG, Smith P, Ai J, Zheng XL. Inhibitory autoantibodies against ADAMTS-13 in patients with thrombotic thrombocytopenic purpura bind ADAMTS-13 protease and may accelerate its clearance *in vivo*. *J Thromb Haemost* 2006; **4**: 1707–1717.

49 Franchini M, Lippi G. Acquired von Willebrand syndrome: an update. *Am J Hematol* 2007; **82**: 368–375.

50 Mohri H, Motomura S, Kanamori H, Matsuzaki M, Watanabe S, Maruta A, *et al*. Clinical significance of inhibitors in acquired von Willebrand syndrome. *Blood* 1998; **91**: 3623–3629. Erratum in: *Blood* 1999; **93**: 413.

51 Nitu-Whalley IC, Lee CA. Acquired von Willebrand syndrome: report of 10 cases and review of the literature. *Haemophilia* 1999; **5**: 318–326. Review.

52 Siaka C, Rugeri L, Caron C, Goudemand J. A new ELISA assay for diagnosis of acquired von Willebrand syndrome. *Haemophilia* 2003; **9**: 303–308.

Index

Page numbers in *italics* represent figures, those in **bold** represent tables.

abciximab 111
accreditation 9, 49, 55
accuracy 10–11
activated clotting time, point-of-care
    testing 76–7
activated partial thromboplastin
    time 9, 23, 32
    anticoagulant monitoring 194–5,
        194, **195**
    factors affecting assay **68**
    heritable thrombophilias 147
    lupus anticoagulants 162–3
    method selection 67–9, *68*, **68**
    minimum evaluation 69
    point-of-care testing 76
    single/multiple factor deficiency
        68
    systemic lupus erythematosus 161
    von Willebrand disease 126
activated protein C resistance 147,
    153–4
    testing for 153–4
activated protein C sensitivity
    ratio 153
ADAMTS13 138
    deficiency 204–5
afibrinogenemia 95
aggregometry 115–16, *115*
Alphanate 26, **27**
ancrod, International Standards **20**
annexin V 161
anti-β₂-glycoprotein I antibodies 160
    assays 167
        performance 167
anticardiolipin antibodies 160
    assays 165–6
        performance 166–7

anticoagulants 33–7, **33**
    blood to anticoagulant ratio (fill
        volume) 33–5
    calibration for measurement
        accuracy **191**, *191*
    clotting factor assays 81
    direct thrombin inhibitors **191**,
        193–4
    factor Xa inhibitors **191**
        direct 192–3
        indirect 191–2, *192*
    factor Xa/thrombin inhibitors 193
    global monitoring tests 194–5, *194*,
        195
    hematocrit 35
    heparin *see* heparin
    new 190–7
    oral *see* oral anticoagulant therapy
    see also individual drugs
antiphospholipid antibodies 147,
    160–1
antiphospholipid syndrome 160
    clinical/laboratory criteria **161**
antithrombin 11
    assay 149–50, *150*
    EQA **53**
    heparin cofactor activity 148–9
    heritable deficiency 148–50,
        150
    International Standards **20**, 28
antithrombin Cambridge II 149–50,
    150
antithrombin Wobble 149
anti-von Willebrand factor
    antibody 84
APCR *see* activated protein C
    resistance

apixaban **191**
aPTT *see* activated Partial
    Thromboplastin Time
ardeparin **172**
argatroban **191**, 195
    standard curve *191*
Arrhenius equation 22
aspirin 111
    resistance 114
atherosclerosis 110

barcoding 64
batch analyzers 63
Bernard-Soulier syndrome 110
best-fit 17
between-run error 46
BIBT 986 **191**
    monitoring 193
bivalirudin **191**
Bland-Altman plot 17
bleeding time 112
blood to anticoagulant ratio (fill
    volume) 33–5
blood samples 32–7
    refrigeration 37–8

C4b-binding protein 152
CARDIAC D-dimer assay 78
carrier diagnosis 94
centrifugation 38–9
Chédiak–Higashi syndrome 111
chorionic villus biopsy 94
chromogenic assays
    Coamatic FVIII 85
    factor IIa inhibition *191*
    factor VIII 87
    factor Xa inhibition 174, *192*

citrate, theophylline, adenosine and dipyridamole 34–5
Clinical Laboratory Standards Institute (CLSI) 6, 16
  evaluation of clinical laboratory tests 65
  frequency of testing 45
Clinical Pathology Accreditation 49
clinical sensitivity 17–18
clopidogrel 111
clot formation, in vitro studies 120
clot retraction 119
clotting factor assay 81–9
  dose-response curves 82
  factor IX 81–4, 82, 83
    lupus anticoagulant 83–4
    post-clotting factor infusion 87–8
    sensitivity 67
  factor VIII 81–4, 82, 83
    chromogenic 87
    elevated levels 85–6
    lupus anticoagulant 83–4
    post-clotting factor infusion 87–8
    sensitivity 67
    two-stage 86–7, 87
  one-stage components 84–5
  pretest variables 81
  severe deficiency 85
  see also individual clotting factors
clotting time 33
CoaguCheck 57
CoaguCheck S 73, 74
CoaguChek XS 73, 74
CoaguChek XS Plus 73, 74
Coamatic chromogenic FVIII assay 85
coefficient of variation 11, 17, 46
collaborative studies 21–2
collagen, platelet adhesion to 120
collection containers 32
College of American Pathology 55
comparative statistics 17
complement control proteins 161
confidence intervals 17
conformation sensitive gel electrophoresis 93
consumers 2
coumarins, interference with lupus anticoagulant assay 165
cryoprecipitation 44

dabigatran etexilate 191
Dale, Sir Henry 19
dalteparin 172
DAPTTIN reagent 84

D-dimer
  heterogeneity of 99–100
  specificity of monoclonal antibodies 100
D-dimer testing 99–109
  calibrators for 100–2, 101
  harmonization 102–6, 103–6, 105
  point-of-care 72, 77–8
  practical problems 106–7
  standardization 102
deemed status 56
deep venous thrombosis 100
Deming principles of quality management 2
denaturing gradient gel electrophoresis 93
descriptive statistics 17
developing countries, EQA 58–60
  challenges of 58–9
  India 59–60
    extension to other developing countries 60
    impact of program 60
    profile of participants 59–60
    samples 59
    target value 59
dilute Russell's viper venom time 163–4, 193
discard tubes 36–7
disseminated intravascular coagulation 99
DNA sequencing 93
DU-176b 191
DX-9065a 191
  monitoring 192–3
dysfibrinogenemia 95, 154

Ecarin time 163, 165, 193
EDTA 33–4
educational role of EQA 56
electron microscopy 112–14, 113
ELISA 17, 200
  D-dimer assay 102
  heparin assay 172
  protein S 152
  von Willebrand antigen 127–8
endogenous thrombin potential 194
enoxaparin 172
eptifibatide 111
EQA see external quality assessment
error correction 5–6
error detection 5–6
error logs 49
error sources 40

European Concerted Action on Thrombosis Foundation 105
European Department for the Quality of Medicines 22
evaluation of laboratory performance 53–5, 53
expert laboratories 52
external quality assessment 4–5, 13, 51–62
  advantages of 56–7, 57
  developing countries 58–60
  educational role 56
  evaluation of laboratory performance 53–5, 53
  limitations 57
  molecular genetics 97
  monitoring results 55–6
  recent developments 57–8
  samples for 51
  target values 52–3, 52
  von Willebrand disease testing 143–4
external quality assurance 3–4
External Quality Assurance in Thrombosis and Hemostasis (EQATH) 54

F8 gene 92
F9 gene 92
factor II
  assay sensitivity 67
  deficiency 94
  International Standards 20
factor IIa inhibition assay 175, 191
factor V
  deficiency 95
  EQA 56
  inhibitors 204
factor V Leiden 147, 153–4
  detection of mutation 154
  EQA 54
  International Standards 20
factor VII
  cold activation 44
  deficiency 95
  International Standards 20
  spurious results 31
factor VIIa, International Standards 20
factor VIII 11, 32
  activation 91
  assay 81–4, 82, 83
    chromogenic 87
    elevated levels 85–6

lupus anticoagulant 83–4
post-clotting factor infusion 87–8
sensitivity 67
two-stage 86–7, **87**
deficiency *see* hemophilia A
EQA *56*
inhibitors 198, **203**
International Standards 19, **20**,
  24–7
  British Plasma Standards 24
International Unit vs. normal
  plasma 25
plasma and concentrate units 25–7,
  27
spurious results 31
types of concentrate 24–5
von Willebrand disease 127
factor IX
activation *91*
assay 81–4, *82*, *83*
  lupus anticoagulant 83–4
  post-clotting factor infusion 87–8
  sensitivity 67
deficiency *see* hemophilia B
inhibitors 198
International Standards **20**, 27
factor IXa, International Standards
20
factor X
assay sensitivity 67
deficiency **95**
International Standards **20**
factor Xa
inhibition assay 174, *175*, 192
inhibitors **191**
  direct 192–3
  indirect 191–2, *192*
factor Xa/thrombin inhibitors 193
factor XI
deficiency 94, 95–6
inhibitors 198–9
factor XII, assay sensitivity 68
factor XIII
deficiency 94, **95**
inhibitors 204
fibrin 100
high molecular weight 100
low molecular weight 100
fibrinogen 32
assay 4, *4*, 7, 11
  abnormal test samples 45
  method selection 69–70
  minimum evaluation 70
deficiency **95**

heritable thrombophilias 154
International Standards **20**, 28
fibrinogen equivalent units 100
fibrinogen inhibitors 204
fibrinolysis, International Standards
  20, 29
fill volume 35
filtration of plasma 38
flow cytometry 117–19, *118*
fluorescein isothiocyanate 117
fondaparinux 190, **191**
monitoring 191–2
Food and Drug Administration,
  Centre for Biologics Evaluation
  and Research 22
freezers 44
frequency of testing 45–6
frozen IQC materials 44
frozen samples, thawing of 39–40
Fruit Fly 96
functional inhibitors of hemostasis *see*
  hemostasis inhibitors

G20210A mutation 154
International Standards **20**
Gaussian distribution 14, 46
gene mutations *see* molecular genetics
gene sequencing 121
genetic counseling 93–4
genomics 120–1
GGCX 96
Glanzmann thrombasthenia 110, *118*
β₂-glycoprotein I 162
antibodies 160, 167
good laboratory practice 9
gray platelet syndrome 111, 113

Haemophilia B Mutation database 92
HAMSTeRS database 92
hematocrit 35
Hemochron Jr II 74
Hemochron Jr Signature+ **73**, 77
Hemochron Response 77
Hemochron Signature 57
Hemofil M 26
hemoglobin 7
hemolysis 38–9, 70
hemophilia A 58
clotting factor assay 81
gene mutations 92–4, **92**
genetic counseling, prenatal and
  preimplantation diagnosis 93–4
genotypic-phenotypic
  relationship 93

molecular genetics 90–2, *91*
severe 8
hemophilia B
gene mutations 92–4, **92**
genetic counseling, prenatal and
  preimplantation diagnosis 93–4
genotypic-phenotypic
  relationship 93
molecular genetics 90–2, *91*
severe 8
hemophilia C *see* factor XI, deficiency
Hemophilia Federation (India) 59
hemostasis inhibitors 198–207
assays
  methods 200–2, *201*, **202**
  pitfalls/limitations 202–5, **203**
clinical manifestations 199
screening tests 199–200
see also individual inhibitors
heparin 33, 170–8
EQA 52–3
interference with INR
  determination 186
International Standards **20**, 23
limitations of 170–1
low molecular weight 21, 171, *171*,
  172
  characteristics of **172**
  International Standards **20**
  monitoring 177
  point-of-care testing 77–8
  preparation 171
measurement 172–5
  chromogenic Xa inhibition
    assay 174
  hybrid assays 175
  IIa inhibition assays 175
  one-stage assays 174–5
  protamine sulfate assay 174
  recommended protocol 173–4
  Xa inhibition clotting assays
    175
mechanism of action 170, *171*
pharmacokinetics 170–1
point-of-care testing 72
quality control and assurance
  175–7
  blood processing 176
  calibration curves 176
  control plasmas 176
  specimen collection 175
side-effects
  osteoporosis 171
  thrombocytopenia 171–2

heparin cofactor II 149
heparin neutralizing agents 65
Heptest 192
Hermansky–Pudlak syndrome 111
hirudin **195**
  standard curve *191*
"home-brew" assays 9, 10
homocysteine assay 154
Human Genome Variation Society 96
hyperhomocysteinemia 147
hypofibrinogenemia 95

icteric samples 38–9, 70
ideal sample **40**
idiopathic thrombocytopenic
  purpura 111
idraparinux 190, **191**
  monitoring 191–2
immunoreceptor-tyrosine-based
  activation motif (ITAM) 119
Impact Cone 115
imprecision 46
India, EQA 59–60
  extension to other developing
    countries 60
  impact of program 60
  profile of participants 59–60
  samples 59
  target value 59
initial evaluation of hemostasis 63–71
  instrument selection 63–4, **64**
  method evaluation 65
  method selection
    activated partial thromboplastin
      time 67–9, *68*, **68**
    fibrinogen 69–70
    prothrombin time 65–7, *66*, **67**
    thrombin time 8
Innovin 165
INR *see* International Normalized
  Ratio
Institute for Reference Materials and
  Measurements (IRMM) 181
instrument selection 63–4, **64**
internal quality control 2–4, *3*, **4**, 13,
  43–50
  acceptable limits 46
  accreditation 49
  frequency of testing 45–6
  materials 43–5
  molecular genetics 96–7
  out of limits results 47–9, **48**
  regulatory bodies 49
  storage/processing of results 46–7

troubleshooting **48**
von Willebrand disease testing 143
International Normalized Ratio 4, **4**,
  17, 23, 24, 52, 102, 165
  conversion of PT to INR 65–6, *66*,
    183
  factors affecting 183–5
    ISI 185
    mean normal prothrombin
      time 184
    patient's prothrombin time 183–4
  implementation of 186–7
  limits of 185–6
International Reference
  Preparations 19, 23
  thromboplastin 180, *180*
  hierarchy 181–3, *181*, *182*
International Sensitivity Index 23–4,
  60, 65, 74, 165, 173
  determination of 180
  local calibration 181–3, *182*
International Society on Thrombosis
  and Haemostasis (ISTH) 21, 99
International Standards 19–30
  choice of materials 21
  collaborative study 21–2
  establishment of 20–3
  "like vs. like" 21
  physical attributes 21
  stability studies 22
  usage 22–3
  see also ISO; and individual
    standards
International Standards Organization
  (ISO) 6
International Units 20
IQC *see* internal quality control
ISI *see* International Sensitivity Index
ISO 15189 6, 49
ISO 17025 6
ISO 22870 78, 79

Jewish populations, mutations in 96

kaolin clotting time
  lupus anticoagulants 162–3
  systemic lupus erythematosus 161
kininogen, high molecular weight,
  assay sensitivity 68
Kogenate 26, *27*

laboratory cycle *3*
LAT 119
lepirudin **191**

Levey–Jennings chart 46–7, *47*
"like vs. like" 21
limit of detection 11–12
limits of quantitation 12
linearity 12
linear regression 17
linkage analysis 94
lipemic samples 38–9, 70
livedo reticularis 160
LMAN1 96
local method quality 4
low molecular weight heparin 21,
  171, *171*, *172*
  characteristics of **172**
  International Standards **20**
  monitoring 177
  point-of-care testing 77–8
  preparation 171
lupus anticoagulants 161–2, 199, 203
  assays 68–9, 162–4
    activated partial thromboplastin
      time 162–3
    in coumarin-treated subjects 165
    dilute Russell's viper venom
      time 163–4
    kaolin clotting time 163
    performance of 164–5
  in clotting factor assay 83–4
  EQA 54
  interference with INR
    determination 186
LY517717 **191**
lyophilization 44

material for IQC 43–5
  frozen 44
  lyophilization 44
  stability of 44
matrix effect 51
May–Grünewald–Giemsa stain 112
MCFD2 96
mean 17, 46
Medtronic ACT Plus analyzer 77
megakaryocytes 110
methylene tetrahydrofolate reductase
  mutation 147
Minquant 78
molecular genetics 90–8
  external quality assessment 97
  factor XI 94
  hemophilia 90–2, *91*
    gene mutations 92–4, **92**
  internal quality control 96–7
  rare bleeding disorders 94–6, *95*

reporting 97
testing 58
monitoring 55–6
monoclonal antibodies, D-dimer 100
Montreal platelet syndrome 112
multiplex ligation-dependent probe amplification 93
mutation analysis 137, 140–2, **142**
  missing mutations 141–2
  necessity for 141
  too many mutations 141–2
  what to analyze 141, **142**
myocardial infarction 110

nadroparin **172**
National External Quality Assessment Scheme UK (NEQAS) 51–3, **52**, 56, 59, 82, 97
  see also external quality assessment
National Institute for Biological Standards and Control (NIBSC) 21, 102
national method quality 4
national total quality 4
near-patient testing *see* point-of-care testing
needle gauge 32
NetGene2 96
Nijmegen-Bethesda assay 201, *201*
nomenclature 97, 144
null hypothesis 17

oral anticoagulant therapy 65
  monitoring 179–89
    conversion of PT to INR 183–5
    implementation of INR 186–7
    limitations of INR 185–6
    thromboplastin calibration 180–1, *180*
    WHO International Reference Preparations 181–3, *181*, *182*
  patient self-monitoring 75–6
  point-of-care testing 72–4, **73**
  see also anticoagulants
osteoporosis, heparin-induced 171
otamixaban **191**
  monitoring 192–3
out of control tests 48
outliers 46
out of limits results 47–9, *48*
outwith consensus 60

overfilling
  activated partial thromboplastin time 69
  thrombin time 70
Owren's disease 95

parahemophilia 95
Paris–Trousseau syndrome 113
patient self-monitoring 72, 75–6
peer group analysis 56
  see also external quality assessment
performance 13
  persistently outwith consensus 54
PFA-100 126–7
D-phenylalanine-proline-arginine-chloromethylketone 35
phospholipase 119
phospholipid reagents 84
phycoerythrin 117
plasma samples
  frozen, thawing of 39–40
  stability 39
  storage 39
plasmin, International Standards **20**
plasminogen activator inhibitor-1, International Standards **20**
platelet adhesion 110
  to collagen 120
platelet aggregation 9, 110
  ristocetin-induced platelet agglutination 128–9
platelet aggregometry 115–16, *115*
platelet count 7, 112–13
  von Willebrand disease 127
platelet factor 4, International Standards **20**
platelet function 110–24, *111*
  aggregometry 115–16, *115*
  bleeding time 112
  clot retraction 119
  counting and morphology 112–14, *113*
  flow cytometry 117–19, *118*
  gene sequencing 121
  platelet secretion 116–17
  point-of-care testing 72, 114–15
  proteomics and genomics 120–1
  prothrombin consumption 112
  signaling pathways 119–20
  in vitro studies 120
  von Willebrand disease 127
Platelet Function Analyzer-100 57, 114
PlateletMapping System 114–15

platelet neutralization 163
Plateletworks system 114
point-of-care monitors **74**
  quality assurance of 74–5
    amperometric measurement 74–5
    electrical impedance method 75
    electromechanical detection 75
    integral onboard controls 75
    iron oxide particle/photo-reflection method 74
    optical clot detection 74
point-of-care testing 57, 72–80
  activated clotting time 76–7
  activated partial thromboplastin time 76
  D-dimer 72, 78
  low molecular weight heparin 77–8
  oral anticoagulation therapy 72–4, **73**
  platelet function 72, 114–15
  quality assurance 79
  service management 78–9
  thrombelastography 78
  thrombin time 77
policies 6
polymerase chain reaction 93, 154
pool consensus value 102–3, **103**
pool harmonized values 103
preanalytical testing phase 31
precision 11, 46
preimplantation diagnosis 93–4
prekallikrein, assay sensitivity 68
prenatal diagnosis
  hemophilia A 93–4
  hemophilia B 93–4
  von Willebrand disease 142–3
Primer Design-Exon Primer 96
process descriptions 6–7, *7*
Proficiency testing *see* external quality assessment
protamine sulfate assay 174
protein C 11, 161
  assays 150–1, *151*
  heritable deficiencies 150–1, *151*
  International Standards **20**, 28
protein S
  assays 152–3, *153*
    inter-method variability **156**
  heritable deficiencies 152–3, *153*
  overdiagnosis 155
  International Standards **20**, 28
proteomics 120–1

prothrombin 161
  consumption 112
  deficiency 95, **95**
  G20210A mutation 154
    International Standards **20**
  see also platelet function
prothrombinase-induced clotting
    time 192, *192*
prothrombin complex factors,
    International Standards 28
prothrombin time 4, **4**, 7, 10, 23, 179
  anticoagulant monitoring 194–5,
    194, **195**
  assay 84
    factors affecting **67**
  conversion to INR 183
  heritable thrombophilias 147
  insensitivity to lupus
    anticoagulants 154
  method selection 65–7, 66, **67**
  minimum evaluation 67
  single/multiple factor deficiency 66
  von Willebrand disease 126
  see also International Normalized
    Ratio
Protime III **73**, 74
protocol 13
PRT-054021 **191**
PT *see* prothrombin time
PTT *see* activated partial
    thromboplastin time
purpura fulminans, neonatal 150
P value 17

quality, definition of 1
quality assurance 4
  heparin measurement 175–7
  point-of-care monitors 74–5
  point-of-care testing 79
quality control 1
  external *see* external quality
    assessment
  heparin measurement 175–7
  internal *see* internal quality control
quality improvement 1
quality management systems 1–2, **2**
quality planning 1–8
quality system essentials 6–8, **6**
Quality System Essentials (QSE) 6
Quebec platelet syndrome 115

random error 46
random variation 46
range 12

receiver operator characteristics
    (ROC) curves 18
Recombinate 26, **27**
ReFacto 26
reference distribution 14
reference individuals 14
reference intervals 10, 13–15
  definition of **14**
  establishment of **14**
reference population 14
reference sample group 14
refrigeration of whole blood 37–8
regression 17
regulatory bodies 49
reviparin 172
ristocetin-induced platelet
    agglutination procedure 128–9
rivaroxaban **191**
robustness 12–13
Russell's viper venom time 154, 193

samples
  blood 32
    refrigeration 37–8
  for EQA 51, 59
  frozen, thawing of 39–40
  icteric 38–9, 70
  ideal **40**
  lipemic 38–9, 70
  plasma
    stability of 39
    storage of 39
    thawing 39–40
  thrombophilia testing 155
sample acquisition 32–7, **40**
  discard tubes 36–7
  heparin assays 175
  order of draw 37
  specimen collection system 33–5
  tourniquets 36, **36**
  vascular access device 37
sample consensus value 103
sample processing 39–40
Scott syndrome 112, 119
sequential analyzers 63
significance 17
SimpliRED 78
single nucleotide polymorphisms 121
Six Sigma control process 3, **4**
  coagulation tests **4**
skin bleeding time 126–7
snake venoms 150
sodium citrate collection tubes 34–5
Spearman rank correlation 103

Spearman rho coefficient 103
specificity 10
specimen collection *see* sample
    acquisition
specimen processing 38–9
  centrifugation 38
  hemolyzed, lipemic and icteric
    samples 38–9
Splice Site Finder 97
stability studies 22
standard deviation 11, 17, 46
standard operating procedures 7–8, 7,
    13
  point-of-care testing 78–9
statistics 16–18
  comparative 17
  descriptive 17
streptodornase, International
    Standards **20**
streptokinase, International
    Standards **20**, 29
stroke 110, 160
Student's *t*-test 17
systemic lupus erythematosus 160, 161
systemic variation 46

Taipan snake venom time 165
test validation 9–18
Textarin time 163
thrombelastography, point-of-care
    testing 78
thrombin 110
  International Standards **20**, 28
thrombin antithrombin complex 36
thrombin inhibitors 204
  direct **191**, 193–4
thrombin receptor activating
    peptide 114
thrombin time 10
  heritable thrombophilias 147
  method selection 8
  minimum evaluation 8
  point-of-care testing 77
Thrombi-Stat CD501WB **73**
thrombocytopenia 110, 160
  heparin-induced 171–4
thromboelastography 194
thromboelastometry 194
β-thromboglobulin, International
    Standards **20**
thrombophilia, heritable 58, 147–59
  screening for 147–57, **148**
    activated protein C
      resistance 153–4

antithrombin 148–50, *150*
  factor V Leiden 153–4
  protein C 150–1, *151*
  protein S 152–3, *153*
  prothrombin G20210A
    mutation 154
  sampling 155
  who to test 1576
  screening results 155–7
    patient-specific
      interpretation 156–7
    physiologic and pathologic
      variability 155–6
    reference ranges 156
thromboplastin 163
  calibration 180–1, *180*
  International Reference
    Preparation 179, 180–1, *180*
  International Standards 20, 23–4
  variability of preparations 179
thromboplastin generation test 86
thrombotic thrombocytopenic
  purpura 204
thromboxane A$_2$ 110
tinzaparin **172**
tirofiban 111
"tissue juice" 36
tissue plasminogen activator 100
  International Standards **20**
tourniquets 36, **36**
transportation of specimens 37–8
transverse myelopathy 160
"two-syringe" technique 36

underfilling
  activated partial thromboplastin
    time 69
  fibrinogen assay 69–70
  thrombin time 70
units of activity 19

Vacutainers 25
validation 9, 10–13
  accuracy 10–11

limits 11–12
linearity 12
precision 11
protocol 13
range 12
robustness 12–13
specificity 10
vascular access device 37
venipuncture 32
venous thromboembolism 99, 160
VerifyNow system 114
vitamin K 66, 66, 90
vitamin K antagonists 179
VKORC1 96
von Willebrand disease 125–36
  assay limitations 126
  clotting factor assay 81
  diagnostic laboratory process 129–
    33, **131–2**
    DDAVP challenge 133
  exclusion of 130
  heterogeneity 126
  history 126
  molecular analysis 137–46
    external quality
      assessment 143–4
    external quality control 143
    internal quality control 143
    mutation analysis 140–2, **142**
    prenatal diagnosis 142–3
  phenotypic assays 126–9
    factor VIII testing 127
    PFA-100 126–7
    platelet counts/morphology 127
    platelet function analysis 127
    ristocetin-induced platelet
      aggregation procedure
      128–9
    routing coagulation tests 126
    skin bleeding times 126–7
  preanalytical variables 126
  type 1 125
    diagnostic laboratory process 130
    molecular analysis 140

  type 2 125
    diagnostic laboratory process
      133
    molecular analysis 138–40
    type 2A 137
    type 2B 137–8
    type 2N 139
  type 3 125, 137
    diagnostic laboratory process
      133
    molecular analysis 137–8, *138*
von Willebrand factor 9, 11, 32, 90,
  110, 125
  acquired deficiency 205
  external quality assessment 54
  International Standards 20, 27–8
  testing for 127–8
    ELISA 127
    factor VIII binding assay 129
    functional assays 127–8
    multimer assay 129
VWF 137

WAS 112
Westgard rules 49
WHO 19
  International Reference Preparations
    see International Reference
    Preparations
whole blood specimens,
  transportation 37–8
WHO standards *see* International
  Reference Preparations;
  International Standards
Wiskott–Aldrich syndrome 110
within-run error 46
World Federation of Haemophilia 45,
  56
World Health Organization *see* WHO
Wright's stain 112

YM150 **191**

"z" score 53